LEPROSY IN CHINA

Weatherhead East Asian Institute,
Columbia University

Studies of the Weatherhead East Asian Institute, Columbia University

The Weatherhead East Asian Institute is Columbia University's center for research, publication, and teaching on the modern East Asia. The Studies of the Weatherhead East Asian Institute were inaugurated in 1962 to bring to a wider public the results of significant new research on modern and contemporary East Asian affairs.

Leprosy in China

A History

Angela Ki Che Leung

COLUMBIA UNIVERSITY PRESS New York

Columbia University Press
Publishers Since 1893
New York Chichester, West Sussex

Library of Congress Cataloging-in-Publication Data
Leung, Angela Ki Che.
Leprosy in China : a history / Angela Ki Che Leung.
p. cm. — (Studies of the Weatherhead East Asian Institute, Columbia University)
Includes bibliographical references and index.
ISBN 978-0-231-12300-6 (cloth : alk. paper)
1. Leprosy—China—History. I. Title. II. Series.
[DNLM: 1. Leprosy—history—China. 2. Stereotyping—China.
WC 335 L653L 2009]
RC154.7.C5L48 2009
362.196'99800951—dc22 2008002450
∞

Columbia University Press books are printed on permanent and durable acid-free paper.
This book was printed on paper with recycled content.
Printed in the United States of America

To Charlotte Furth,

for her unstinting dedication to nurturing

the study of late imperial Chinese medicine

Contents

Acknowledgments

My interest in the history of leprosy in China and its sufferers grew out of my earlier study on philanthropic institutions and a developing curiosity about the history of medicine. It is perhaps a strange topic for many historians, and had it not been for the encouragement of my friends and colleagues, I might not have carried the project through. I would like to express my special gratitude to Charlotte Furth, whose unfailing support over the years and critical comments on my work at its various stages have been indispensable for the completion of this book. I am also much indebted to Richard von Glahn for his astute suggestions on earlier versions of the manuscript, which helped me tremendously in my revisions.

I also benefited greatly from the insightful comments of Ruth Rogaski on a later version, and from Benjamin Elman, Susan Naquin, John Shepherd, and Michael Nylan during and after my research stay at the Institute for Advanced Study, Princeton, in the spring of 2004, when I started writing this book. A special thank-you to Dorothy Ko, who gave me most helpful suggestions on both the content of the book and strategies for having it published. I also remember with gratitude my conversation with Nathan Sivin in that same year, in which he pointed out some pertinent issues in the history of Chinese medicine.

In the course of the project, I gained from the comments and criticism of a long list of learned colleagues at my home institution in Taipei, Academia Sinica: Lin Fu-shih, Hsiao Fan, Liang Keng-yao, Li Jianmin, Chiang Chu-shan, Lee Jender, Li Shang-jen, Sean Lei, Kevin Chang, and others, who, if not named here, are nonetheless remembered for their help and generosity.

Over the years, I also presented my research outside Taiwan: in France, at the Collège de France at the kind invitation of Pierre-Etienne Will, at the China Center of the École des hautes études en sciences sociales, under the direction of Françoise Sabban and, later, Isabelle Thireau. The series of talks given at the École pratique des hautes études, organized by the much-respected Michèle Pirazolli-T'serstevens, were particularly memorable for me. Patrice Bourdelais' collegial workshop at the Institut Pasteur allowed me to exchange views with Europeanists and present a paper published in a volume he edited in 2003. A paper I presented at a meeting of Chinese historians from the People's Republic of China (PRC), Taiwan, and Hong Kong at the Chinese University of Hong Kong in 2002 resulted, in 2003, in the publication of an article in *Lishi yanjiu,* one of the most important history journals of the PRC. In the United States, Charlotte Furth and Marta Hanson gave me the opportunity to present my ideas at the University of Southern California and at the University of California, San Diego, when the idea of writing a book was taking shape.

My talks at Pennsylvania State University, Johns Hopkins University, and Bard College at the beginning of the book project helped me greatly to conceptualize some of the issues. I am grateful to my good friends Ronnie Hsia, William T. Rowe, and Robert and Katherine Martin for having invited me and for their great hospitality. I also had the good fortune of being able to present parts of my work at its more advanced stage at the East Asian Studies department of Princeton University thanks to the invitation of Benjamin Elman, and at Osaka City University thanks to Wakimura Kōhei and Iijima Wataru.

At different stages of my research, friends and colleagues provided me with precious materials and information related to the topic. Dr. Jiang Cheng, of the National Resource Center for STD and Leprosy Control, China CDC, Nanjing, received me most graciously in the summer of 2005. His decades of work in leprosy control in the PRC and his painstaking collection of texts and materials related to the disease make him a most resourceful person on the topic, and it was thanks to him and his colleagues that I was able to visit two asylums in Zhejiang province. Dr. Zheng Jinsheng, of the Academy of Chinese Medical Sciences, Beijing, gave me precious help with traditional Chinese materials over the years, and I will never forget the inspiring interview he arranged for me in the summer of 2002 at the Friendship Hospital with Dr. Li Huanying, a charismatic leprologist in China.

Li Yushang collected materials for me in the archives in Shanghai, Shandong, Yunnan, Jiangsu, and Zhejiang with amazing efficiency. Wu Tao assisted me graciously during my stay in Guangzhou during the last stage of my research. Ronnie Hsia and Lee Yu-chung provided me with interesting Spanish missionary materials (often with translations) of the sixteenth and seventeenth centuries. Liu Cheng-yun, Ding Yizhuang, and Lai Hui-min drew my attention to interesting Chinese imperial archival documents, and Pierre-Etienne Will, Chang Chia-feng, Jo Robertson, and Ma Tai-loi kindly indicated special texts to me. Wang Wen-ji showed me his wonderful materials related to Mission to Lepers. Sarah Elman and Amy Leung photocopied useful materials for me from the libraries at Yale and Hong Kong. I also learned a great deal from Heinrich von Staden, Amneris Roselli, and Tzvi Abusch on early Greek and Babylonian medicine and texts.

The bulk of the materials consulted for this book were obtained in the collections, archives, and databases of Academia Sinica, Taipei; Missions étrangères de Paris, Ministère des Affaires étrangères, France; Shanghai Municipal Archives, Shanghai Library; Guangzhou Municipal Archives, the Republican collection of the library of the Sun Yat-sen University at Guangzhou; the Needham Research Institute, Cambridge; the libraries at Princeton University, Columbia University, Yale University, Chinese University of Hong Kong (and its University Service Centre, which keeps a most impressive collection of post-1949 materials on the PRC), Hong Kong University, and the Institute for Advanced Study, Princeton. I am much indebted to the professional assistance of the librarians and archivists at these institutions.

Hung Ching-chün, Lin Fang-ju, Pearl Huang, Pai Yi-chun, Lin Shing-ting, and Sophie Lu helped me with the borrowing, photocopying, and filing of materials at various stages of my research. Their youthful enthusiasm always lightened my days.

Madge Huntington of the Weatherhead Institute and Anne Routon of Columbia University Press assisted me through the final stages of the publication of this book with good humor and admirable patience. Michael Ashby corrected and improved my manuscript with the great precision and assiduousness of a good-natured professional copyeditor. Leslie Kriesel took care of all the technical difficulties during the production process.

This project was supported by research grants from Academia Sinica, the National Science Council of Taiwan, and the School of Historical Studies of the Institute for Advanced Study, Princeton.

Above all, I thank my family and friends, who, over the years, have graciously put up with my unreasonable obsession with one peculiar topic after another.

Introduction

This book offers a story of leprosy over many centuries of Chinese history—one that forms a parallel narrative to the better-known history of the disease in the Mediterranean and European worlds. As in the West, there is evidence for an ancient, feared, and stigmatized disorder that modern researchers identify with leprosy. Literate medicine has left traces of disputes and confusions over its nosology and etiology; the history of Buddhism and Daoism shows how religion played a role in ascribing redemptive meaning and offering solace; the mystery of its mode of transmission provoked popular explanations of contagion and stimulated state and community efforts at segregation. Beginning in the sixteenth century, one can see a clear resemblance between the clinical descriptions of the Chinese *mafeng* and Western observations of leprosy, along with well-documented indigenous Chinese institutional strategies to cope with it. The folklore of leprosy during these centuries linked contagion and heredity, and focused on seductive women as transmitters, figures seen as both bewitching and polluting.

Second, this book puts the history of leprosy in China into a global context of colonialism, racial politics, and "imperial danger" in the nineteenth century. It also shows how a battle to contain and eliminate it was an element in the modernizing state-building projects of the late Qing empire, the Nationalist government of the first half of the twentieth century, and the People's Republic down to today. China, as my research shows, lay at the center of controversies over the perceived leprosy pandemic of the late nineteenth century, as the Chinese diaspora was widely believed to be the source of its global spread. This not only exacerbated racial stereotypes impacting Chinese overseas migration, but it also made the question of disease an especially sensitive one for Chinese Nationalist elites. Leprosy control became inextricably integrated into the state-building policies of a succession of modernizing regimes throughout the twentieth century.

Finally, by linking the premodern and modern, the local and the global, this book shows the centrality of the Chinese experience to the history of disease, public health, and the spread of biomedical regimes of power around the world. The social and cultural formations surrounding leprosy as an endemic disease were specific to China, and the historical record surrounding it is particularly rich and detailed. Even after missionary and colonial agents brought nineteenth-century science to China, strategies to deal with it were shaped by traditional ways of considering this mysterious and horrifying affliction that was believed to have haunted the civilization since time immemorial. This specific history in turn determined Chinese reactions to the late nineteenth century health crisis leprosy presented as it emerged in the context of both colonialism and a growing biomedically governed global public health movement. It is a history that reveals Chinese agency in understanding and attempting to control the disease in the face of the growing hegemony of Western science and medicine. While the modern story casts a critical eye upon public health movements as regimes of power, Chinese engagements with the curse of leprosy also reveal the allure of "hygienic modernity" for elites in societies struggling to overcome the stigma of backwardness with which the disease came to be identified.

Before I go into the Chinese story of leprosy, it is perhaps appropriate to give a brief account of the Western version of the history of leprosy, as it has constituted the most influential discourse on the disease. The Judeo-Christian understanding of the disease was largely coined by the book of Leviticus, which claims that the leper should be sent "without the camp," as he is unclean and must dwell alone. On this basis, the Third Lateran Council, of 1179, ordered lepers to be segregated from the rest of society. From then on, the religious pronouncement of the patient as a living dead, deprived of all his earthly rights, forms an indelible impression on the Western mind. The flourishing of leprosaria all over Europe in the twelfth and thirteenth centuries also bolstered the impression of a serious epidemic situation and the popular fear of its contagion. The medieval history of leprosy has more recently been revised by scholars, who point out that the fear of contagion was in fact a relatively late development, with probably influence from Arabic medicine and the onset of plague epidemics from the thirteenth century onward. The earlier leprosaria have also been redefined as not really an institution for segregating contagious patients but as a locus for religious sanctification, redemption, and demonstration of charity. Many began as small groupings or communities of lepers and had significant local variations. They were not at all homogeneous church-controlled institutions, as popular imagination has perceived them to be. The decline of the prevalence of the disease after the fourteenth century is also no longer considered a result of segregation but of changing socioeconomic conditions and better diagnostic skills able to distinguish between real leprosy and various skin diseases.[1]

The "disappearance" of leprosy became a focus in Michel Foucault's classic analysis of the madhouse, an institution that he considered as having replaced the medieval leper asylum, marking European modernity. The decline or disappearance of the disease was for Foucault, as for many classic historians but for different reasons, an indication of the end of the Middle Ages. Rod Edmond recently revised this view as an overstatement, showing the disease's uninterrupted presence in modern Europe and the continuous manifestation of the profound "ambivalence that was intrinsic to Judeo-Christian responses to the disease" in Western medical discourse and literary representations in the colonial period.[2]

As in Judeo-Christian civilization, leprosy in China has a unique and important place in the long religious and medical traditions. In its frustrating interaction with the West during the colonial period, China also saw in the leprosy problem a powerful metaphor for the difficult national struggle toward modernity.

LEPROSY IN TRADITIONAL CHINA

As in the West, leprosy in China has a long history and was explained and perceived differently in medical texts and popular traditions of different historical periods. It has been believed, until the 1970s, that leprosy is an old disease recorded in most ancient civilizations, including Egypt, India, China, and Mesopotamia.[3] Using the Chinese medical classic the *Inner Canon,* compiled in the second century B.C., many historians of Chinese medicine, including Lu Gwei-djen and Joseph Needham in the 1960s, concluded that leprosy, then called *li/lai* or *dafeng* (big Wind), was found in ancient China. Such a claim was, however, questioned as early as in the 1970s.[4] It is clear that evidence in the old medical classic and other, contemporary literary classics does not fully support the hypothesis of the existence of true leprosy in ancient China. In the mid-1970s archaeological findings revealed a legal document considered to have been compiled between the fourth century and 217 B.C. describing an illness called *li* manifesting symptoms suggestive of leprosy.[5] Despite such important findings, however, there is simply not enough evidence to support the claim that the *li* (also pronounced *lai* in ancient China) or *dafeng* described in ancient Chinese texts refers to a single specific disease corresponding exactly to what we understand today as Hansen's disease or true leprosy. It is perhaps fair to say that these old terms included diseases with various skin symptoms, some of which closely resemble those of leprosy. The problem of identification of true leprosy in early China is similar to that in the rest of the ancient world. Leprosy was for a long time associated with the disease known in the Judeo-Christian world as *ṣāra'at,* mentioned in the famous chapter 13 of Leviticus, the very source of stigmatization of leprosy in the Christian West for more than a thousand years. Recent research, however, indicates that these claims are based on rather inconclusive evidence. Either the old terms considered to have designated leprosy in fact include various types of skin diseases that may or may not include some kind of leprosy, or terms like *ṣāra'at* could not have meant leprosy at all.[6]

The modern Chinese term for Hansen's disease, *mafeng* (numb Wind), a term that highlights the loss of sensitivity as the major symptom, appeared commonly in medical and nonmedical texts sometime before the fifteenth century.[7] One century later the first medical book devoted to the disease was written.[8] From this time onward there were clear continuities between the clinical descriptions of *mafeng* in traditional Chinese medical texts and the modern and Western observations of leprosy from the mid-nineteenth century onward. We are more confident that the same disease is being discussed, even though the term *mafeng* is still used interchangeably with *lai,* a term that late imperial doctors believed to be the old term for *mafeng.* In other words, the apparent connection, however complex, between what the terms *li*/*lai*/*dafeng* and *mafeng* signify establishes a long, continuous history of a disease later on identified as leprosy in its modern biomedical sense. In sociological or cultural terms, therefore, it is no longer essential whether *li*/*lai*/*dafeng* mean true leprosy, as what they represent automatically forms part of the broader sociocultural history of leprosy in China. The complex and rather technical aspects of the medical history of the disorder is discussed in chapter 1.

Leprosy is sociologically and culturally significant in Chinese history, especially from the perspective of the *longue durée.* It will become apparent, in chapters 1 and 2, how the *li*/*lai* disorder was singled out already in the ancient period as a socially and legally problematic disease. Thereafter, throughout China's long history, the disease was not only the focus of discussions in medical texts but also in religious, legal, and literary ones. The evolution of the conceptualization of *li*/*lai* revealed that stigmatization of the disorder in China was a mixture of religious, popular, legal, and medical interpretations formulated during a very long historical period. The negative image of the sufferer of a fatal, contagious, and polluting disease was further enforced and stereotyped in the late imperial and modern periods. From the fifteenth century onward, medical doctors came to an increasingly pessimistic prognosis of *li*/*lai*/*mafeng*, coinciding with the spreading popular fear of the contagiousness of the disease that was also revealed in legal documents, a question that is dealt with in length in chapter 3.

The damned nature of the ailment, on the other hand, made it a favorite object of redemption in different religious traditions. As will be seen in chapter 2, in early medieval religious texts the disorder was described as redeemable by religious faith, an idea sometimes incorporated into contemporary medical discussions. Many medieval Buddhist and Daoist ideas of the *lai* ailment remained at the backbone of the perception of the ailment throughout the imperial and even the modern periods, especially ideas related to its moral causes and ritual cures. In the later imperial period, redemption by extraordinary performance of Confucian virtues, such as female chastity and filial piety, became increasingly visible. The developments of the perception of the disorder in late imperial China subsequently helped to reinforce the Western Christian one brought by nineteenth-century missionaries. By the turn of that century, the leprous body became the symbol of the sick and crippled body politic of a China weakened by an incompetent government and battered by Western powers. Redemption was then considered possible only with political modernization and intervention of modern "science" and medicine. China probably provides the richest and most complete historical account, other than the Christian West, of the construction of *li*/*lai*/leprosy as a medical, social, and political ailment throughout history. Leprosy in China was both a condemned and redeemable disease, first in the context of personal, religious suffering, and later in the context of the collective anxiety of an emerging nation-state.

In chapter 3, I discuss two main traditional perceptions of leprosy in China, formulated during the late imperial period, that are of interest: first, that the illness was a highly contagious disease, communicable sexually and congenitally. This idea was often combined with the popular belief that the "poison" of the disease of a patient could be gotten rid of by passing it to another, healthy person by sexual intercourse, especially from women to men. Second, that it was most rampant in the hot, humid south, on the periphery of Chinese civilization, especially among the semicivilized national minorities. Such perceptions made it necessary to segregate sufferers of the ailment from society, and China began to build leprosaria to accommodate *mafeng/lai* patients in the sixteenth century. These ideas and institutions remained die-hard well into the early twentieth century, strangely echoing certain Western etiological explanations of the disease. It is fascinating to see how Western medical doctors picked up some of these traditional Chinese ideas on leprosy to support their own views of the mysterious disease in the early twentieth century. Many of them did not find the Chinese medical or popular interpretations of the disease outlandish.

CHINA AND LEPROSY IN THE MODERN GLOBAL CONTEXT

The question of leprosy in the nineteenth and early twentieth centuries has been abundantly examined in the past several decades as one of race, colonial medicine, or "imperial danger," especially in the context of ex-colonies such as British Africa, India, Australia, the Philippines, and so on.[9] It has also been a subject of compassionate discussion related to human rights and the question of identity, as it highlights stigmatization and enforced segregation, especially in noncolonies, such as the United States and Japan.[10] Indeed, the leprosy question in the modern period provokes investigations on two fronts: on the international or global front as a complex colonial medical and racial problem, and on the national front and in relation to the control of the disease as a constituent in the process of state building, often related to the Foucauldian discourse of exclusion.[11] In both discussions, China should be at center stage, but the lack of publications on the question related to China has left a remarkable lacuna in the modern history of leprosy as a global question.

China indeed played a central role in the perceived global pandemic of leprosy beginning in the mid-nineteenth century, as it was believed to be the main exporter of the disease. The incrimination was particularly blatant in Australia. To this day, many believe that leprosy was brought to northern Australia by Chinese immigrants.[12] The association between leprosy and the Chinese diaspora was indeed a strong one, as China was commonly considered to be a global reservoir of the disease.[13] Chinese immigrants were believed to be at the source of the leprosy epidemic in Hawaii and California in the late nineteenth century,[14] even though individual specialists considered these accusations ungrounded.[15] One of the most important consequences of such accusations was in the area of international human migration. As Alison Bashford recently stated, "If the cholera epidemics drove much of the 19th-century international quarantine measures, the sudden concern about leprosy and especially its connection with the Chinese diaspora from about the 1880s coincided with the new (but related) immigration and emigration restrictions which appeared classically in the Australian colonies, but also in many other contexts."[16] She quotes in particular laws restricting Chinese immigration in Canada, New Zealand, and the United States beginning in the 1880s. While considerable ink has been spilt on the global panic over the threat of the perceived pandemic originating from China, the situation of the disease inside China during this critical period remains grossly understudied. To clarify the situation in China from a historical point of view is thus one main purpose of this book.

On the other hand, from China's perspective, the international accusation of being the main exporter of leprosy, and the presence of concerned medical missionaries on its soil, inevitably made it much more sensitive to the issue than ever before. While the imperial government remained fairly impervious to the problem traditionally considered to be endemic to the deep south,[17] the Republican regime of the early twentieth century gradually redefined leprosy to be a national public health problem. Indeed, as John Fitzgerald has so eloquently pointed out, the first generation of Republican Nationalists of this period, represented by Sun Yat-sen, were convinced during this period of the "indissoluble connection between the state of personal ethics, hygiene, and deportment among the Chinese people and the deficiencies of Chinese social organization and imperial administration." To remake the state was to "remake the Chinaman."[18] The struggle thereafter toward achieving "hygienic modernity," as Ruth Rogaski pertinently puts it, became an intrinsic part of the Nationalist state-building project. The New Life Movement, launched by Chiang Kai-shek in the 1930s to reform "the way Chinese looked and acted in public," was directly in keeping with Sun's line of thought.[19] Such an idea prepared for the eventual acceptance and popularity of the idea of racial hygiene, of improving the "breed" of the sickly Chinese race.[20] None other than the Chinese leper, now increasingly noticeable and under scrutiny, could better personify the lack of hygiene, morality, public tidiness, and, in brief, the inferiority of the Chinese race and nation. It was not an accident that the fear and disgust caused by patients of the disease grew in a period when the epithet "sick man of East Asia" became the most popular self-imposed humiliating depiction of the physical body of the Chinese citizen.[21] The "remaking," or sometimes even the "eradication," of the leper became one of the most urgent public enterprises of the Chinese state since the turn of the twentieth century, albeit with much participation of Chinese Christians and Western medical missionaries before the establishment of the People's Republic of China (PRC) in 1949.

After the failure of the Republican government, the PRC state doubled the effort of putting patients of leprosy under control by reinvigorating the segregation policy on an unprecedented national level. For more than four decades, leprosy control policies were inextricably integrated into the complex state-building programs of the regime: the setting up of a vertical control system that mobilized resources on all administrative levels, adoption of the production village as the model of segregation, and application of traditional Chinese herbs and treatment during the first three decades, followed by a more "open" policy of collaborating with global organizations in the 1980s. Every stage of leprosy control fit perfectly into the major political movement or orientation of the time, until the official declaration of the eradication of the disease according to China's higher norm in the 1990s. In a sense, "fighting" the disease constituted a unique and significant part in the history of the formative years of the PRC state. The leprosy control strategies reflected the characteristics of the new nation-state and its unique "modernization" features, and at the same time responded to China's specific historical memory of the disease.

This last point—addressing the specific history of leprosy in China—constitutes, consciously or unconsciously, an essential part of modern China's public health strategies in controlling the disease. In this sense, China is not unlike colonial India, a civilization probably most scrutinized by nineteenth-century European colonialists.[22] Both civilizations had a long and rich history of diseases and medicine. In other words, China's strategies to deal with the disease were determined not only by its understanding of biomedicine or the reaction to its international image as the main exporter of the disease, but above all by its own traditional management of this mysterious and horrifying disease.

EPIDEMIOLOGY

One of the reasons leprosy became a focus of medical discussions in the nineteenth century was that it was, and remains, a mysterious disease, as its channels of transmission remain unclear to epidemiologists. This characteristic, together with the frightening external symptoms of some patients, rather than the mortality of the disease, largely explain the universal stigmatization of patients. Even though the causal organism for leprosy, *Mycobacterium leprae,* was identified by the Norwegian scientist G. H. A. Hansen as early as 1873, much of the mystery surrounding the disease remains unexplained to this day, even though the disease is now curable. Modern epidemiology traditionally classifies leprosy into two main types: lepromatous, the most severe form, and tuberculoid, with indeterminate and borderline forms in between. A more recent classification scheme divides cases into paucibacillary and multibacillary active types according to the bacteriological index (BI), an expression of the extent of bacterial loads observed on skin smears taken from patients. The paucibacillary type, with a BI of less than 2, includes tuberculoid and some indeterminate leprosy, and the multibacillary type, with a BI of 2 or greater, includes lepromatous and borderline leprosy. The bacillus typically provokes destruction of cells, and of the neurological system, resulting in the loss of sensation, disfiguring nodules, destruction of the nasal cartilage, damage to the vocal cords, and weakness of the muscles. Patients may lose eyesight, and eventually the use of their limbs. Leprosy, however, is not considered a fatal disease, as it is rarely an immediate cause of death, though the death rate for lepromatous patients can be three to four times higher than that for the general population.

Even though *Mycobacterium leprae* was one of the first bacilli affecting humans to be identified under the microscope, the disease is still mysterious in many ways. For one thing, even after its identification in 1873, the bacillus has not yet been successfully cultivated in an artificial medium despite numerous trials, making it impossible to develop a vaccine. Above all, for centuries the question of the transmission of the disease has remained a puzzle. The identification of the bacillus, curiously, has not given any clue to specialists for understanding the exact mechanism of its transmission. For a long time, the most widely held belief was that leprosy was transmitted by contact between patients and healthy persons. More recently, the possibility of transmission by the respiratory route and even by insects has been considered. It is generally accepted that there are two portals of exit of the bacillus: the skin and the nasal mucosa. It has been found that the bacillus from the nasal secretion can survive up to thirty-six hours, or up to nine days under tropical conditions. This suggests the possibility of contaminated clothing, bedding, and so forth as sources of infection. However, transmission remains a mystery, as the roles of dosage and the portal of entry of the bacillus into the human body remain unclear, even though the skin and the upper respiratory tract are believed to be the likely routes. At present, one thing that experts can be sure of is that individuals who are in prolonged and close association or proximity with patients have a greater chance of acquiring the disease.[23]

There have been many myths surrounding the disease, coming from popular beliefs from different cultures, and even from modern Western medical research of not too long ago. A most popular one was that leprosy was a tropical disease, a finding upheld notably by the father of British tropical medicine, Patrick Manson, in the late nineteenth century. In fact, the disease has actually been observed over a broad range of altitudes, humidity levels, and temperatures. Similarly, the beliefs that the disease was hereditary, congenital, and transmissible by sex, strong in modern Europe and in China, have been shown to be ungrounded.

The disease was basically incurable before the late twentieth century but was increasingly put under control. Chaulmoogra oil, an old remedy used in India and China for centuries, was still the major drug used in the nineteenth and early twentieth centuries, rather as a palliative. Since the 1930s, and especially during the 1940s, sulfonamides and diaminodiphenylsulfone (DDS), strong and toxic chemicals, were tested and developed to control leprosy more effectively. It was also found that vaccinating with BCG (Bacillus Calmette-Guérin) also provided certain immunization to leprosy. However, the continued use of dapsone (DDS) later proved to have provoked the emergence of drug-resistant strains of *M. leprae,* accounting for relapses. It was the development of multidrug therapy (MDT)[24] to treat leprosy in the early 1980s that made the eradication of leprosy a feasible goal for the World Health Organization (WHO). It was first used in 1982–1985 and had been applied worldwide by 1990. This therapy has until now improved the problem of dapsone resistance and dramatically reduced the number of patients all over the world. The therapy was introduced in China in 1982 in three areas and was implemented on a national level in 1987. However, China was in fact considered to have eliminated leprosy on the national level in 1982 when MDT was introduced, and on the subnational level by 1992.[25] Despite the apparent success of MDT, medical research on the disease continues today, especially on the total deciphering of the bacillus in order to design a better-suited drug that will avoid all possible danger of drug resistance.[26] Clearly, scientists do not think that the "war" against leprosy is won and the fight over.

Today, according to WHO statistics, there are still a dozen countries with leprosy as an endemic, even though, between 1985 and 2003, the global prevalence had fallen by almost 90 percent and more than 13 million patients had been cured. By the end of 2003 there were still ten countries that had not been able to reach the elimination target at the national level, meaning with prevalence at or above one case per 10,000 population: Angola, Brazil, the Central African Republic, Congo, India, Liberia, Madagascar, Mozambique, Nepal, and the United Republic of Tanzania. Of these countries, India was said to have the largest number of patients (more than 400,000 at the start of 2003).[27] In many other countries, even though prevalence seems to be below the WHO norm or statistics are not viable, leprosy is still a visible public health issue and stigmatization is still strong, despite the progress in treatment.

Leprosy has been a major global problem in the nineteenth and twentieth centuries because of its long history loaded with complex cultural meanings, its mysterious biomedical character, and its inextricable relations with the questions of race, nation, religion, and modernity. It was considered a major threat to civilizations also because of its visibility. Despite the significant progress made in drug treatment during the latter half of the twentieth century, however, its presence and its stigma have not disappeared in the twenty-first century. Many experts talk about its "comeback" together with tuberculosis.[28] If the development of a vaccine remains unsuccessful, the disease is doomed to coexist with humanity as long as rural poverty and political instability persist. Moreover, Hansen's disease remains in the camp of the most feared and stigmatized human diseases long after it has ceased to be a real threat to humanity. A look at China's long history of leprosy, from the premodern to the modern and then postcolonial periods, and in a global context but from a non-Western perspective, probably helps us to understand better the modern fear of any real or imagined scourge on a global scale.

PROBLEMS OF CONTAGION AND SEGREGATION

The belief in contagion of leprosy inevitably highlighted the question of segregation. As in Europe, the idea of *li/lai* as a contagious ailment emerged relatively late, sometime in the thirteenth century. The institutional segregation of sufferers of the ailment began in southern China only in the early sixteenth century, a development treated in chapter 3. These nonreligious institutions organized and financed by local governments were different from early Buddhist asylums for *lai* patients in the sense that they were mainly a means of prevention of contagion and not a locus of purification rituals or demonstration of religious charity. Indeed, *lai/mafeng* was the only chronic disorder known in traditional China necessitating institutional exclusion. Exclusion was, however, not a national but a regional phenomenon that was, moreover, forced out from modern public memory despite the continued presence of asylums into the twentieth century. The question of segregation came under the spotlight again when modern Chinese elites were taught that the disappearance of leprosy in Europe was largely due to the systematic exclusion policy during the medieval period, as I shall describe in chapter 4.

However, even among modern Western experts, the question of exclusion was ambiguous. To say the least, the prevalent hereditary theory before the 1890s and British liberal rule were incompatible with enforced segregation of patients. Even after the general acceptance of leprosy as a contagious disease from the last decade of the nineteenth century onward, not all Western leprologists saw segregation as a rational strategy, for both practical considerations of the actual social conditions of these "backward" countries and for medical reasons.[29] In India, for instance, even after the 1898 Lepers Act calling for the confinement of sufferers, only paupers with the disease were interned, and without much enforcement by the police, with the result that "most leprosy sufferers of South India escaped confinement."[30]

For Chinese elites, the visibility of leprosy in China was totally incompatible with the ideal of "hygienic modernity," and its eradication was urgent. While traditional asylums, if mentioned at all, were dismissed as grossly underequipped and ideologically backward, perpetuating the inmates' antisocial mentality and behavior, a stricter, more "scientific" segregation policy was idealized by many. They imagined a situation where all lepers would be interned and disciplined systematically, treated medically, and allowed to live and die inside, leaving public space free of their loathsome sight, and above all, of further contamination. They saw strict segregation as a necessary step toward elimination of the disease. Indeed, as chapter 4 will show, in the Republican period, a few asylums taken over from missionaries were guarded by the military, and identified patients were arrested and forcibly interned. Probably many Chinese elites shared the belief of the American doctor G. Woods, who declared in 1887 that, "by separation—shutting him [patient of leprosy] off from all the rest of mankind, and so letting the infected and the disease die out together; and making a public opinion which should consider this work of ostracism a religious and civil duty . . . The results show the wisdom of this policy."[31] Such an attitude was not an exceptional one in the late nineteenth and early twentieth centuries.

Australia, for example, adopted drastic policies to rid the country of leprosy, by two means: deportation and enforced segregation. From the 1880s until the 1950s, nearly all people with leprosy were removed and detained, sometimes for their whole lives, in northern Australia. Chinese and Aborigines, especially, were strictly isolated. Moreover, as Chinese were thought to be mostly responsible for the introduction and spread of the disease in Australia, these "foreign" patients were, whenever possible, repatriated or deported, mostly to Hong Kong. These "explicitly racialized practices of segregation" ran counter to the liberal principle of British colonial rule.[32]

In Japan, where the question of mixed races was not a problem, patients began to be forcibly interned during the Meiji period, when the "governmental and civic elite wanted to establish their country as part of the modern world and to distance it from 'backward' Asian societies such as India and China." With some figures suggesting that Japan was "the most leprous country in the world" in the beginning of the twentieth century, drastic measures of isolation were believed to be necessary to rid Japan of "the sign of an uncivilized country."[33] The Leprosy Prevention Law was passed in 1907, legalizing the confinement of "wandering lepers," followed by a campaign in 1915 to encourage sterilization of patients (ending only in the 1960s), enforced abortion, and, finally, a lifetime exclusion law in 1931, with the new goal of confining all of Japan's "lepers."[34] The "modern" leprosaria, it was well understood, had as a model not the hospital but the prison. The Kyushu Leprosarium, set up in 1909 and accommodating more than 1,500 patients by around 1960, for instance, was encircled by concrete walls with policemen stationed outside and deep moats surrounding its walls. Patients had to wear special striped uniforms and use special money within the compound. It was estimated in 1941 that the percentage of segregated patients in Japan was at 78 percent, a ratio that eventually rose to almost 90 percent, a most astonishing figure.[35] Clearly, the concern for the purity of race and nation was behind such drastic measures, intriguingly corresponding to Foucault's premodern exclusion model. Japan's enforced exclusion of patients of leprosy ended legally only in 1996.[36]

The Chinese Republican state, on the other hand, did not have enough political muscle to impose stringent segregation measures on a national level. The Christian colonial style of "soft" segregation, combining medical treatment and productive activities of inmates aimed at uplifting their moral and spiritual characters became a more common model in China. The images of the colony in Molokai, Hawaii, rendered famous by the Belgian Father Damien, who ended up contracting the disease, and Culion, in the Philippines, as a showcase for American colonial rule, were probably the best known in China and greatly admired by concerned elites. Both "myths" have been much deconstructed and critiqued in recent research,[37] but in the early twentieth century they were understood as examples and models of ideal "modern" leper colonies. The premises of such models, of course, were that the inmates fell ill partially due to weaknesses in their physical and spiritual natures that could be reformed. These model colonies, for elites aspiring to total Westernization, would be miniatures for the spiritual and corporal modernization of China.

Indeed, the idea of salvation through productive labor had, in the early twentieth century, somehow replaced the traditional idea of redemption by religious charity or miracle in many parts of the world. As Robert Muir, of the British Empire Leprosy Relief Association, said in the 1920s, "The modern leper colony was no longer an almshouse or lazaret, but rather it was analogous to an agricultural or industrial settlement." It should be "educative, self-supporting, and a model community for the outside world—an ideal first stage on the path to civilization."[38] However, during the entire Republican period, the Chinese government was too weak to mobilize with success the necessary resources for the organization of such colonies. As a consequence, only a small number of missionary-run colonies in the early half of the century made some attempts to realize such an ideal. It was the Chinese Communist regime that finally achieved a version of the Christian liberal model. By establishing a nationwide network of economically self-supporting and politically educative "leper villages," as part of the agricultural cooperative movement of the 1950s and 1960s (described in chapter 5), the PRC state realized a dream that had never been reached by Republican activists. Unlike the more urban-oriented Republican government, the RPC regime deliberately integrated leprosy control as part of its complex rural reform program. For the Chinese organizers of these villages in the late 1950s and early 1960s, the model they adopted was the "Latin-American model" transmitted to them by an Argentine specialist who came to China to train workers in the 1950s.[39] The transformation of the originally Christian liberal colony of isolation into a socialist village seemed to be a smooth process in China, showing close ideological affinities with the Foucauldian "inclusive" model for controlling and reforming the socially undesirable in modern societies.

Another question drawing increasing scholarly interest is that of the self-identity of the incarcerated patients. For Megan Vaughan, the prevalent Christian liberal model imposed on many British colonies in Africa, such as Basutoland, encouraged patients to identify with the lepers of the Bible, for example. Even though such an identity often conflicted with other identities of patients as wives, husbands, and members of tribes, inmates did self-consciously take on the biblical identity so as to "exploit all the ambiguities of the European Christian tradition in an attempt to improve their unhappy situation." In fact, all recent worldwide campaigns to eliminate leprosy have "rested on the perpetuation of the figure of *the* 'leper.'"[40] For non-Christian societies not colonized by any Christian country, such as Japan, identity created by systematic isolation was another matter. Susan Burns shows that, through a special literature known as "leprosy literature" (*rai bungaku*), Japanese interned patients of the early twentieth century developed a new identity embracing the life within the leprosarium and the "ethos of resignation."[41] China went through several decades of Christian influence on the leprosy question in the early twentieth century, before the PRC adopted the "leper village" model. Little research has been done on the problem of identity created by modern leprosaria during the twentieth century, although we know that there is a certain amount of literature by patients in China, including a magazine published in the Shanghai asylum in the 1940s, recent romanticized accounts by ex-inmates of the hard lives inside leprosaria, and an unknown number of archival materials in a Taiwan asylum.[42] Most of these primary sources, however, have not yet been systematically classified and analyzed, rendering the question of identity little more than a speculative issue. On the other hand, as parts of chapter 2 show, patients in traditional hospices in the southern regions of late imperial China created their own pseudolineages, with a new group identity emerging from their self-empowerment as a result of the general fear of their pollution in society. Such an image contrasts interestingly with the attitude of resignation that many modern patients manifest in some of their writings. Was there a continuity or discontinuity in the identity construction of patients from the late imperial to the modern periods? Was there a new identity emerging in the twentieth century with the rise of the modern nation-state? If so, how was it related to the past? How did the type of isolation models affect the construction of patients' identity and subjectivity? These are some of the questions that scholars may want to address in the future.

A POSTCOLONIAL HISTORY OF MEDICINE

China was indeed in a unique position in the colonial era of the nineteenth and early twentieth centuries. Unlike India, British Africa, Korea, or the Philippines, China was never a truly colonial state. The Chinese state in this period was marked by its political weakness, and Chinese society was obsessed by the question of modernization and nationalistic sentiment, but the nation was never totally colonized by the Western powers or Japan. The urge for modernization in the face of imperialist threat inevitably made the question of health, hygiene, and medicine a major issue on the Nationalist agenda. It is in this context that a biomedical subject formation of the Chinese citizen can be analyzed. The new identity was therefore not promoted by a strong colonial state and subaltern agency, as in India, Korea, or the Philippines, or even perhaps in British Africa. The construction of modern Chinese subjectivity was shaped by the interplay of three elements born of nineteenth-century colonialism: a weak but indigenous state, a dominating elitist nationalistic discourse on radical Westernization, and a strong, popular memory of the indigenous (imperial) past that often resisted effectively the Westernization discourse. What the present study emphasizes is the last element: the overwhelmingly rich historical memory, much transmitted by texts, and a robust and living tradition of popular knowledge and beliefs in medicine and health practices, reinforcing the Chinese agency in the modern and global story of disease control.

Unlike Japan, which had a strong modern government with an effectively eclectic Westernization agenda, and where the quest of racial purity was integrated into the building of a strong nation-state, China was restrained not only by its political and economic weaknesses but also by its ethnic complexities and sheer size in building a modern and idealized biomedical regime. There are more similarities between the experiences of Japan and Europe in the construction of an imperial regime based on a "colonial medicine." Recent research on Taiwan, Korea, and Manchuria shows the effects of Japanese colonial experiments in building its biomedical empire.[43] Japan was, after all, a colonizer on the European model. China, on the other hand, despite its relative autonomy and the elites' aspiration for a totally Westernized regime based on science and democracy, was held back not only by its various "weaknesses" but also by its own strong traditions and social realities. Its choices were inevitably different from those of Japan and various colonized states in Asia and elsewhere.

China's history of leprosy provides a particularly informative alternative to the master narrative of modernity as defined by "European" experience. In this sense, this book is an attempt of "provincializing Europe."[44] The history of the Chinese understanding of the ailment and the changes in its strategies to control it should thus be read as one of the "dynamic, multisited histories" of postcolonial medicine, an agenda well described by Warwick Anderson.[45] For a civilization such as China, to appreciate its construction of a hybrid modern regime of health management requires not only the grasp of the nature of its unique political regime since the late nineteenth century, but, above all, an understanding of its long and complex medical, religious, and social traditions since antiquity. The long and unbroken story of *mafeng/lai* certainly provides one of the most useful keys for such an appreciation.

ONE

Li/Lai/Dafeng/Mafeng

History of the Conceptualization of a Disease/Category

In the early twentieth century, when China was obsessed by its leprosy problem, medical doctors and historians alike looked back in history in order to identify evidence of true leprosy in ancient classics and medical texts.[1] The mentions of *dafeng*/*lifeng* (big Wind, Wind of *li*) in the *Huangdi neijing* (*The Yellow Emperor's Inner Canon*), the most important medical classic in China,[2] and the famous episode in the *Lunyu* (*Analects*) on Confucius lamenting the "malignant ailment" (*eji*) of his disciple Ran Boniu were probably the most quoted examples in modern articles written on the Chinese history of leprosy to illustrate the early existence of the disease. These mentions were made famous in Western literature by Joseph Needham and Lu Gwei-djen in the 1960s in their effort to show the occurrences of true leprosy in ancient China.[3] The approach of describing the history of leprosy by equating certain early terms with Hansen's disease, or taking as proof of its existence the mention of a few suggestive symptoms seems outdated nowadays. This approach was legitimately challenged, notably by Nathan Sivin, already in the 1970s.[4] As it is practically impossible to judge from texts if a recorded case was indeed true leprosy, determining the moment when leprosy first appeared in China is doomed to be futile and controversial. What is of greater interest to today's historians is the historical development of the conceptualization of the disease, or rather, a category of diseases called *dafeng* or *li/lai*[5] in early China that late imperial doctors reanalyzed as a single category called *mafeng* (numb Wind), a name that is still used today to translate Hansen's disease. This approach would at least reveal the complexities of old Chinese disease categories, which are not easily analyzable by familiar modern biomedical ones. The historical conceptualization of *dafeng/li/lai/mafeng* would also provide a concrete case of the historical construction of medical knowledge in China in the past. In other words, by avoiding imposing modern biomedical meanings onto old Chinese disease names, I attempt to reveal the rich history of old Chinese disease categories on their own terms, a better way to grasp the nature of the old Chinese nosological system. The history of *mafeng* provides an excellent example for such an understanding.

Ancient disease names in China were of two broad types: those describing symptoms, and others that refer to broad configurationist etiological patterns that were considered to be responsible for producing disorders. These patterns were mostly cosmological or environmental, such as yin/yang, the five phases (*wu xing*) that constituted the basis of ancient Chinese thought,[6] and the six *qi* (atmospheric influences, or "energetic configurations"[7]): Wind, Cold, Summer Heat, Dampness, Hot Dryness, Fire, a notion derived from the five atmospheric influences described in the *Inner Canon.*[8] These six *qi* were later sometimes also called the six excessive influences or external pathogens (*yin*). The terms *dafeng* or *lifeng* thus designated disorders caused by the intrusion of Wind as a cosmic or atmospheric influence. *Li*[9] or *lai,* on the other hand, were names describing symptoms: essentially sores on the skin. Throughout the ancient and medieval periods, ailments with symptoms suggestive of leprosy were described in either symptomatic or configurationist terms in a variety of eclectic combinations: *dafeng, li, lai, lifeng, efeng* (malignant Wind), *zeifeng* (vicious Wind), and so on. In the later imperial period, after the eleventh century, there was the gradual emergence of a term combining a single new symptom-related descriptor, *ma* (numb), with the configurationist concept of Wind in the more modern compound terms *mafeng* and *damafeng* (big numb Wind). Along with the new, stable nomenclature gradually emerged new images and conceptions of the disease. In the same period, speculations about the transmission of the disorder by human contact, that is, a medical model of contagion, also came into place.

ETIOLOGY OF THE DISEASE CATEGORY: A HISTORY

The Early Imperial Period (Fourth Century B.C.—Eleventh Century A.D.)

A Wind-Induced Disorder: Dafeng/Efeng

In the *Inner Canon, feng* (Wind), the first of the five atmospheric influences, the other four being Cold (*han*), Dampness (*shi*), Hot Dryness (*zao*), and Fire (*huo*), was described as the "origin of the hundreds of disorders."[10] Since then Wind was indeed considered the cause of many serious and dramatic ailments that constituted the dominant class of disorders in subsequent mainstream medical texts.[11] One such disorder occurred when Wind and Cold resided inside the circulation channels of the human body. In section 42 of the "Suwen" (Plain Questions) part of the *Inner Canon* (see n. 2), where the various detrimental effects of Wind are explained, the disorder called *lifeng* (Wind resulting in the *li* disorder), also known as Cold Heat (*han re*), is described as having the following sequence and symptoms: "The [Wind-] heated constructive energy digresses [from the channels deep in the body's interior] into the skin, polluting the [patient's] *qi,* leading to the degeneration of the bridge of the nose, and the deterioration of the color of the skin that would eventually erupt into sores."[12] In the same section, various disorders caused by Wind entering into or stagnating inside different parts of the body are described as having common symptoms such as numbness, paralysis, corruption of the complexion, loss of appetite, sweating, fatigue, and so on. In other words, there are a number of symptoms shared by various Wind-induced disorders. Terms like *dafeng* or malignant, vicious Wind (*efeng, zeifeng*), not necessarily names of specific disorders, also appear in different sections in the *Inner Canon* usually referring to serious cases of Wind intrusion with various clusters of symptoms.[13]

In section 55 of the *Lingshu* (*Divine Pivot*) in the *Inner Canon, dafeng* is described as causing symptoms such as "the swelling of bones and joints, and the falling out of hair and eyebrows," curable by acupuncture, first applied on the flesh, then on the bones.[14] The compilers of the *Inner Canon* were apparently describing what were for them two categories of pathogens, *lifeng* and *dafeng,* in two distinct sections, one affecting essentially the skin, the other, the bones. From the brief descriptions in the medical classic, it is difficult to tell if these two broad types of Wind-induced symptoms were considered by the compilers as related. Also hard to fathom is the range of these two types, as the symptoms described could be common to various Wind-induced disorders. Nonetheless, due to these two passages, *li,* in *lifeng* (which could in fact be pronounced as *lai* in this case), and *dafeng* have frequently been cited by modern historians of medicine as early terms for leprosy, as well as proof that true leprosy existed in China before the first century A.D.

The discussions on Wind-induced disorders in the *Inner Canon* were elaborated more systematically in the seventh-century classic on etiology by Chao Yuanfang (550–630), *Zhubing yuan hou lun* (*General Treatise on the Origins and Symptoms of Disorders* [ca. 610]). In this medical classic, names and categories of disorders are expressed and discussed more methodically and in more concrete terms. Chao begins the book with two chapters on Wind-induced disorders, fully indicating their dominant position in the nosological hierarchy already implied in the *Inner Canon.*[15] The two chapters listed fifty-nine types of symptoms caused by the effect of Wind. Of these, the last eleven types, beginning with type forty-nine, were related to the *dafeng* category as described in *Divine Pivot* of the *Inner Canon.* In brief, Chao labeled this group of symptoms the "falling out of the beard and eyebrows caused by *efeng*" and discussed in detail different symptoms caused by Winds "from the eight directions."[16] In general, the author considered these as the results of "Wind, Dampness, and Cold" entering the skin and flesh and into the viscera. In this context, Chao provided more concrete interpretations of the causes by saying that the disorder was "caused either by water entering the body of a sweating person, or cold water entering into his skin and flesh." He went on to explain, "[Someone could catch the disorder by] lying on wet ground after having taken alcoholic drinks, or confronting wind, or sitting under a tree, or on wet grass. [He could also catch this] by scratching his itchy body, which slowly develops sores. If not cured, [the ailment] will turn into the *feng* disorder after a few years."[17] Clearly the opening up of pores under the effects of alcohol and scratching was considered the immediate cause of the introduction of Wind and other bad atmospheric influences into the body.

The final three types of Wind-induced disorders caused by *efeng,* types fifty-seven through fifty-nine, were called *lai* (for a more detailed discussion of *lai* in this text, see the following section), clearly defined by the skin symptoms. In fact, most of the *efeng* and *lai* symptoms were related to the skin, including itchiness, eruption into sores, deterioration of the complexion, and loss of sensitivity of the skin, but there were also other serious symptoms, such as the falling out of hair, collapse of the bridge of the nose, hoarseness of the voice, deterioration of eyesight and hearing, and death. Chao explained the more serious *lai* symptoms and elaborated on the complex nature of the disorder by evoking the five Winds attacking the five viscera, causing the five main symptoms of the falling out of the eyebrows, the collapse of the bridge of the nose, the voice becoming hoarse, a ringing or roaring in the ears, and, finally, death.[18] Even though the author repeats many similar symptoms in the last eleven types of Wind-induced disorders, he nonetheless deems it necessary to distinguish the *dafeng* from the *lai* category, with emphasis on skin symptoms for the latter.

The ambiguous relations between the two categories of related disorders, with one highlighting the Wind factor and the other skin symptoms, persisted in Tang medical texts, as shown notably by Sun Simiao's (581–682) *Beiji qianjin yaofang* (*Essential Recipes for Urgent Use Worthy of a Thousand Gold Pieces* [ca. 650–659]),[19] and Wang Tao's (670–755) *Waitai miyao fang* (*Secret Essentials from the Imperial Collections* [ca. 752]),[20] the most important medical texts of the period. Sun discusses *lifeng* and *eji*/*dafeng* in two separate chapters. *Lifeng* is discussed in chapter 8 as a serious category of Wind-induced disorders, whereas *eji*/*dafeng* is described, more lengthily, in chapter 23, together with disorders such as hemorrhoids and tinea. In chapter 8, Sun elaborates on the various symptoms of and especially the recipes for disorders caused by the intrusion of Wind, which he called *lifeng* or *efeng,* into the skin and flesh, including those with symptoms such as itchiness, deafness, and the loss of eyebrows. The *eji*/*dafeng* category, with multiple symptoms, is described more lengthily in chapter 23, where other skin disorders are also described.[21] In his account of *eji*/*dafeng,* Sun specifies that a patient may have some but not all the symptoms, including the falling off of the limbs' extremities, sensation of extreme cold or heat in the body, dehydration or constant sweating, dry itchiness, white flakes or painful sores on the skin, or total anesthesia, and so on. The colors on the deteriorating skin also varied. According to his own experience as a doctor, people affected by the disorder would usually die in no more than ten years, or even in five or six years. Sun never uses the term *lai* for the *eji*/*dafeng* category. In another work, he uses the term *ebing* (malignant disorder) to indicate the same symptoms.[22] It is in fact difficult to distinguish clearly between the disorders he describes in chapters 8 and 23, as both were considered Wind-induced and shared many similar symptoms. Wang Tao, on the other hand, basically combined Chao's and Sun's descriptions. Chapter 30 of his synthesis begins with a section called *eji*/*dafeng,* repeating almost word for word Sun's account under the same title, followed immediately by three sections on *lai,* summarizing Chao's account of *lai.* In brief, despite the confusion in the naming of the disorders, Sui-Tang medical experts continued to describe separately two related groups of disorders, with one sharing many similar symptoms of other serious Wind-induced disorders, and the other with more conspicuous skin symptoms.

Disorders with Skin Symptoms: Li/Lai

Li (which, as mentioned, could also be pronounced *lai*[23]) was a popular term in early China for a disease with serious skin symptoms, or an ugly sick person. Even though it did not appear in the *Inner Canon,* it was frequently mentioned in a number of nonmedical early classics. The story concerning Yu Rang, the famous assassin recorded in the *Zhanguo ce* (*Record of the Warring States*) and *Shiji* (*Records of the Grand Historian*), of the first century B.C., also mentions *li/lai* as an ailment with skin sores and the falling out of hair and eyebrows.[24] In the *Zhuangzi* (Master Zhuang, ca. 369–286 B.C.) a "person of *li*" is contrasted with the famous beauty Xishi. The Tang philologist Cheng Xuanying (seventh century) thus rendered *li* as an "ugly sick person."[25] Since the late Qing, these stories in nonmedical texts have been cited as illustrations of early occurrences of *mafeng* leprosy. In fact the term *li/lai* should be dated even earlier. Thanks to archaeological findings in the 1970s, we have a text, dated between the fourth century and 217 B.C., recorded on bamboo strips, about a case of a *li/lai* patient being diagnosed by a doctor. This was a legal interrogation of a villager brought before justice because of being suspected of having *li/lai.* The villager confessed, "At the age of three, I became sick with sores on the head; my eyebrows swelled up; it could not be ascertained what sickness it was." The prosecutors ordered a physician to examine him, and the latter reported, "C has no eyebrows; the bridge of the nose is destroyed; his nasal cavity is collapsed; if you prick his nose, he does not sneeze; elbows and knees down to the soles of both feet are defective and are suppurating in one place; his hands have no hair; I ordered him to shout and the *qi* of his voice was hoarse. It is *li/lai.*"[26] This physician, active in a period before the compilation of the *Inner Canon,* might have studied earlier medical texts, such as the *Mai shu* (*Book on Vessels*), excavated in Zhangjiashan in the early 1980s and dated to the early Han period (ca. third century B.C.). In this text a section on the symptoms of sixty-seven disorders describes a *li/lai* disorder with symptoms such as sores on joints that looked like buffalos' eyes, and loss of eyebrows.[27] Clearly in this early period, *li/lai* was already used to mean a person with a disease strongly suggestive of Hansen's disease. However, evidence is still too patchy to allow us to say that *li/lai* exclusively meant true leprosy, even though it is clear that the term was popular and was used in both medical and nonmedical contexts meaning a person with a repulsive physical appearance characterized by skin lesions.

The fluidity and popularity of the term *li/lai* is shown in one of the first important and popular medical texts that mention *lai:* the *Zhou hou beiji fang* (*Handy Recipes for Urgent Use*), by the Daoist doctor Ge Hong (283–343). Ge Hong employed the term *lai* for a disorder having the following symptoms: "At the beginning, there is numbness of the skin, or a feeling of agonizing itchiness as if worms were creeping [on the skin]. Or the vision is blurred by lines like falling silk. Persistent red or black skin eruptions may appear."[28] In this fifth chapter on essentially skin diseases and various kinds of swelling, Ge Hong considers numbness of the skin a specific symptom of *lai,* but he makes no mention of the corruption of bones and limbs, or of the falling out of hair and eyebrows. Doctors after Ge Hong considered this as a development of the *Inner Canon*'s discussions on *lifeng* and *dafeng* and compiled as annexes to that passage recipes for the *dafeng/li/lai* disorders analyzed in the later, especially Sui-Tang periods.[29]

As mentioned, the first extant detailed medical descriptions on *li/lai* was provided by Chao Yuanfang, of the Sui dynasty. Similar to Ge Hong, Chao considered *lai* disorders as mainly related to the skin and caused by "vicious Wind and violation of taboos." For Chao, even though *lai* disorders, like *efeng,* were basically Wind induced, there were differences in the specific causes. While *efeng* disorders were caused by Wind, Dampness, and Cold intruding into the body after alcohol or while lying on wet ground, or sitting under trees in windy conditions, the *lai* disorders were caused by "excessive physical exertion, unhealthy diet, and excessive sexual activities," which opened the pores, allowing the intrusion of conflicting Cold and Hot Winds into the viscera.[30] Wind trapped inside the flesh, he continued, would prevent sweating, cause pain in the limbs, insensitivity of the skin even when pricked by needles, itchiness, sores, different forms of swelling in the face, and various types of sores, and ringworm, abnormal colors of the urine and of the skin. He also distinguished two types of *lai:* one spreading from the head down, and the other from the lower limbs up. Different forms of *lai,* according to him, had incubation periods varying from three to twenty years. A black *lai* and a white *lai,* moreover, were also mentioned, the former closer to the classic *lai* form, and the latter appearing to be a less-serious form. For the first time, *lai* disorders obtained systematic clinical descriptions, and in sociological terms, Chao seemed to imply that people from the laboring classes were more likely to suffer from *lai* disorders.

It is thus important to note that, until the eighth century, mainstream medical writers closely followed the classification in the *Inner Canon,* distinguishing the more complicated *dafeng* category, with symptoms of corrupted bones, from the *li/lai* category of disorders, with essentially more visible skin symptoms, even though both were considered to be primarily provoked by the intrusion of noxious Wind. The similarity to medieval Arabic medicine is striking. It appears that in medieval Arabic medicine, there were also two categories of disorders related to leprosy, *judhām* and *bara;* the former was similar to *dafeng,* implying some kind of destruction of the limbs, whereas the latter seemed to indicate skin disorders that were divided into the "black" and "white" types.[31] It is fair to say that, for doctors of the Sui-Tang periods, *dafeng* and *li/lai* did not clearly indicate a single disorder but a variety of diseases affecting the skin and corrupting extremities of the limbs, including probably some form of Hansen's disease. Doctors of this time were obviously interested in the complexities of the two disorders, between which they attempted to establish some connections. Many symptoms of both categories of ailments are strongly suggestive of Hansen's disease as we understand it today, but they may also apply to other skin diseases, such as psoriasis, various forms of tinea, pellagra, and so on, or diseases with similar apparent symptoms at various stages of development, such as forms of diabetes, syphilis, yaws, and others. This ambiguous understanding and classification of the ailments was similar to that in other ancient civilizations. No historical evidence supports the claim that certain terms specifically indicated Hansen's disease in the ancient world.[32] What early Chinese medical experts identified as *li/lai, lifeng/dafeng/efeng* were probably two related categories of diseases with overlapping symptoms, some defined by their cause, others by their symptoms, probably including some forms of leprosy, but not exclusively Hansen's disease as defined today.

Merging of the Dafeng *and* Li/Lai *Categories*

The ambiguous differentiation between the two broad categories of *dafeng/efeng* and *li/lai* disorders finally disappeared around the tenth century, and the two merged into a single group of disorders while still being considered as Wind induced. In two of the most representative medical compilations of the early Song period, the *Taiping shenghui fang* (*Recipes of the Imperial Grace During the Great Peace* [992]), and especially the *Shengji zonglu* (*General Record of Imperial Charity* [eleventh century]), the two classes of disorders finally became one. The compilers of the *Taiping shenghui fang* were the first to use the term *dafeng lai* for the category. However, as they still discussed the *dafeng* and *lai* categories separately, albeit in the same chapter devoted to disorders caused by *feng,* the merging was not yet complete.[33] It was the *Shengji zonglu,* compiled a century later, that finally came up with a single category combining all symptoms of *dafeng/efeng* and *li/lai,* containing ten subgroups. This voluminous compilation, sponsored by the Northern Song government, begins with fourteen chapters on Wind-induced ailments. *Efeng, dafeng,* and *lai* were all included in the last of the fourteen chapters, focusing on Wind-induced disorders with skin symptoms. The six subtopics in this chapter, *efeng, dafeng* causing the loss of eyebrows, *dafeng* with emerging *chong* (creeping worms),[34] *dafeng/lai,* black *lai,* and white *lai,* synthesized discussions of *dafeng* and *lai* in earlier medical classics. More important still, the compilers explain specifically that disorders with symptoms of eyebrow loss due to *dafeng* were in fact *lai* disorders: "Wind, Dampness, noxious *qi* imbued the flesh, causing the excessive pathogen to spread and overflow. The itchiness would develop into sores, corruption of the skin, the collapse of the bridge of the nose, and the falling out of hair and eyebrows."[35] It became clear by the eleventh century that *dafeng* and *lai* disorders should belong to the same category. Medical doctors especially of northern China thereafter all tended to discuss *dafeng* or *li/lai* disorders together in the same category.[36] The interpretations of the relevant passages in the *Inner Canon* by Jin-Yuan medical masters showed this point quite clearly.[37] Liu Wansu (1120–1200), for instance, explained *lifeng* by saying, "[*Lifeng*] is also called *maifeng* [vessel Wind], which finishes by developing *li*, which is what the common people call *lai*." He also considered the treatment by acupuncture for *dafeng* described in the *Divine Pivot* of the same canon as the appropriate cure also for the *lifeng* disorder. Clearly for him, as for the compilers of the *Shengji zonglu, dafeng, lifeng, li/lai* unquestionably referred to the same category of ailments.[38] One should also note that most medical doctors, especially those of the northern tradition, still considered Wind intrusion as the main cause of the disorders.[39]

The Late Imperial Period (Twelfth to Nineteenth Centuries)

During the Song-Jin period, from 1127 to 1279, when China was divided into the northern, Jurchen, Jin and the southern Chinese, Song, regimes, medical knowledge underwent significant development.[40] On the *dafeng/lai* disorders, while northern experts combined *dafeng* and *lai* into a single category of Wind-induced disorders, southern experts started to question the validity of Wind as the essential cause. Chen Yan, one of the most innovative medical writers of the Southern Song and the author of the influential work on etiology *San yin ji yi bingzheng fang lun* (*A Treatise on the Three Categories of Pathogenic Factors of Disorders* [1174]), clearly disagreed with classifying *lifeng, dafeng,* and *lai* as simply "Wind-induced diseases." He said, "*Lifeng* described in the *Inner Canon* is actually *dafeng* and malignant *lai* described in recipe books. Even though the category is called *feng* [Wind], the disorders are not necessarily all caused by Wind."[41] Chen was thus one of the first medical writers who did not situate the *dafeng lai* disorders within the Wind-induced class of disorders. Instead, he discussed the category in a separate chapter that dealt with scrofula and malignant sores and scabies, disorders related mostly to the skin and later classified under *waike* (external medicine), a specialty emerging after the Song on disorders with "external" symptoms, that is, on the body's surface. It was from this point onward that *dafeng lai* as a single category of disorders was increasingly discussed and treated as a skin disease.

This reclassification of the *dafeng lai* disorders as *waike,* or ailments with distinct external symptoms, was parallel to the gradual loss of interest by most elite Confucian doctors in them. While Wind-induced disorders remained as the dominant nosological category deserving sustained attention of elite doctors, specialties such as *waike,* eye disorders, those involving acupuncture, surgery, and so on requiring hands-on expertise, were increasingly snubbed by highly literate elite doctors.[42] Daoist healers, on the other hand, became the more innovative practitioners and authors on *waike* ailments, including *dafeng/lai.* In a fourteenth-century Daoist medical compilation on therapeutics for external ailments, *Xianchuan waike bifang* (*Secret Formulas of External Medicine Transmitted by Immortals*), a passage on the *dafeng* ailment attributed to the Northern Song master Zhang Jixian (1092–1127) combined classical analysis as explained in the *Inner Canon* with new Daoist conceptions of disease transmission developed from the Song dynasty onward. Causes of the ailment now included bad geomancy of ancestral tombs, transmission within the lineage (blood-related relatives), and careless behavior outside the household. The author of this fourteenth-century Daoist passage added that "famous doctors and intelligent literati dread the filthiness [of the ailment] and do not pay much attention to it, whereas ignorant people pass on nonsensical methods,"[43] showing quite accurately the marginalization of medical interest among elite Confucian doctors and the importance of Daoist interpretation and healing related to this ailment by this time. It is thus possible that Daoist views on the ailments were already known by mainstream doctors such as Chen Yan of the twelfth century, who, however, remained silent on his sources.

One has to wait until the mid-sixteenth century for fuller analyses of the ailment. By this time, the dividing line that elite Confucian doctors (*ruyi*) wished to draw between themselves and other medical practitioners was more visible. Scholar-physicians began to take Confucian learning as a model in the Song/Yuan period, and their learning and practice were characterized by a return to old classics, an emphasis on sophisticated diagnostic strategies, and erudition in materia medica, allowing them to prescribe precisely. They also began to distance themselves from hands-on technology and strong drugs, and to condemn ritual and witchcraft healing. Consequently, these specialties, formerly essential parts of healing in the classic age, including acupuncture, moxibustion, various kinds of surgery, the application of strong drugs and magic were increasingly left in the hands of the "others": marginal, popular, or even itinerant, illiterate healers. Many of them were from the Daoist tradition, some were authors of anonymous popular medical texts. From the point of view of mainstream, scholar-physicians, marginal doctors and quacks were almost the same, as they were both ignorant of Confucian and medical classics and their methods were considered too dangerous.[44]

The influential Ming palace doctor Xue Ji (1487–1559) was one of the rare late imperial mainstream doctors who discussed *li*/*lai* at length. Xue was from an important medical lineage of the Jiangnan region and author of major works on external medicine. His three-chapter book on the *li*/*lai* disorders, entitled *Liyang jiyao* (*Keys and Essentials to Skin Disorders of the* Li *Category*) and published in 1528–1529, was probably the first integral book on the disorder. Other than Xue's work, much of the new understanding of *dafeng lai* in the late imperial period was introduced by marginal doctors, less constrained by learned theories and more receptive to popular beliefs and practices, often with a Daoist background. Two such experts were Shen Zhiwen, of the sixteenth century, and Xiao Xiaoting, of the eighteenth century.[45] Shen Zhiwen, the author of one of the first extant books on the disorder, *Jiewei yuansou* (*Sources of Relief* [preface dated 1550]), was definitely a marginal doctor. Other than information contained in this book, published long after his death, in 1816, there is no other extant information about him. We know from the preface that his grandfather was a bureaucrat interested in medicine, and who, however, did not seem to have frequented elite Confucian doctors. Instead, he befriended "hermits dwelling in mountains and forests, eminent men within the four seas," implying Daoist and other marginal medical practitioners. Shen inherited his grandfather's medical learning through his father. He himself also followed the family's tradition of seeking advice and knowledge from "immortals and extraordinary men of the rivers and lakes." The reason for his not publishing the book during his lifetime was that, "after more than thirty years roaming in the rivers and lakes, I have not met the kind of man [to whom I would entrust this book]."[46] The book existed in manuscript form for some 250 years before it was discovered by chance by Huang Zhong, a doctor from Wuxi, a specialist of *waike* and acupuncture with a good reputation in the Jiangnan area. Huang edited and published the manuscript in 1816.[47]

We know a little more about Xiao Xiaoting, author of the *Fengmen quanshu* (*A Complete Work on the Feng Disorder* [preface dated 1796]). A native of Jiangxi province, where he practiced medicine in the late eighteenth century, Xiao specialized in treating *mafeng*. Like his father, from whom he learned medicine, Xiao attempted the civil examination, but without success, at least until 1796, when he wrote the preface for his writings on *mafeng*. On his deathbed, he entrusted the manuscript to a scholar friend, who was also an unsuccessful candidate in the civil examination but who finally got the manuscript published in 1836 as a charitable act "to save the lives of thousands of patients."[48] From Xiao's own descriptions of his unsuccessful scholarly career, and those of his friends with a similar fate, we know that medicine was not his main pursuit, and his reputation as a specialist of *mafeng* was based mostly on his rich experience in treating a large number of such cases in his native place—more than a thousand, as he claimed. In other words, neither Xiao nor Shen could call themselves Confucian doctors or doctors from a respectable medical lineage, nor could they consider themselves heirs of any master or prestigious school of medicine. The content of their unique medical works, characterized by few references to classical theories, in contrast to the rich descriptions of popular concepts and practices, also shows their nonscholarly training in medicine.[49] They were precursors of the leprosy specialists who were active in the late nineteenth century. It was by interviewing these "old leper physicians" in Canton who "had practiced the cure of leprosy for 20 or 30 years" that Wong Foon (Huang Kuan [1829–1878]), a Cantonese doctor trained in Edinburgh and medical officer of the Imperial Maritime Customs in the 1870s, reconstructed and reported on the situation of the disease in the Canton area in 1873.[50]

Together with a small number of mainstream doctors who briefly discussed *mafeng* in their more general medical works, Xue, Shen, and Xiao elaborated on a new understanding of the disorder in the Ming-Qing period initially introduced by Daoist healers and liturgists in the Song period. These other Confucian doctors included Liu Chun (1358–1418), a palace doctor, Xu Chunfu (sixteenth century), Zhang Jiebin (1563–1640), and Qi Kun (mid-seventeenth century), all influential medical doctors and writers of the period. There were, in brief, six major new developments in the understanding of *dafeng* in medical texts on *lai* in this late period: (1) decline of Wind as the external pathogen of the disorder, (2) reclassification of the disorder as a skin disease belonging to the *waike* category, (3) basic symptom being anesthesia of the skin (which explains its new popular term, *mafeng* [numb Wind]),[51] (4) subdivision into two types, one being more serious than the other, (5) disorder considered essentially a disease of the south, and (6) differentiation between a male and a female *mafeng* body. While most of these new ideas were elaborated in concrete detail by marginal doctors often inspired by Daoist healers, the reclassification of the disorder in the nosological structure was brought about mainly by mainstream Confucian doctors.

The dethroning of *mafeng/li/lai* from the Wind-induced category of disorders was obvious in the writings of mainstream doctors from the twelfth century onward. As mentioned, the influential Southern Song doctor Chen Yan was one of the first to challenge the classical etiological explanation of *dafeng/li/lai,* claiming that the disorder was not necessarily caused by Wind. He wrote in his influential work on etiology that disorders under the category of *dafeng/li/lai* "are caused by excessive sexual activity or overexertion on the *qi* and Blood. Such acts generate [internal] heat that provokes sweating. [If the person under such conditions] does not avoid perverse Wind, Cold, and Dampness, excessive *qi* will counteract the defensive *qi* [of the body]. . . . The bodily *qi* will stagnate, and anesthesia of the muscles will follow. When the constructive and defensive *qi* are polluted, they digress [from their respective channels] into the skin and the flesh and corrode their colors, causing their degeneration into sores, and the collapse of the bridge of the nose."[52] While respecting the *Inner Canon*'s descriptions of the mechanism of the digression of constructive *qi* out from its channel into the skin, provoking the external symptoms, Chen rejected the abstract configurationist etiological pattern of Wind as the cause, and provided here the concrete causes of excessive sex and physical exertion, provoking an internal heat that triggered the lethal digression of the body's defensive *qi*.

By the thirteenth century, even the most orthodox doctors no longer considered the disorder a Wind-induced one. Zhu Zhenheng (1282–1358), the most influential Confucian doctor of the Yuan dynasty,[53] reinterpreted *feng* in *dafeng/li/lai* as a special "deadly *qi* between heaven and earth" that was "extremely violent, ferocious, and fearsome."[54] Like Chen Yan, he transformed the abstract configurationist Wind factor of antiquity into a specific notion of a noxious, local *qi*, which became a powerful idea by the Ming period. The important doctor Xu Chunfu, of the sixteenth century, echoed this transformation of the Wind factor. He considered the cause of *lifeng* to be internal heat accumulating into a toxin that he compared with Fire : "[The process] is like a dried object being rapidly inflamed by a fire. One cannot deny that it is not [due to] Wind."[55] The replacement of external Wind by internal heat (Fire), resonant with Chen Yan's explanation in the twelfth century, was a growing medical concept after the Jin-Yuan period.[56] Wu Youxing, the mid-seventeenth century doctor famous for his discussions on impure *qi* (*zaqi*), explicitly rejected the Wind pathogen as presented in the *Inner Canon* as a cause of *li* and suggested "impure *qi*" as the original cause of *li*. In his influential *Wenyi lun* (*Treatise on Epidemics Caused by the Warm Factor* [1642]), Wu explains, "The impure *qi* causes most ailments. But the entire world mistakes it to be the six pathogens [configurationist patterns]. Those ailments mistaken to be caused by Wind, including, for instance, *da mafeng* . . . etc. are actually not caused by Wind but by impure *qi*." This impure *qi*, moreover, entered the body by the mouth and nostrils, unlike Wind , which entered the body through the pores.[57] Wu's position was more radical than that of Zhu Zhenheng three centuries earlier. The idea of impure *qi* emanating from a delimited local region, especially from the ground, causing deadly ailments was increasingly current and continued to influence medical thought in the eighteenth and nineteenth centuries, especially in southern China.[58]

Dislodged from the Wind-induced category, *dafeng/lai* disorders were systematically discussed in chapters or books on skin diseases or *waike* from around the thirteenth century onward. This is the second major change regarding the new understanding of the disorders in the late imperial period. The most important example of this change is the publication of Xue Ji's *Liyang jiyao.* Here, Xue begins his discussion by quoting the mentions of the *lifeng* disorders in the *Inner Canon* and by Zhu Zhenheng without any elaboration on the causes of the disorders, which he clearly categorizes as "*yang,*" skin disorders with sores. Specialized in *waike* disorders, Xue was interested more in discussing the complex symptoms of various types of *liyang* and the corresponding therapeutic methods.[59] For him, there was no longer a need to justify the naming and classifying of the disorders under *waike.* Later mainstream works on external medicine, including Dou Menglin's *Chuangyang jingyan quanshu* (*Complete Book on Sores and Skin Diseases Based on Experience*) and Qi Kun's *Waike dacheng* (*General Work on External Medicine* [1665]), all devoted special sections to discussions of the *dafeng lai* disorder under the topic *da mafeng.*[60] Qing palace doctors concluded this development in the important imperial medical compendium *Yizong jinjian* (*Golden Mirror of Medical Orthodoxy* [1742]), in which *da mafeng* is briefly discussed in the *waike* section, one of the last chapters emphasizing hands-on therapeutic techniques.

This major development in the late imperial period was, in my opinion, closely related to an important new understanding of the disorders: that the primary symptom was anesthesia of the skin, explaining the popularity of the term *mafeng,* in this late imperial period. Even though the loss of sensation (*buren*) had been described as a symptom of Wind-induced disorders in general in the *Inner Canon,* and the Daoist Ge Hong of the fourth century also mentioned numbness of the skin in his discussion of *lai,* the symptom was neither specifically associated with the *dafeng* disorder nor taken seriously in major medical texts until the Ming. Before that, I suspect that Daoist healers were again among the first to elaborate on Ge Hong's observation on numbness of the skin as an important symptom of the *lai* ailment. In the mentioned fourteenth-century Daoist compilation on *waike,* the *Xianchuan waike bifang,* the author of the passage on *dafeng* described the progression of the *dafeng* ailment as "five deaths": the first death was that of the skin, causing numbness, followed by the death of the flesh, then of the Blood, the tendons, and last, the bone, manifested by the collapse of the bridge of the nose. Numbness of the skin was thus the first significant symptom of the ailment.[61]

Later, the sixteenth-century palace doctor Xue Ji, in his *Liyang jiyao,* also mentions five main symptoms, of which anesthesia of the skin came first, followed by insensitivity of the flesh, degeneration of the skin and flesh, falling off of the limbs, and finally, collapse of the bridge of the nose. The logic was that the disorder aggravated progressively from the skin, to the flesh, blood, tendons, and finally the bones, causing specific symptoms at different stages.[62] It is obvious that Xue's understanding of the ailment was similar to that expressed in earlier Daoist texts. Shen Zhiwen, who was explicit on this Daoist background, further elaborated on this symptom: "[At the beginning], when one touches the skin [of the body and hands], it feels as if there were a sheet of paper placed between, there is an irritating numbness. Gradually the flesh will also lose sensation, so that the patient will no longer feel anything, even if cut by a knife."[63] In a way, Shen further stressed the symptom of numbness, as he now discussed the disease as *da mafeng.* The late eighteenth-century expert of *mafeng,* Xiao Xiaoting, considered the great Yuan Confucian doctor Zhu Zhenheng the first to identify this particular symptom, anesthesia of the skin, as the basic one for the *mafeng* disorder, although, as we have seen, the idea was already present in a passage attributed to a Song Daoist and incorporated in the early Ming Daoist canon.[64] This concept soon spread with the popularization of the term *mafeng.*[65] Zhang Jiebin, of the late Ming period, thus wrote, "*Lifeng* is the same as *dafeng,* it is also called *laifeng,* and the popular name for it is *da mafeng.*"[66] Contemporary mainstream works on external medicine, including Qi Kun's *Waike dacheng,* clearly stated in their sections on *da mafeng* that all patients of this disorder "certainly first experience numbness."[67] The new terms *mafeng* and *da mafeng* gradually replaced the older terms *dafeng/lifeng* and are still used as the most common translations of Hansen's disease. The modern understanding of *mafeng* in China was formulated largely in the late imperial period, roughly from the fourteenth century onward, before it incorporated concepts from Western biomedicine of the nineteenth century.

The fourth innovation in the understanding of *mafeng/lai* was the distinction between two types of *lai* according to curability. In a sense, doctors were rationalizing the ancient division of the disorder into two types: *dafeng* and *li/lai,* now that there was only one category, *mafeng.* On this, Shen Zhiwen was most explicit: "In former times, the disorder was divided into *feng* and *li.* If [the pathogen] enters deeply into the body, it is called *feng;* and if it remains on the surface, it is a superficial infection and is called *li. Feng* is more serious than *li.* . . .

Feng, after entering the viscera and having resided several years inside the vessels, manifests itself on the flesh and skin, and there are progressive mutations. A patient harmed by *li* will have filthy sores, until his physical appearance degenerates. So one says that the *feng* disorder manifests late but death comes sooner, whereas *li* manifests itself sooner but death comes later. Yet both can be equally damaging." In another passage, Shen repeated, "The difference between *feng* and *lai* is their relative gravity, though the damage is the same. A cured *lai* patient can still restore his physical appearance, whereas a cured *feng* patient loses his original vital energy forever. Those who die of *lai* are few whereas most die of *feng*."[68] Here Shen seems to imply that patients of *feng* will have *li* symptoms at a later stage, whereas patients of simple *lai* and not *feng* had a less-serious case and could survive longer. One can say that by the sixteenth century, medical experts agreed that *dafeng lai* was of the same category but having two main subtypes of similar apparent symptoms, one being more serious than the other. This view was fully adopted by Qing specialists. The important early Qing doctor Zhang Zhicong (1610–1695), in his interpretation of the related passage in the *Inner Canon*, indicated that the serious form of *li*, caused by the digression of the constructive energy out of its vessels into the skin, will have symptoms like the collapse of the bridge of the nose and the corruption of the skin, whereas a lighter form of *li*, caused by Cold Wind residing inside the vessels, has symptoms like purplish or white patches on the skin.[69] Similarly, Xu Dachun (1693–1771), made the following comment on the section on *lai* in a work on external medicine by Chen Shigong (fl. 1617), "There are cases appearing to be *da mafeng* but that are curable. It is when the toxic *qi* has not penetrated too deeply and remains mostly in the flesh."[70] By the mid-nineteenth century, at least in the Canton area, specialists of leprosy claimed that they could distinguish five or six different types.[71]

The fifth new development was that the disorder was gradually perceived to be a southern disease. This idea might already have been implied in Zhu Zhenheng's proposition of a specific violent local *qi* as the main cause of the disease. We know that the southeastern region of Lingnan, covering Fujian, Guangdong, and Guangxi provinces, had been considered as infested with noxious epidemic *qi* since antiquity,[72] and the idea developed into a commonplace by the mid-Ming period. It became natural to state that the miasmic region of southern China was nurturing this noxious *qi* that caused *li*/*lai*. By the sixteenth century, the idea was dominant in medical texts. Xue Ji stated that the *li* category of skin diseases were found mostly in areas to the south of the Huai River, the Lingnan region and Fujian province.[73] Shen Zhiwen, in various chapters of his text on *mafeng*/*lai*, repeated the belief that Fujian and Guangdong provinces were the most affected. Later Ming medical texts even distorted older texts on *dafeng lai* in order to conform to the belief that it was indeed endemic in the warm regions. The *Shouyu shenfang* (*Miraculous Recipes for Achieving Longevity* [of Chongzheng's reign, 1628–1644]) quotes the well-known Tang story of a leper, who, after having drunk a viper wine known to be an effective cure, melted into water, with only his hair remaining intact. The author of this late-Ming text twisted the original version by adding that the leper had been infected with the disease while visiting Guangdong province.[74] This distortion was in line with many other contemporary and later texts that considered the *li/lai* or *mafeng* disorder as a southern endemic, such as Chen Shidou's *Shishi milu* (*Secret Record of the Stone Chamber* [1689]). Chen gave a new name to the disorder, *zhangli* (miasmatic *li*): "It is due to a *qi* metamorphosed from the steaming of the thick *qi* of the Guangdong and Guangxi regions. This *qi* is all hot and not cold . . . as *da mafeng* is purely a hot and noxious *qi*, residing in the skin."[75] This popular concept departed greatly from the original one in the *Inner Canon*, where Wind and Cold were said to be the main pathogens of *dafeng*. Indeed, from the mid-seventeenth century onward, *dafeng lai*, alias *mafeng* or *da mafeng*, was commonly perceived to be a disease rampant in the hot and damp Lingnan regions, including Fujian, Jiangxi, Guangdong, and Guangxi provinces.

The new conceptualization of *dafeng lai* or *da mafeng* as a class of disease crystallized in the seventeenth century was summarized in the imperial medical compendium of the mid-eighteenth century, the *Yizong jinjian*, mentioned in the preceding. In this medical encyclopedia, still in use today as a textbook in colleges of Chinese medicine, under the section "Essentials of Authentic Methods in External Medicine" (*waike xinfa yaojue*), the disorder is named *da mafeng*, anesthesia being its primary symptom, and described as an ailment common in the "miasmatic regions" of the empire, "rarely seen" elsewhere. A milder form, with symptoms appearing slowly and eventually curable, is mentioned, otherwise the disease was described as fatal.[76] This understanding of *da mafeng* would remain in effect until the modern period.

Finally, one last important idea emerged in nonmainstream medical texts regarding the *mafeng/lai* disorders, and that is the differentiation between the female and the male bodies in their receptivity to the disease. The female body was believed to be more "resistant" to the ailment, with its menstrual blood regularly expelling internal poison, and it was also thought to be able to retain the poison without manifesting the usual symptoms. The female body was thus a particularly dangerous contagious body, as its healthy appearance could be deceptive. The idea, never addressed in mainstream medical texts, was greatly elaborated by marginal doctors. This idea was in fact also present in late medieval medicine in Europe.[77] Shen Zhiwen wrote that women retaining the toxin inside their viscera

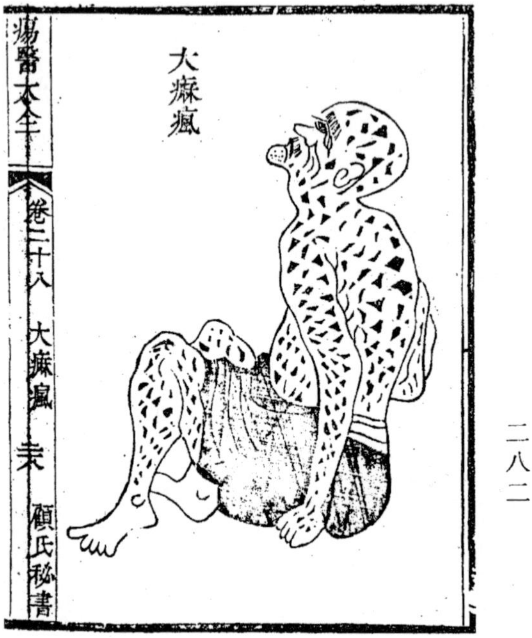

Representation of a leper in the *Yangyi daquan* (*Complete Book on the Medicine for Sores* [1760]), by Gu Shicheng.

could pass the disorders onto men with whom they had intercourse, or to their children. He demonstrated his point by quoting the example of the daughter of a patient who appeared without illness but gave birth to a son with the disorder.[78] Xiao Xiaoting was even more systematic in his declaration of the differences between male and female patients of the disorder: "It is rare that men pass the disorder to women, but often women pass it on to men. Why is this so? It is because women release the toxin by their monthly menstruation, and fewer are those who suffer from the disease."[79] The emergence of the idea of a contagious and dangerous and southern female body retaining an unmanifested toxin in the late imperial medical texts introduced the fear of "careless" sexual intercourse, and corresponded with the growing popular belief of the "passing on of *lai,*" that virgins of southern China with the disease in the incubatory stage could get rid of the toxin by passing it on to men, usually those from the north, whom they seduced (see chap. 3).

The changes of the *mafeng*/*lai* category in the general nosography according to symptoms over the centuries reflect significant developments in the etiological analyses of the disorder in different historical stages. While it is impossible to be certain if the diseases conceptualized under the headings of *dafeng, li/lai, dafeng lai,* and *da mafeng* of different historical periods were the same, especially since medical texts described a great variety of symptoms, the etiological analyses of them throughout history did allow a line of development to be drawn going through all of them, making the reconceptualization of these categories into a single one, now generally called *mafeng,* in the late imperial period understandable.

The Factor of Magic: The *Chong* Agent and *Gu* Magic

Another important etiological explanation for *dafeng* and *li/lai* is related to the idea of *chong* (creeping or flying worm) and *gu* (witchcraft using *chong*). The idea of harmful *chong* inside the human body was present in an important ancient medical text, *Wushi'er bing fang* (*Recipes for Fifty-two Ailments* [ca. 300 B.C.])[80] though it was absent in the *Inner Canon*. Briefly, this idea is associated with an eclectic tradition closer to ancient witchcraft and medical folklore. Extant materials of the early period contain scarce information on *chong* as a cause of disease, and writings by Chao Yuanfang and Sun Simiao of the seventh century are the earliest extant ones that provide details on the phenomenon of *chong.* For Chao, *chong* was an important cause of *lai:* "Various Winds can harm the human body. The five Winds create five kinds of harmful *chong* to human beings. . . . They are called Winds of ailments [*jifeng*]. When they enter the five viscera, [the *chong* associated with these Winds] gnaw them away. [The *chong*] become numerous inside the body, and enter the marrow of the bones, and nothing will stop them from going around the body."[81] How did these *chong* damage the body and cause *lai*? "When they gnaw at the depot of the Liver [*gan*], the eyebrows fall out; when they gnaw at the depot of the Lung [*fei*], the bridge of the nose collapses; when they gnaw at the depot of the Spleen [*pi*], the voice becomes coarse; when they gnaw at the depot of the Kidney [*shen*], the ears ring; when they gnaw at the depot of the Heart [*xin*], as the Heart cannot be touched, the patient dies."[82] For Chao, *chong* was at the same time a constitutive part of the human body and its potential destroyer. "There are 80,000 corpse *chong* [*shi chong*] constituting the human body, which would be incomplete without them. Then there are various vicious evils and ailments and Winds harmful to the human body. The so-called five Winds stimulating the five *chong* can do harm to a person. . . . [Winds of ailments] can enter the five depots and [stimulate the *chong* to] gnaw them away. Then the *chong* reproduce and become numerous inside the human body. They enter the marrow of the bones, and nothing stops them from traveling back and forth."[83]

Sun Simiao further elaborated on such an idea with the notion of the nine *chong* (a multiple of the Daoist "three corpses" forming the human body) constitutive of the body but also potentially harmful to it. These *chong*, according to Sun, had a head and a tail, measuring three *cun*. Each of the nine *chong* had a name and different colors and shapes. They attacked different parts of the viscera, causing different ailments to the person. One of them could cause *lai* in a person.[84] Chao's and Sun's views perhaps reflected contemporary Buddhist and Daoist notions of the human body.[85] *Li/lai* was simply one of the ailments that were caused by vicious Winds triggering a series of actions of some *chong* already residing inside the body, especially inside the viscera.

The idea of *chong* apparently did not draw much interest from Song-Yuan mainstream medical writers.[86] It reemerged as an important cause of *mafeng/li/lai* only in the late imperial period, when the disorder was at the same time increasingly associated with the southern miasmatic regions, which were also known for *gu* witchcraft, whereby mysterious ailments were transmitted. This point was most clearly brought out by Shen Zhiwen, who wrote, "In the regions of Fujian and Guangdong, there are witchcraft techniques involving vipers [*she gu*], and poison spread by magic water, talismans, and incantation in the miasmatic region is most harmful. Poisonous *chong* emerge from the seven orifices of corpses of people who have just died of the malignant ailment [*eji*] and fly toward any living human passing by, and conceal themselves as *gu* that will do him harm later on."[87]

Shen's description reflects a long and complex history of *gu* magic that was associated with *chong*. The ideogram for *gu*, "at least as ancient as the Chinese script itself," is composed of two parts: the upper part is the ideogram *chong*, and the lower part, the ideogram *ming*, meaning a vessel. The magic consisted precisely of putting *chong* in a vessel.[88] The *chong* used in this magic consisted not only of creeping worms but also of vipers, toads, and other vermin. Extant early texts do not describe details of how the magic was carried out, though it was definitely closely related to diseases. Ge Hong, of the fourth century, included recipes for the treatment of *gu* ailments in his famous book on prescriptions for urgent uses.[89] As far as we know, the first extant account of *gu* magic was given by Chao Yuanfang: "There are several kinds of *gu*, which are all bewitching. People sometimes deliberately manipulate them. They take snakes and worms and other similar creatures and put them together in a vessel. They allow these creatures to devour each other until only one is left, and the survivor is *gu*. It can transform itself and bewitch. When put in food and drink, it harms [the person who takes the food and drink]. It does harm to others but is beneficial to the manipulator of the *gu*. . . . There are also flying *gu*; they travel back and forth without trace. . . . He who is attacked by them become gravely sick. Whoever becomes sick because of *gu* usually dies, because the poison of *gu* is extremely strong. Therefore it is called *gu* poison." In another passage, Chao writes that a person attacked by *gu* will die from his viscera being eaten up. After his death, "the ailment is poured onto [*liu zhu*] those nearby. This is called the 'pouring of *gu*.'"[90] *Gu* as a witchcraft inducing disease was also associated with female seduction since ancient times.[91] One point that should be stressed here is that, from the earliest appearances of the character *gu* until the medieval period, as Feng and Shryock have pertinently pointed out, "the practice of *gu* seems to have been a specific cultural feature which the ancient inhabitants of the Yellow River valley shared with inhabitants of more southern areas."[92] *Gu* was therefore a practice common in most regions in ancient China.

After the Tang dynasty, mainstream Confucian doctors no longer dealt with *gu* as a cause of disease as did Chao Yuanfang. Daoist liturgists of the Song period, especially after the twelfth century, became the leading innovators in the description and prevention of *gu*. The most representative is Lu Shizhong, founder of the Great Method of the Jade Hall (Yutang dafa) in Daoist ritual tradition. Rituals dealing with various types and stages of *gu* and *chong*, as well as epidemics, were described in great detail in his compilation. This text, interestingly, also contained descriptions of symptoms of ailments, in particular *lao* consumption, caused by *gu* and *chong* comparable to earlier medical texts such as Chao's. In this sense, there was no clear boundary between such Daoist ritual texts and medical texts.[93] Lu's tradition became especially influential in the Southern Song period (1127–1279), a time when the *gu* belief had found more fertile ground in southern China.

There are indications that, since the early medieval period, the central authorities had passed laws that punished practitioners of *gu* by drowning.[94] The practice was probably suppressed in many parts of central China before and during the Song but somehow survived in peripheral southern China, and it was considered from then on as a practice of that region, particularly among the semicivilized peoples of China's periphery. In addition, the idea of *gu* magic was readily associated with the climatic and ecological characteristics of the south. In the famous collection of recipes for ailments of the Lingnan region, the *Lingnan weisheng fang*, of the latter thirteenth century, one section is devoted to a description of *gu* that largely repeats Chao's ideas. According to the compilers of the volume, the region was so rampant with vipers and worms of all kinds, that *gu* was a common practice.[95] Nonmedical texts of the Song also record *gu* practice as specific to south or southwestern China, especially among women of the non-Chinese minorities. Zhu Zhenheng wrote simply, "The poison of *gu* is rare in the center of the empire [*zhong tu*]. There are more than a hundred that transmit the practice, most of whom are people from the deep mountains in Fujian and Guangdong."[96]

The idea became commonplace in late imperial texts of the Ming and Qing. The Miao and Dong women were often believed to be practitioners of *gu,* which was executed usually on the fifth day of the fifth moon, the time for confronting the gods of pestilences.[97] The interpretations of the practice of *gu* magic in the late imperial period show its association with semicivilized peoples and the polluting female of hot regions, interpretations that were absent in early records on *gu,* but they also confirm its ancient role as a mysterious cause of horrifying and deadly diseases.

It was in this context that Shen Zhiwen wrote his text on *mafeng/lai* in the mid-sixteenth century. The text contained many of the ideas already recorded in earlier texts, with the new idea that *gu* was now clearly a southern Chinese magic practice. Medically speaking, there are two other new ideas in Shen Zhiwen's passage on *gu* in relation to the *mafeng* ailment. It was the first time that the *mafeng/lai* ailment was related to *gu,* the use of magic *chong* from outside the patient's body. In early medieval texts, by which time *chong* was already viewed as an agent, it was, however, the innate, constitutive part of the patient's body that had gone bad under the influence of vicious Wind. Chao Yuanfang and Sun Simiao did not relate *gu* to the *li/lai* ailment. Second, the ailment was therefore logically considered to be specific to the southern region. This new idea of *chong,* an evil, vicious, disgusting, and terrifying witchcraft agent, contributed greatly to the reconstruction of the *li/lai* disorder as perhaps the most dreaded disease in late imperial China, in a region not quite civilized by Chinese culture, as *gu* magic was by then considered as something alien to Chinese civilization. In the words of Zhang Jiebin, the influential late Ming doctor, *lifeng* "is the foulest, the most dangerous, and ugliest of all disorders." It is significant that he wrote these words right after he explained the effect of *chong* as a cause of the disorder.[98] The *chong* element also led to a new etiological analysis of the disorder, that of *chuanran* contagion (contamination by transmission).

The Notion of *Chuanran* Contagion and the Association with Guangdong Sores (Syphilis)

The concept of disease transmission in traditional China was not purely medical. Closely associated with the idea of retribution and taboo violation in the ancient and medieval periods, it was appropriated by "Confucian medicine" only in the later imperial period. As in many cultures, leprosy or diseases with ugly external symptoms were often understood in China as a retribution for prior sins or wrongdoing, or a violation of taboos. During the medieval period, a nonmedical equivalent term for the disorder was *tianxing* (punishment from heaven). Chao Yuanfang's work contains abundant information on taboo violation as a cause of *lai:* "All *lai* ailments are due either to [the intrusion] of vicious Wind [*efeng*] or to the violation of taboos [*fan chu jihai*]."[99] Sun Simiao later wrote that many patients of the "vicious disease" were literati who, when asked the reason for their having fallen ill, answered that they had been "doing unkindly [*bu ren*][100] things for a long time, and had committed extremely despicable sins." Sun further commented that "words of regret without sincere repentance" would not help the curing of the disease. Wang Tao repeated Sun's recommendations almost word for word.[101] For all of these major medieval doctors, immoral behavior and its retribution were certainly one major cause of *dafeng* or *lai.* These ideas of retribution persisted in later medical texts, including Chen Yan's treatise on etiological categories of the thirteenth century, and most Ming-Qing texts on the ailment.[102] I give, in the next chapter, examples of people contracting *lai* after having committed serious crimes, as narrated in nonmedical texts. These ideas were echoed in most late imperial medical texts analyzing the ailment.

Moral transgression was, moreover, often not a problem only for the individual; the guilt of serious wrongdoing was believed to be borne not only by the responsible person but also by his household, descendants, and people dwelling in the same area. The transmission of disease, often called *zhulian* (the "pouring" of an ailment onto a succession of victims), was often linked to such an idea of collective responsibility, as already clearly expressed in the early Daoist classic *Taiping jing* (*Scripture of the Great Peace*), an early-Han text (ca. third century).[103] Based on this and other contemporary texts, Yang Lien-sheng and, later, Li Jianmin highlighted this idea of shared fate in the concept of disease transmission, essentially within the lineage and household.[104] Such ideas developed greatly during the medieval Sui-Tang periods, with the agents *chong* or *gu* magic seen as the main media of transmission. Chao Yuanfang's text is particularly rich in descriptions of disease transmission within a lineage or among people living under the same roof.[105] Chao described in several places two stages of transmission, a primary one within the same household and a secondary one extending to "bystanders."[106] The underlying idea was obviously a shared guilt among lineage members. Even though these ideas are rarely seen in Song Confucian medical texts, they occurred in religious texts. An important example is the passage referred to previously on the *dafeng* ailment attributed to the Northern Song master Zhang Jixian included in the early Ming Daoist medical text *Xianchuan waike bifang.* The author of the passage puts forth bad geomancy of ancestors' tombs and transmission within the same lineage as the leading causes of the ailment.[107]

It is thus likely that sometime during the Song-Jin-Yuan period, through such religious texts, the transmission of the *lai* ailment within a lineage was considered similar to that of *lao* consumption.

Shen Zhiwen further developed these ideas, claiming as the first of the four major causes of *mafeng/lai* "damage done by [bad] geomancy and yin/yang astrology," including the undesirable position of one's dwelling or ancestors' burial ground, bad stars under which one was born, violating the gods, offending bad spirits, and so on.[108] Contemporary mainstream doctors such as Gong Tingxian also identified bad geomancy as a main cause of the disease: "Bad geomancy of [ancestors'] tombs will provoke the appearance of strange sores and symptoms [of the skin]."[109] More important is that both Ming doctors mentioned "biological transmission" as the second major cause, implying that ill omens resulting from immoral behavior and violation of taboos would be borne not only by the responsible person but also by his descendants. Similarly, one had to suffer the consequences of the immorality of one's ancestors and relatives. This ancient idea of transmission by *zhulian* was the basis of the new idea of *chuanran* contagion that emerged in the Song and matured in the Ming-Qing period. For late imperial specialists of *li/lai,* the ailment was transmitted not only within the family but also *outside* the household.

The term *chuanran* first appeared in medical and nonmedical texts in the Song period, and it referred to contamination (*ran* [literally, to dye]) by transmission (*chuan* [to transmit, to pass from one place to another]), usually specifically person-to-person transmission. Other composite terms with *ran* referring to the spread of disease by various means appeared in earlier texts, only some of which vaguely implied contamination by personal contact.[110] Chen Yan was the first medical doctor to use the term *chuanran* as one of the causes of the *dafeng/lai* disorder. Before his time, neither the Wind nor the *chong* factor as causes of the disorder was associated in any way to the idea of transmissibility from one person to another. Chen's idea of transmission was nonetheless vague: "And *chuanran* is also a cause. One is not, in this case, accountable for [contracting the disease], as one is only being careless. The transmission through *qi* and Blood is not quite the same as retribution for former sins."[111] Chen here was probably deliberately vague concerning this new idea of transmission, about which he was uncertain. My speculation is that the "carelessness" he mentions in this passage referred to careless behavior while traveling, including careless sex, my reason being that the idea of the transmissibility of the ailment by sexual intercourse was already popular in southeastern society by his time. I will elaborate on this point in chapter 3. Chen was obviously at a loss in attempting to explain and elaborate on the idea of *chuanran.*

This emerging idea of *chuanran* in Southern Song medical texts was very probably introduced by contemporary Daoist liturgists. The twelfth-century Daoist ritual handbook *Wushang xuanyuan santian yutang dafa,* compiled by the influential master Lu Shizhong and his followers, includes the emerging idea of disease transmission in relation to *lao zhai* consumption, perceived to be transmitted by *chong* (creeping bugs). The text describes rituals for preventing contagion by clothing, bedclothes, beds, utensils, or by entering the house of a patient or sharing his food. Things used by the sick or by the dead were believed to be impregnated with corrupt *qi,* or polluting *gu* toxin.[112] While disease transmission by *gu* or *chong* mentioned in Sui-Tang medical texts was typically described within the household context, this Southern Song Daoist text recognized contagion "irrespective of family relationship," as observed by Michel Strickmann, for whom this text marks a break in the traditional Daoist understanding that the chain of disease transmission was a consequence of shared guilt or genetic predisposition of the same lineage. According to the new understanding (see also my discussion on Daoist redemption in chap. 2), anyone in proximity to the sick or the dead was prone to *chuanran* contagion.[113] Contagion was thus no longer uniquely a hereditary moral cause of disease, it could simply be the consequence of "being careless," as stated by Chen Yan.

This new Daoist idea on disease transmission had yet to be defined and incorporated in the Confucian medical tradition, as the established medical canon did not provide any easy theoretical framework for its development. This is the main reason for the long reticence after the term *chuanran* was coined in Chen Yan's text. The idea was, however, inevitable, as old etiological categories were no longer satisfactory for explaining all the observable features of many ailments, especially epidemics, and person-to-person contagion outside the household was already a popular idea. One of the first reactions to Chen Yan's idea of *chuanran* regarding *lai* was uttered by the early Ming palace doctor Liu Chun. In an interesting comment on the etiological explanation of *lifeng* by Xu Yanchun (?–1384), a disciple of the great Confucian doctor Zhu Zhenheng,[114] Liu expressed his skepticism about the idea of *chuanran* while accepting the ancient idea of transmission within a family: "As for cases caused by *chuanran,* there may be a few. However, even though [through] Blood and the channels, eating and drinking [in the same place], [sharing the same] habitat and temperament [*qiwei*] [of members] within the same family, mutual transmission [*xiangchuan*] [could be facilitated], there will be no infection [*ran*] if there is no accumulation of internal poison by excessive heat."[115]

Liu's comment reveals several interesting ideas around the term *chuanran* as applied to *mafeng/lai* in the early fifteenth century in mainstream medical thought. First, the idea remained of essentially transmission within a lineage or among blood-related persons, as was prevalent in texts of the seventh century. Second, within this general idea, a few interesting details were specified: there were several possible paths of transmission, of a very different nature, including physiological relationships (Blood and channels), close physical contact (sharing meals and habitat), and a shared psychological predisposition (same temperament). More interesting still is Liu's reluctance to confront the idea of contagion outside the family, as already described in Song Daoist ritual texts and suggested by Chen Yan. However, one can nonetheless say that implications of congeneric, congenital, or hereditary transmission and contagion by close contact with the sick can be read in Liu's comments. Liu remained skeptical, however, of the importance of *chuanran* as a major cause of the *lai* disorder.

It was again marginal doctors such as Shen Zhiwen who further elaborated on the notion of *chuanran* and *li/lai* in the late imperial period. More clearly than the Daoist ritualists of the Song, Shen distinguished two modes of *chuanran* transmission: the traditional one within the lineage, and a new one occurring outside the lineage. The former, which Shen referred to as "affected by transmission [*chuanran*] at the [biological] origin" (*yuanliu chuanran suo xi*), is described as follows: "Human beings are formed by the essence and Blood of one's father and mother and activated by heaven and earth and nature. Thus, if [one is] in contact with unharmonious *qi* between heaven and earth, one will fall ill. If [one's] parents are longtime patients of the malignant ailment [*eji*], their Essence and Blood certainly contain poison. [Sexual] intercourse [will produce] an infected fetus, and the disease will thus be transmitted to the child." Shen continued to elaborate on such a hereditary transmission by emphasizing the different clinical expressions after infection of male and female children. We have seen that by Shen's time, the female body was already considered to have a distinct receptivity to the *mafeng* disorder. Its monthly discharge of blood was believed to have the function of ridding it of internal poison, thus preventing the woman from getting the full disease. Women were also said to be able to pass the disease, it will be recalled, to their sexual partners without showing the symptoms themselves.[116] Based on such an understanding, Shen further enriched the idea of *chuanran* by adding to the notion of congenital transmission the possibility of contagion by sexual intercourse, mostly from women to men. He used the magic notion of the "pouring of poison [onto]" (*zhu*) to explain the process of contagion from women to men through sexual intercourse, thus avoiding reference to the more conventional physiological notions of Blood and channels: "A poison obtained during intercourse of excessive lust could be eliminated during [another act of] intercourse of excessive lust. Is this not dreadful?"[117] While congenital transmission from parents or ancestors to descendants was unquestionably within the same lineage, sexual transmission, especially from women to men, was ambiguous, as the sexual partners were not necessarily from the same lineage. Thus careless sexual behavior outside the household was a possible channel of *lai* transmission.

The second mode of *chuanran* transmission, outside the lineage, which Shen described as "infection by filthy *qi* and the pouring of *gu*" (*qi hui guzhu*). Here Shen borrowed directly from the magic *gu* transmission of *lao zhai* consumption depicted previously by the Song Daoist liturgist Lu Shizhong:

> The process by which the poison of one is poured onto another is called *zhu*. . . . If a person with depleted Blood and *qi*, and a weak Spleen and Stomach, encounters by chance someone with the malignant disorder, he might inhale the filthy *qi* of the latter. The poisonous *qi* from the patient might force its way into the mouth and nostrils of the healthy person while talking to him, and [this *qi*] will enter the five viscera and develop into an illness. Another possibility is that when a weak or hungry person uses a toilet visited by a patient . . . , the filthy and poisonous *qi* excreted by the latter, not yet dissipated, will force its way up and enter the healthy person's mouth and nostrils and into his viscera. . . . This belongs to the same kind of transmission by sweat, as in cases of diarrhea epidemics.[118]

Here, as is clear, contagion by close contact with a patient, not genetically related, through the upper respiratory system or by bodily discharge is described. However, one must note that, even if the breath of the patient, his excrement, and sweat are seen as the contagious elements, the physical constitution of the healthy person is also a determining factor. Depleted and weak persons are more likely to be infected when in close contact with a sufferer. Shen here adds a few very interesting new channels of transmission to Lu Shizhong's description: the mouth and nostrils, bodily fluid like sweat, and the toilet, which was now seen as a particularly dangerous place of infection.

Shen's borrowing from *lao zhai* consumption continued the idea of *chong* as an agent in the process of *zhu* transmission. *Chong* was described as transmitting the disease in several ways: it could, for example, fly out of corpses toward healthy people and infect them, seen mostly in the "miasmatic regions of Fujian and Guangdong," famous for *gu* witchcraft poison. For Shen, corpses of people dead for a long time could still be dangerous, and he cited examples of healthy people infected with the disorder while walking by old tombs or cemeteries. *Chong*, moreover, was also responsible for cases of the sort of congenital transmission described previously. Besides the possibility of being infected by the poison of one's father's Essence and mother's Blood at the moment of conception, one could also be infected by the disease by vicious *chong* residing in the parents' viscera, just as the *lao* (consumption of the lungs) disorder was transmitted from parents to children.[119] The danger of *chong* as a contagious agent, therefore, was closely associated with the living bodies of progenitors and the dead bodies of *lai* patients, especially in China's deep south. These magic ideas on disease transmission, once prominent in medical texts in the medieval period, were again described in this late imperial text penned by a marginal doctor clearly influenced by Daoist medicine.

Ming mainstream doctors after Shen soon picked up some of these ideas on contagion and provided interesting clarifications. The palace doctor Gong Tingxian (fl.1577–1593) said in one of his works, under the heading of *da mafeng*, that there were three main causes: "One is due to [bad] geomancy, another is transmission and mutation, and the third one is poor bodily discipline [*shi tiaoli*]." He then elaborated on the idea of transmission and mutation: "[The disorder can be] transmitted from one to another [*huxiang chuan zhe*], from ancestors [to descendants] or parents, from husbands and wives or other members of the family; or [it can be] transmitted, if one is careless *outside* [my emphasis], in toilets, bedrooms, by bedding, clothes, and covers."[120] Gong clarifies for us here the phrase "being careless" already used by Chen Yan three centuries earlier by adding the adverb "outside," explicitly indicating the second mode of transmission outside the lineage context, independent of wrongdoing by ancestors and parents. Gong implies here traveling men's imprudent behavior, including particularly the search for carnal pleasure, resulting in their contracting the disorder in chambers, toilets, and from bedding. From there, of course, the ailment could be transmitted from husband to wife and from ancestors to descendants and so on. Congenital and sexual transmission with sexual partners other than one's wives and concubines is clearly evoked in Gong's short description.

However, the theoretical aspect of the contagiousness of *mafeng* was not resolved. Chen Yan's reticence and Liu Chun's doubt were never addressed by mainstream doctors. What Gong Tingxian and the Qing imperial compendium described as processes of contagion were more in the realm of magic than properly medical in the Confucian sense. The issue of Blood and *qi* raised by Chen was never discussed. The problem was finally tackled directly, albeit awkwardly, by the late eighteenth century marginal doctor Xiao Xiaoting. After having further elaborated the various channels of contagion of the *mafeng* disorder already mentioned by his predecessors, he added his own observations,[121] writing, "People might ask that, since the *qi* and Blood [of a person] each follows its respective channel [*jing*], how can [any disorder] be transmitted from one to another? Do they not realize that even psoriasis and tinea can be contagious [*chuanran*], not to mention leprosy."[122] Xiao's statement suggests the reason behind the mainstream doctors' reluctance to elaborate on the process of contagion more fully. It is obviously difficult to explain body-to-body *chuanran* when each body is seen as an enclosed structure with its own distinct circulatory system of Blood and *qi*. Xiao's "solution" was to explain by analogy with less serious skin diseases of similar external symptoms.

This development of the idea of person-to-person transmission, especially congenital contagion and through sexual intercourse, in the mid-sixteenth century was definitely related to the appearance of a disease considered to be new in the sixteenth century, the "Guangdong sores" (*Guang chuang*). Most historians of Chinese medicine consider this to be some form of syphilis, and with good reason. The terms *Guang chuang* or *yangmei chuang* (*Myrica*, or bayberry, sores) first appeared in medical texts of the early sixteenth century. One of the first doctors who mentioned this disease was Yu Bin, in a work published in 1522: "During the end of the Hongzhi reign [1488–1505], there were people who suffered from malignant sores. The Cantonese were the first to suffer from them. People of the Wu region [Jiangnan area] do not know this and call the disease 'Guangdong sores.' Sometimes they also call them *yangmei* sores, as their shape looks like *Myrica* type berries."[123] A few decades later, Li Shizhen, author of the influential pharmacopoeia *Bencao gangmu* (1579–1593), provided a more detailed account of the disease: "*Yangmei* sores were not recorded in old recipes, there were no patients of such a disease. It began recently in the southeastern region [Lingbiao] and spread all over the empire. It is because the southeastern region is low and warm. There are mountains emanating miasmatic vapor that steams under the heat. People there like to eat spicy and hot food. Men and women are lascivious and immoral. Dampness and heat accumulate thickly to form a pathogen that causes the development of malignant sores that are mutually contagious among people [*huxiang chuanran*] [and spread] from the south to the north, so that the disease is now everywhere. But then all those who fall victim are lascivious people."[124] In other words, soon after the spread of the ailment was visible in southern China, it was seen as a sexually transmitted disease. It was precisely during this period that Shen Zhiwen wrote his book on *mafeng*/*lai*.[125]

The full impact of *yangmei chuang* would be felt from the seventeenth century onward, as shown by the publication of Chen Sicheng's book *Meichuang milu* (*Secret Account of the Rotting Sores Disorder* [1632]), which was even taken to Japan. In this work, Chen provides details on the different ways in which the disease could be passed on from one to another, especially on hereditary and sexual transmission within the lineage context: "This ailment is not transmitted only through sexual intercourse. When people with weak constitutions go to use toilets in town, or talk with patients with the disorder, they are sometimes infected with the toxic *qi*. . . . The disease can also be transmitted [by a husband] to his wife or concubine [*neishi* (literally, inner chamber)]. Even if the wife or concubine does not fall ill, the disease can be transferred [*yi*] to the children, nephews, or grandchildren." Guangdong sores were obviously considered to be transmitted similarly to *mafeng*/*lai* as described by Shen Zhiwen about a century earlier. But Chen, like Li Shizhen, was particularly emphatic on transmission by sex: "Recently customs have deteriorated, numerous are those who indulge themselves in brothels and do not take precaution while doing so. . . . Before they realize [that they are infected], they have already passed the disease on to their wives and concubines, or to their pretty boy servants."[126] Again, carelessness was associated with sexual behavior.

The strikingly similar ways of transmission of *mafeng*/*lai* and Guangdong sores described in Ming-Qing medical books reflects the frequent confusion of the two ailments. The confusion can be read in Shen Zhiwen's work, written several decades after the recorded "appearance" of the new disease. Immediately following his general analyses of the causes of *feng* and *lai*, he adds, "People north of the Yangzi River call the *li* disorder 'blister sores [*paochuang*],' and southerners imitate the name and call them *yangmei chuang*, or Guangdong sores."[127] The confusion, I think, was due largely to two factors: first, both diseases were considered, even by mainstream doctors of the sixteenth century, as endemic to the south, and second, both had similar external symptoms. We have already seen how important sixteenth-century doctors like Xue Ji classified the *li* disease as a southern disease. That *li*/*lai* was now seen as a disorder caused by accumulated internal heat mutated into toxin (ideas of Zhu Zhenheng and Xu Chunfu) greatly encouraged doctors to view it as specific to the hot, damp south. For the same reason, Li Shizhen and others considered Guangdong sores, the new disease, as originating in hot, damp, miasmatic Guangdong. Chen Sicheng echoes Li's explanation of Guangdong sores: "In the Lingnan region, the ground is low, damp, and warm; it never snows nor freezes, snakes and insects do not hibernate. All filth accumulates there. When the first *yang*[128] arrives, damp poison and miasma [*zhangqi*] steam [under the sun]. Things in contact with it easily rot and perish. Human beings in contact with it are easily infected with rotting sores."[129] Ming-Qing doctors tended to consider the south, with its particular topography, climate, and customs, as a breeding ground for particular kinds of disorders with similar etiological explanations, linked especially to *du* toxin generated internally due to an immoral lifestyle or introduced externally by poisonous or magical agents. These ailments had similar external symptoms: ugly sores and rotten skin. These regions were, of course, inhabited by populations considered as not quite civilized by the Han culture of the central plains.

The contagiousness of Guangdong sores through sexual intercourse, physical contact, and hereditary relations, observed and confirmed by doctors early on in the sixteenth century, was soon grafted onto *li/lai,* already suspected to be somewhat contagious from the late twelfth century onward. It is therefore not surprising that, in the Qing period, even though the two disorders were no longer easily confused, as they once were in the sixteenth century, they were still strongly believed to be closely related. Major medical *waike* texts often grouped them together in the same chapter, as in a mid-eighteenth-century imperial compendium on medicine, the *Yizong jinjian,* which quoted Gong's passage on *mafeng/lai* almost word for word on its contagiousness, followed by descriptions of Guangdong sores, in the same section of the chapter on *waike.*[130] More interestingly, in the late Qing text *Fuxie xinshu* (*A New Book for Overcoming Pathogens* [1911]) the author, Liu Jiren, describing the *da mafeng* disorder, writes: "This *feng* disorder is called *mafeng* in Guangdong, which is the origin of cases transmitted to all other provinces. It is like the sores of *Myrica* berries, also named Guangdong sores, originating equally from Guangdong province. The ultimate and external symptoms of the two disorders are in general similar. This is because they are ailments of the same climate. Their origin is the same though their developments are different. . . . They [are caused by] the same epidemic *qi.*"[131]

The classic medical frameworks for etiological explanations could not easily accommodate the idea of person-to-person transmission as a cause of ailments. The history of the conceptualization of *dafeng/lai* reveals this point in compelling ways. The perception of the contagiousness of the ailment emerged at the same time as it was no longer classified as a Wind-induced disease, but one belonging to the area of *waike,* external medicine, a specialty snubbed by most mainstream doctors since the Song. *Waike* specialists, until the late imperial period, were mostly not equipped with classical medical theory and tended to treat external symptoms with hands-on techniques based on practical experience, without the refined diagnostic procedures developed since the Northern Song.[132] Such a "vulgar" practice of *waike* became the target of severe criticism from mainstream doctors beginning in the Song.[133] Innovations in the analysis and therapeutics of *dafeng/lai* following the Song were gradually left in the hands of marginal doctors well versed in Daoist medicine and rituals. New concepts

Table 1.1 Highlights of Discussions on *Li/Lai/Mafeng* in Major Medical Texts

Author or Text	Disease Name	Causes	Symptoms	Special Features
The Yellow Emperor's Inner Canon (ca. second century b.c.)	*Dafeng* (big Wind); *lifeng* (Wind causing li)	Wind intrusion	*Dafeng:* swelling of bones, falling out of hair; *lifeng:* collapse of bridge of nose, degeneration of complexion	
Handy Recipes for Urgent Use (third to fourth century)	*Lai*	Not specified	Numbness of skin, itchiness, blurred vision, skin eruptions	
General Treatise on the Origins and Symptoms of Disorders (ca. 610)	*Efeng* (vicious Wind); *lai*	*Efeng:* Wind, Cold, Dampness; *lai:* excessive physical exertion, bad diet, taboo violation	*Efeng:* beard and eyebrow loss; *lai:* itchiness, sores, loss of eyesight, deterioration of complexion, hoarseness of voice	Mention of *chong,* creeping bugs inside the body interacting with Wind, causing internal corruption
Sun Simiao (518–682)	*Jifeng* (Wind ailment); *eji dafeng/ebing* (malignant ailment)	Wind intrusion, retribution	Similar to General Treatise	Mention of *chong*
General Record of Imperial Charity (eleventh century)	*Dafeng lai*	Wind intrusion	Collapse of bridge of nose, skin corruption, itchiness, eyebrow loss, hoarseness of voice	Considers *dafeng* the same as *lai*

A Treatise on the Three Categories of Pathogenic Factors of Disorders (twelfth century)	*Dafeng/lai*	Excessive physical activity and desires, retribution, *chuanran* contagion	Loss of complexion, numbness of skin, sores, collapse of bridge of nose	Refutes Wind intrusion as a cause; proposes contagion as a cause (without description)
Secret Formulas of External Medicine Transmitted by Immortals (fourteenth century, quoting a twelfth-century Daoist text)	*Dafeng*	Excessive sexual activity, depleted body, intrusion of toxic Wind, Dampness and Cold, bad geomancy, transmission within lineage, carelessness outside the household, *chuanran* contagion through shared utensils, bedding, toilet	Numbness of skin and flesh, sores, falling off of limbs, collapse of bridge of nose, loss of voice, falling out of hair, death (five-stage progressive development of symptoms)	First detailed descriptions of *chuanran* contagion; accuses elite doctors of not being interested in the ailment because of its filthiness
Keys and Essentials to Skin Disorders of the Li Category (1528–1529, by a palace doctor)	*Liyang* (skin disorders of the *li* category)/*da mafeng* (big numb Wind)	Collapse of defensive *qi*, excessive physical exertion, Dampness and Heat	Same as Secret Formulas	Considers disease endemic to south of the Huai River, Lingnan and Fujian regions; no mention of contagion
Sources of Relief (1550)	*Da mafeng/fenglai*	Same as Secret Formulas; inevitable congenital transmission, body fluids as contagious, transmission by *chong* creeping bugs flying out of corpses, contagion related to *gu* magic	Corruption of skin and muscles, sores, falling out of hair, numb and shrunken limbs, falling off of limb extremities, itchiness	Endemic to Fujian and Guangdong; female patient at incubation stage capable of passing the disease on to her male sexual partner (*guolai*); menstruation makes women less receptive to manifesting symptoms; confusion with Guangdong sores (syphilis)

Table 1.1 continued

Author or Text	Disease Name	Causes	Symptoms	Special Features
A Complete Book to Save the World (late sixteenth century, by a palace doctor)	*Da mafeng*	Same as Secret Formulas	Same as Secret Formulas	
Golden Mirror of Medical Orthodoxy (1742, imperial compendium)	*Da mafeng*	Endemic to miasmatic regions, contagion through patient or within lineage; same as Secret Formulas	Same as Secret Formulas	Southern endemic disease
A Complete Work on the Feng Disorder (1796)	*Mafeng/da mafeng*	Dampness and Heat, contagion especially from women to men	Same as Secret Formulas	Southern disease; tobacco smoke as medium of contagion; confirmed *guolai* transmission; menstruation makes women less receptive to manifesting symptoms

related to *chuanran* contagion and even the application of drugs for the ailment now came mostly from Daoist liturgic and medical texts. These were later picked up and elaborated upon by marginal practitioners in the Ming-Qing period. Confucian doctors remained reticent or laconic on the new concepts, as they became uninterested in research on the ailment altogether, probably repelled by the "filthiness" of the symptoms.

The evolution of the conceptualization of *daifeng/mafeng/lai* closely parallels the development of the *waike* specialty after the Song. To a great extent, it shows some of the most profound characteristics of Confucian medicine since the Song, and especially in the Ming-Qing period. Too little is known of the history of *waike* and Confucian medicine of the late imperial period to permit making conclusive remarks here. Regarding *mafeng/lai* of the late imperial period, however, we can say that the discourse on this *waike* disorder, with its ugly external symptoms and now considered highly contagious, was almost entirely monopolized by marginal doctors such as Xiao Xiaoting, of the late eighteenth century, who observed: "The *li* ailment separates father and son, husband and wife, drives away relatives, invites the loud curses of passers-by. It is not like the other ailments that only affect the patient himself, as *li* is very contagious. It can harm relatives and friends, or even the entire family, and numerous are those who are [thus] refused marriage and are without posterity."[134] This was also how Chinese society, especially in the southern regions, looked at *li/lai* in the late imperial period.

THERAPEUTICS

There were basically two main types of therapeutics throughout the long history of *dafeng* and *li/lai:* acupuncture and treatment with drugs based on herbs or minerals. The principle of treatment by acupuncture, and also that of fumigation using certain drugs, was to induce sweating to release the stagnating Wind or internal heat accumulated inside the body. Treatment by herbal or mineral medicines had more complex therapeutic implications. Medicines could be applied externally to treat skin symptoms. They could be taken internally for the purpose of expelling pathogenic Wind or excessive Heat or noxious *chong.* Certain methods or drugs were "fashionable" during certain historical periods but were condemned as being too risky or ineffective in others. The general trend seemed to be that stronger drugs and methods used in earlier times gradually gave way to milder methods from the late medieval period onward. A brief look at the history of therapeutics for *dafeng* and *li/lai* will also give us an idea of the extent to which these disorders were considered as separate or the same categories.

Acupuncture, Fumigation, Baths

The *Inner Canon* essentially suggested acupuncture as the main treatment for *dafeng* and *lifeng*. "[When] one is attacked by big Wind, the bones and their joints swell, the hair and eyebrows fall out. [The disorder] is called *dafeng*. [In such cases] acupuncture of the flesh is applied for one hundred days to induce sweating. [Then] acupuncture is applied to the marrow of the bones for [another] hundred days to induce sweating. [After] two hundred days, [the treatment can] stop when the hair and eyebrows grow again."[135] As for *lifeng*, the classic proposed a different acupunctural remedy: "Apply acupuncture directly on the swollen part. Once done, apply a sharp needle to the [same] part, press it to allow the exit of bad *qi*. Stop when the subsidence of swelling is complete. Follow the usual diet, and do not have other food."[136] Clearly, the *lifeng* disorder was, unlike *dafeng*, considered essentially a skin or flesh ailment.

Acupuncture as a treatment for *dafeng* or *lifeng* disorders somewhat fell out of fashion after the early period, but it became the preferred method again of northern medical experts of the Jin dynasty, in the twelfth and thirteenth centuries. By then, *dafeng, lifeng, li/lai* were seen as constituting one category. Liu Wansu (1120–1200) recommended as therapy acupuncture on the flesh for one hundred days, and moxibustion (three times, with seven moxa cones each time), supplemented with drugs consisting of birch bark, licorice root (*gan cao*), almond, bitter orange (*zhiqiao*), rhubarb, and honey locust thorn (*zaojiaoci*).[137]

The same principles of applying acupuncture to provoke sweating were later applied to diaphoretic therapy using drug fumigation or hot baths. Such recipes became current from the Tang. Wang Tao mentioned a diaphoretic therapy for *dafeng* based on the fumigation of *xiaoshi* (mirabilite, sodium sulphate) and sesame oil.[138] Chen Yan suggested that *dafeng* patients should take a series of two to three hot baths with ephedra root (*mahuang gen*), wolfberry bark (*di gu pi*), and wild aconite root (*cao wutou*) mixed with pepper, green onion, *Artemesia argyi* leaves (*aiye*), and rice vinegar. Patients were to bathe until profuse sweating resulted.[139] Again, northern experts of the Jin period further highlighted the effectiveness of sweating. Zhang Congzheng (ca. 1156–1228) recorded a case where he refused to treat a *lai* patient in the early spring, preparing for the patient medicines including garlic only in the fifth and sixth months of the year. He explained, "One sweats little in the spring cold, whereas one does so readily in the summer months." He also judged the curability of a *lai* case by seeing if the patient could still sweat. His preferred method was to use medicines to provoke a patient's abundant sweating in a hermetic room several times. The sweat and the saliva of the patient should, according to him, stink badly.[140]

It seems that before the Song, when *dafeng* and *li/lai* were considered as separate categories of disorders, different acupuncture methods were applied to the two disorders. After the Song-Jin periods, however, as the two categories were gradually reclassified as one, diaphoretic therapy incorporating acupuncture, fumigation, and hot baths was applied to *dafeng lai* together with other recipes based on drugs.

Drugs

Treatment using drugs, though not recorded in the extant version of the *Inner Canon,* appears in various ancient texts discovered in recent archaeological excavations. The drugs in recipes for treating *dafeng* and *li/lai* disorders generally have one of the following qualities: they are toxic, as strong, toxic drugs were believed to be effective for serious ailments caused by accumulated poison; they are efficacious for repelling pathogenic Winds, as the disorders were considered induced by Wind; or they are known for being *chong* repellants. Mainstream doctors after the Southern Song, however, tended to prefer using milder drugs.[141] Nonetheless, strong, toxic drugs seemed to have been recommended for the *dafeng/lai* disorder for a long time in the earlier periods. In an incomplete medical text dated to the early Eastern Han (ca. 25–89) discovered in Wuwei, Gansu province, in the 1970s, there is a recipe for the *dafeng* disorder that explains as its purpose that of "reviving all that has fallen out, reerecting all that has broken off, and reestablishing sensitivity." Its ingredients included essentially minerals, often of strong, toxic qualities, such as realgar (*xionghuang*), cinnabar (*dansha*), mirabilite, and magnetite.[142]

Ge Hong introduced, in his *Zhou hou beiji fang,* another set of therapeutic drugs for *lai,* based not on minerals and prepared mostly as alcoholic drinks. For the typical *lai* disorder, he suggested a "barbarian alcoholic drink" (*manyi jiu*). The contents of this drink is not mentioned in the text, however, and it could possibly be the same as the one bearing the same name in Sun Simiao's *Beiji qianjin yaofang,* of three hundred years later, which included herbs like *duhuo* (pubescent angelica root), *fangfeng* (*Ledebouriella* root), *mahuang* (ephedra), and others known mostly for their qualities for treating *efeng* disorders with symptoms of eyebrow loss. Making alcoholic drinks from these herbs would have enhanced their capacity for expelling pathogenic Wind.[143] The name of the recipe suggests its non-Chinese origin, though the ingredients were typically part of the Chinese materia medica. Ge Hong's recipe for white *lai, kushen* (flavescent *Sophora* root) in alcohol had similar qualities.[144] *Kushen* alcoholic drinks in fact remained one of the main recipes for *lai* disorders in later ages. Another recipe, probably added in the sixth century to Ge Hong's original text[145] for white *lai* arouses some interest on the possibility of intercultural transmission of medical knowledge. The recipe consisted of a big viper (*da fushe* [Pallas' pit viper]) soaked entirely in alcohol and then heated gently. A small piece of the cooked viper was to be mixed with winter lard and applied externally to sores.[146] The use of vipers in prescriptions for *li*/*lai* comes up frequently in later medical texts, but more often as the basis of an alcoholic drink. It is interesting to note here that there were also recipes using vipers in wine for elephantiasis in second-century Greek texts, such as those by Galen and Aretaeus of Cappadocia. Folk stories about the miraculous curing power of such a wine seemed to be widespread in Asia Minor during the first centuries A.D., and it is possible that such tales found their way not only to Greece but also to China before the sixth century.[147] Even more intriguing is the mention of recipes using the fat of the "great serpent of the open country" to put on the skin of a patient of "leprosy" in an archaic medical text (ca. fourteenth century B.C.) from the Middle Euphrates region.[148] The use of snake or viper in recipes for leprosy-linked skin diseases thus seems to have been common in many early cultures. More than tracing the origin of the idea or the possible routes by which it traveled, interest here is in the cross-cultural use of viper or snake as a reflection of a common idea of cure by analogy, whereby an extremely malignant ailment was treated with an equally venomous drug. The persisting importance of this old recipe is revealed in a text published in a journal in the 1930s on leprosy edited by Western-trained doctors, in which the use of viper in alcoholic drinks was still described as an effective drug.[149]

The early medieval medical experts (Sui-Tang) inherited most recipes of the earlier periods, but they also created new ones. Other than recipes for various alcoholic drinks, in particular *kushen* drinks, *chong*-repelling drugs became fashionable during this period, as the interaction of Wind and *chong* inside the body had come to be seen as a main cause of *dafeng lai.* One frequently mentioned drug in the medical texts, especially those by Chao Yuanfang and Sun Simiao, is *leiwan* (*Polyporus mylittae*), a toxic drug made from a mushroom. The drug was supposed to be effective for expelling poisonous *chong* from the body. This quality of the drug was confirmed by Li Shizhen, the author of the important pharmacopoeia *Bencao gangmu,* of the late sixteenth century.[150] Sun Simiao further recommended a compound based on *leiwan,* called *awei leiwan,* that combined the plant *awei* (*Ferula sinkiangensis*) with a number of minerals, some rather toxic and already mentioned in the early Han formula: realgar, cinnabar, talc, quartz, ox gallstone (*niuhuang*), and others.[151] The use of *awei* is an indication of foreign pharmaceutical influences, as the herb originated in the Persian region and was brought to China probably via India or Mongolia.[152] In fact, both Sun

Simiao and Wang Tao explicitly mentioned Indian influences in some of their prescriptions for *dafeng* and *lai* disorders. Sun recorded the recipe for *awei leiwan* in a passage entitled "Qipo's [Methods] in Treating the Malignant Ailment," Qipo being the Chinese transliteration of the Sanskrit name Jīvaka, a famous Indian doctor. Wang Tao also referred to a diaphoretic therapy based on fumigation as a recipe from "Brahmin monks."[153]

Doctors of the late medieval period seemed to favor drugs for internal use rather than acupuncture for treating both *dafeng* and *lai* disorders. The encyclopedic *Taiping shenghui fang*, of the Northern Song, records recipes for *dafeng* disorders using most of the strong ingredients mentioned in earlier texts, such as cinnabar, realgar, *awei, xiaoshi, kushen, fangfeng,* and often viper. The most frequently mentioned drugs are the rather toxic minerals such as realgar and cinnabar, also essential elements of Daoist alchemy. Recipes for *dafeng lai,* on the other hand, relied less on toxic minerals and more on plants and various animals like vipers. The black viper (*wu she*) was a favorite ingredient, and *fangfeng, duhuo, fuzi* (*Radix aconiti praeparata*), *langdu* (ebracteolate euphorbia root), and *kushen* were often used, with occasional application of realgar and cinnabar. Recipes treating black *lai* were essentially based on animal ingredients, including all kinds of snakes, frogs, centipedes, spiders, insects, hedgehog skin, mixed with cinnabar and other mercuric derivatives, quartz, and others. These mostly toxic drugs were supposed to be effective for expelling *chong* from the body. The more toxic minerals, especially realgar, were then often made into an ointment for external use on the sores.[154] From these recipes, one is tempted to deduce that *dafeng* was seen as a more serious ailment affecting the internal viscera and needing strong, toxic minerals as drugs, whereas *dafeng lai* was be seen as slightly less serious and benefiting from herbal drugs, sometimes mixed with toxic minerals, to expel Wind. *Lai* was treated as a skin disease caused by expellable *chong.*

Strong, toxic drugs gradually fell out of fashion during the Song period. By the twelfth century, when Chen Yan wrote his book, realgar, cinnabar, and vipers were no longer favored drugs for *dafeng* or *lai.* Chen recommended much milder ingredients for both internal and external uses. He proposed, for instance, a series of ointments for external use on sores based on mild elements like ginseng, purple perilla, *kushen,* the dried larva of silkworms, rhubarb, talc, prepared rehmannia root (*shu dihuang*), croton seed (*badou*), almond, *Phaseolus* seeds (*chi xiao dou*), dried tangerine peel, musk, *Agastache* (*huoxiang*), and so on. His proposed recipes for internal use were also based on mild herbs such as angelica root, prepared rehmannia root, *chuanxiong* rhizome, *fangfeng,* red peony root, croton seed, black *Pharbitis* (*hei qianniu*), subprostrate sophora root (*shan dou gen*), *chebula* fruit (*hezi*), and so on; another recipe, which he considered useful for expelling *chong,* consisted of curcuma root (*yujin*), rhubarb, white *Pharbitis* (*bai qianniu*), and honey locust thorn, all of which were of milder qualities. Toxic arsenic ingredients were mentioned only sporadically in his recipes for *dafeng* disorders.[155] Ming doctors still included arsenics and mercuric ingredients, but essentially in the preparation of ointments for external use. By the Qing, doctors clearly disapproved of the use of toxic ingredients to treat the disorder. The mid-eighteenth-century imperial encyclopedia *Yizong jinjian* mentions one or two formulas calling for vipers and scorpions, but realgar and calomel are not recommended. Xiao Xiaoting, of the late eighteenth century, was quite clear: "Even though *li*/*lai* is a malignant ailment, it can be treated effectively with mild drugs. One can, to a certain limit, use vipers and scorpions, but ingredients like arsenic, centipedes, blistering beetle [*banmao*], and calomel should not be used unless the case is extremely serious. They should not be applied on a regular basis."[156] The notion of curing a malignant ailment using toxic ingredients had fallen out of fashion in medical books by then.[157]

One main therapeutic innovation for *dafeng* and *lai* in the thirteenth century was the use of chaulmoogra seeds (*da feng zi*). The herb was first mentioned in various Daoist and medical texts. The *Gengdao ji* (*Collected Texts on the Way of Refining Gold* [twelfth to thirteenth centuries]), a text on alchemy in the Daoist canon, contains a recipe for a pill to cure the big *ma*/*lai feng* composed of some toxic ingredients, such as mercury, scorpion, and also a heavy dose of *da feng zi.* In a slightly later Daoist text already mentioned, the *Xianchuan waike bifang, da feng zi* is again recommended in a recipe for an ointment to treat sores and corrupt skin.[158] In the famous medical text compiled during the Song-Yuan transition, the *Lingnan weisheng fang* (*Life-Preserving Recipes for the Lingnan Region*), the same drug is mentioned as an external application with *qingfen* (calomel) on sores in the case of *yangmei chuan* sores.[159] The growth of trade with Southeast Asia from the Southern Song onward explains the increasing availability of this tropical plant commonly grown in South and Southeast Asia. According to Li Shizhen, Zhu Zhenheng of the Yuan had already warned against the use of *da feng zi,* saying that its nature was too "hot" and an overdose could damage Blood and cause blindness.[160] Zhu Xiu's collection of recipes of the early Ming, *Puji fang* (ca. 1403–1424), also includes a number of recipes using chaulmoogra for *dafeng* disorders, including a few for internal use,[161] showing that prescribing chaulmoogra for *dafeng* and *lai* had already become common by the Yuan-Ming transition, since its introduction in the Song period by Daoist healers, which explains the Chinese popular term for the plant (seed for the *dafeng* ailment). It remained a favorite drug used by doctors to treat *dafeng lai* in the late imperial period, though mainstream Confucian doctors insisted on its danger as a component in remedies for internal application, as had Li Shizhen.

Abstinence and Other Techniques

Besides treatments using acupuncture and drugs, patients were also advised to abstain from sexual intercourse and other worldly activities. As touched on in the preceding, from the medieval period onward, doctors, especially Daoist ones, advised patients to "leave their wives and concubines" in order to be cured, as excessive sexual activity was thought to aggravate the stagnant pathogenic heat inside the body. Certain foods were also to be avoided. For Chao Yuanfang, all cereals, meat, and fish were bad for *lai* patients, who should restrict themselves to a diet based on sesame, pine, and rhizome plants. A healthy person should also avoid eating fish without gills, as it would induce *lai*.[162] For the Daosit doctor Sun Simiao, on the other hand, "The first thing to stay away from is sexual intercourse. Then one should also avoid great anger and heat. As for food, greasy, spicy, cold, and raw food, such as vinegar, sweet paste, white alcohol, the meat of pork, fish, chicken, dog, donkey, horse, beef, and lamb are all to be shunned. These are the major things to be avoided absolutely."[163] Such were the details of the recommended dietetic regime. The main principle was to practice an ascetic lifestyle: "Once one has the ailment, one should abstain from salt, and take pine resin. All public and private things and affairs should be abandoned, as if they were shoes taken off from the feet. The hundred tastes [of delicious food] should be given up, and so should cereals ultimately. Keep away from all worldly affairs, celebrations, or funerals. Live hiding in a cave in the mountains, and in one year, one will be cured. Even if one is cured, one should be prudent about sexual intercourse throughout one's life. The illness can recur if one is not careful."[164] Later doctors often repeated such proscriptions, including Wang Tao and many others. The underlying principle was, of course, the abandoning of all physical and worldly desires and lust, a principle that was perfectly in tune with Daoist precepts for the attainment of immortality and sainthood. For this reason, Sun and Wang told readers of their texts that it was not unusual for patients of *eji* who respected such counsel to the extent they left the world to live alone in isolated mountains to attain immortality.[165]

Doctors after the Song no longer promoted such beliefs, but they still strongly suggested abstinence for *lai* patients. For them, this bodily discipline was a minimal requirement for the patient's slim chances of survival, and not a technique for achieving immortality.[166] As evident in the fourteenth-century Daoist text on *waike,* referred to previously, Daoist healers from the Southern Song onward recommended "living in seclusion, abstaining from wine and sex, leaving aside worries, and purifying thought, trusting the legendary doctor, repenting sincerely, avoiding anger, meat, fish, salt, sauces, and all kinds of cold foods." With the aid of such discipline, and proper medication, "all could be cured."[167] Abstinence and bodily discipline in such cases were simply the proper behavior for the purpose of healing. Immortality seemed now to be a much more remote goal. Moreover, excessive sex, though always considered as immoral and harmful to health, was now popularly thought to be a channel of disease transmission. Abstinence was thus prescribed probably for more than one reason.

Another typical Daoist ingredient worth mentioning was pine resin, yet another reminder of some old Greek remedies.[168] A story recorded in a work by Ge Hong, the *Bao pu zi,* concerns a literatus infected with *lai* who leaves his family to live in a cave in the mountains. Days and nights he wept, until an immortal took pity on him and gave him some medicine from his bag. After having taken the medicine for one hundred days, he was cured. The immortal then told him that the medicine was refined pine resin, one that one should take for life for obtaining youthfulness and longevity.[169] Thereafter, almost all medical texts mentioned pine resin as an important ingredient in recipes for the treatment of *dafeng* or *li/lai.* Sun Simiao, probably inspired by Ge Hong, also mentioned several recipes using pine resin as an ingredient for treating *eji dafeng.*[170] Such use, however, gradually disappeared in medical books after the Song as the idealized myth of *lai* patients transforming into immortals faded from popular memory.

One can see two almost contradictory developments in the long history of the medical understanding of the *dafeng li/lai* disorder in premodern China. On the one hand, one observes an increasingly sophisticated description and analysis of the disease. This finally led to the conceptualization of a clearly distinct disease that no longer belonged to the very broad category of Wind-induced disorders. The same trend occurred in the area of therapeutics. The usage of milder drugs for the purpose of first replenishing the weakened patient rather than that of strong, toxic drugs also suggests a more practical approach to the incurable disease. This trend was most clearly reflected in the appearance of specialized medical works on *mafeng* or *li/lai* from the mid-Ming onward, written by *waike* specialists. On the other hand, one also observes an increasing stigmatization of the *mafeng li/lai* disorder, an ailment relegated to the *waike* department, snubbed by elite doctors. Daoist healers and liturgists, by providing new understanding as to the causes of the disorder, including its contagiousness outside the lineage context through the media of *chong* or *gu* toxin, highlighted its mysteriously dangerous nature. The classification of the disease as a southern, contagious, and venereal disease from the sixteenth century onward quickly turned it into a much-dreaded disease, one that was more visible in low society.

Mafeng/lai, subsequently no longer one of the many "respectable" ailments induced by Wind, became the disease of "the other"—the semicivilized populations of the south. Its ambiguous link, beginning in the sixteenth century, with the sexually transmitted Guangdong sores further stigmatized its victims. While Sun Simiao, of the Tang, wrote that many patients of *dafeng* were respectable literati, late imperial medical texts tended to describe *mafeng* patients as mostly lascivious people of miasmatic southern China. The image of the genteel hermit suffering from *lai* but finally achieving the sainthood of an immortal after having purified his sores disappeared in late imperial medical books. Instead the dangerous, contagious, and polluting female *lai* body emerged in literati writings as well as in marginal medical texts. The disease came to be depicted as the ugliest, most repulsive, and dangerous of all ailments. When informed nonexperts considered *mafeng* as one of "the most tragic, cruel, and contagious diseases, which one cannot bear to look at"[171] in the late imperial period, the disorder had by then incited tremendous anxiety, fear, and disgust among the general population. *Mafeng/lai* clearly became stigmatized as a disease of people with weak or immoral characters, who were either overindulgent in sex or had undisciplined bodies. Doctors wrote that it was only natural that *mafeng* victims were abandoned by their families, friends, and neighbors. From the sixteenth century, patients of *mafeng/lai* were stuck with this extremely negative image, until the coming en masse of Western missionaries in the nineteenth century, who came with yet another set of prejudices that only helped to enforce the traditional stigma.

A Cursed but Redeemable Body

TWO

While the history of social rejection of lepers in Christian Europe is a well-known story,[1] and the relative tolerance of lepers in Islamic society has also been described,[2] we still do not have a general picture of how Chinese society regarded *mafeng/lai* patients. In fact, in both the medical and religious traditions in China, there were two contradictory but coexisting views of *li/lai*. It was at the same time incurable and redeemable. While descriptions in most mainstream medical texts were more categorical, religious or social attitudes toward the ailment were confused, ambiguous, and mixed. Religious and social perceptions of the disorder were often full of contradictions, at times confirming its deadliness, and suggesting that it was curable.

The view that the *mafeng lai* victim was incurable and contaminating has deep historical roots. The religious aspects of malignant diseases, of which *li* was one in early China, though largely suppressed by mainstream Confucian doctors of the post-Song period, lurked in the popular mentality and emerged in individual and collective social practices throughout the imperial period. From roughly the third century onward, the immorality of *li/lai* was defined essentially by Buddhist and Daoist teachings. The belief that malignant diseases, particularly those with conspicuous and ugly external symptoms on the skin, were retribution for unrepented former wrongdoing or sins of the victims or of their ancestors was dominant. It remained so strong that even Confucian doctors of the late imperial period still accepted that retribution was a major cause of the disease. The ailment was also considered transmittable, just as immorality was considered contaminating. Transmission was believed to be carried out essentially by the agent *chong,* thus basically limited to the immediate household of the victim.[3] The influence of Buddhist and Daoist ideas in Chinese medicine in the early medieval period was distinctly clear on the question of *li/lai.*[4] The idea of *chong* as an agent of transmission, and *zhu,* a procedure of such a transmission, was fully developed by doctors between the third and sixth centuries (see chap. 1).[5] However, these early ideas of transmission, often confined within the family context, were closely linked to the religious issue of retribution and did not imply a broader notion of contagion, as during epidemics. Such diseases, in a way, were a necessary reminder to society of what sinful thoughts and immoral deeds could bring, and an indication of the tragic, inescapable human fate. However, despite such deep-rooted negative views of *li/lai* throughout the earlier imperial period, the condemned bodies of *li* patients remained those of wayward or unfortunate individuals, or their relatives or posterity, inside an otherwise wholesome social body of the civilized world.

In this chapter, it will be seen how, especially in early imperial China, *li/lai* victims, considered as personifications of evil spirits or the worst of sinners, were condemned and cursed by the law and in various religious traditions. On the other hand, it also become apparent how these victims became the perfect objects of religious redemption, largely because of their ghastly and horrifying appearance.

LEGAL CONDEMNATION: HUMAN RESPONSE TO A PUNISHMENT FROM HEAVEN

The early religious (pre-Buddhist and pre-Daoist) views of *li/lai* patients were most clearly seen in the harsher than normal legal treatment they received. Their special status in the law reflects two main attitudes toward *li/lai:* that the disease was caused by some evil spirit needing to be exorcized, and that it was also a punishment from heaven. Early laws represented human efforts to counter a threat from the nonhuman world, and also to respond accordingly to the bigger cosmic order.

We saw in chapter 1, in a preimperial legal document in bamboo dated between the fourth and third centuries B.C., and excavated in 1975 in Hubei, that a patient of *li* was interrogated and diagnosed by a physician during a process of prosecution, to make sure that he did have the ailment. This document indicates that being a victim of the disease in this early period called for legal intervention, and that a *li* patient had unusual legal status. Indeed, this is clear in Qin (221–207 B.C.) statutes according to which a patient of *li*, found guilty of a crime, was to be condemned to drowning in still water, or be buried alive.[6] Derk Bodde and Lin Fushi, who have given slightly different interpretations to these early texts, agree that such a severe and particular capital punishment for *li* criminals involves ritual meanings deeper than their apparent legal expression. In other words, it was probably the religious aspect of *li* that required this extreme legal treatment. Lin provides a fuller philological investigation of the texts to show that a patient of *li* in early China in fact embodied three different meanings: a malignant disease with ugly lesions as external symptoms, a ghastly spirit (*gui*), and physical and moral vileness. In brief, the patient personified a vicious, ugly fiend causing malignant disease. The act of drowning a *li* victim, or burying him alive, was a ritual performance to intimidate or subordinate by violent means the embodied evil spirit of *li*, so that it would not manifest itself in the human world again anytime soon.[7] The incriminated *li* patient in Qin times could also be punished in another way according to the law. He could be transferred to "a quarters for *li* [*li suo*], or be drowned in the still water in the quarters for *li*."[8] These early legal practices did not seem to have continued, however, in the imperial period. We do not find them in major law codes and statutes in later dynasties. The ritual aspects of the punishment for *li* victims nonetheless persisted. The drowning, burying alive, and isolation of victims of *li*/*lai* and *mafeng* continued to be practiced in society of the later imperial or even modern periods, often as popular customs. This severe legal treatment of *li* victims in early China largely reflected the fundamental Chinese cultural and religious attitudes toward this category of ailments and also explained related social practices in subsequent periods. If capital punishment of *li* patients was no longer put in later penal codes, authorities continued to carry out massive killings of *li* patients in the medieval period,[9] and even in the modern periods, as we shall see in the following chapters.

The tragic and irreversible fate of *li*/*lai*[10] patients was also fully reflected in the deprivation of their right of marriage, and thus of having a posterity. This was probably the worst thing that could happen to anyone in traditional China, other than punishment by death. According to ancient rites, a woman who had a family history of *eji* (malignant diseases) was not to be taken as a wife, as she was considered to have been "abandoned by heaven."[11] A woman could also be legally divorced if she was found to have a critical ailment after marriage. In early texts, *li/lai,* together with dumbness, deafness, blindness, baldness, lameness, having a hunchback, and barrenness were considered malignant ailments that denied a woman marriage.[12] That one should not marry someone with *eji* was maintained in subsequent laws of the Tang, Song, and Ming. In Tang law, *eji,* together with madness, lameness, and blindness were considered as *duji* (critical diseases).[13] In a bureaucrat's handbook of the Song, the *Lixue zhinan* (*Instructions to Bureaucrats*), the author specifies that one of the legitimate reasons for divorcing a wife is that she has *eji* with a stinking body.[14] In the Qing novel *Xingshi yinyuan* (*Marital Relations Awakening the World*), by the famous scholar Pu Songling (1640–1715), this specific article is mentioned, and a character in the story says, "It is written in Ming law that those who have *eji* will be divorced. And there is nothing more serious than *tian pao chuang*[15] in the category of *eji.*"[16] *Eji* in the law of the later imperial period included serious chronic ailments with conspicuous external symptoms, especially of the skin. *Li/lai, dafeng,* and *mafeng,* together with Guangdong sores, were definitely considered as *eji.* Even husbands were similarly subject to such a stipulation. In other words, men and women engaged or married to someone found to have a malignant ailment could legally annul the engagement or seek divorce.

Concrete examples of the application of the clause were sporadically recorded in medical and other texts throughout the imperial period,[17] particularly in the later period, as this stipulation generated interesting conflict with the growing cult of female virtue. We can find some of the examples precisely in records on virtuous women. Stories of virtuous women relinquishing their legal rights of dissolving an engagement to a sickly fiancé for a greater moral cause is recorded in the famous classic *Lienü zhuan* (*Biographies of Virtuous Women*), compiled by Liu Xiang, of the Han dynasty (ca. 77–6 B.C.). One such story takes place in the Spring and Autumn–Warring States period (ca. eighth to fifth centuries B.C.). The mother of a young wife from the state of Song married to a man from the state of Cai makes plans to have the young woman remarried to someone else when the husband is found to have *eji.* The virtuous young wife refuses such an arrangement, saying, "The misfortune of my husband is also my misfortune. How could I leave him? The principle of marrying a man is to stick to him till the end of one's life."[18] Her example, recorded in this widely read classic, probably inspired numerous later women to imitate the virtuous act and reject remarriage, though permitted by law, particularly in the late imperial period, when the cult of virtuous women became increasingly influential.

One example is a woman from Shanghai of the Ming period. When her husband is found to have *lai,* her mother-in-law plans to have her remarry the husband's younger brother. Aware of the plan, she flees and returns to her own family, with the consent of her dying husband. After his death, against all taboo, she bathes his body and clothes it before committing suicide by drowning herself in the river on the shore of which the body of her husband was exposed according to the local custom.[19] Another virtuous woman of the Qing dynasty, by the name of Yuan Ji, was engaged to a young man Gao. When the fiancé was found to have the malignant ailment, her father wanted to annul the engagement, only to be rejected by the virtuous young woman, who insisted on having only one man in her life even though he had an incurable ailment, and also a most violent temperament, as she later found out. Her sacrifice won her the official honor of virtuous woman.[20] In a way, the dreadful illness of the husband was a great opportunity for an unfortunate woman to achieve the superior status of an officially honored chaste woman, the only way she could have her name recorded in the official history of the empire. The nature of *eji* being an indicator of abandonment by heaven rendered the virtuous act of honoring a legally dissolvable marriage with the patient, meaning the acceptance or even embrace of an escapable tragic fate, a most spectacular moral performance.

The significance of such virtuous acts resided precisely in their relative rarity. Virtuous women in these cases represented only a privileged few who did not have to worry about their livelihood. Under most circumstances, basic material needs necessitated the dissolution of a marriage, especially when the breadwinner became sick. A vivid example is provided by a judicial case of 1736 in a village in Xuyong district, Sichuan province. A poor peasant, having contracted *lai,* is not able to work in the fields to support his wife and his two children of twelve and nine years of age. He had planned, around 1732, to "sell" the wife so that all could have a chance to survive. Eventually he sells his wife to a nearby neighbor as his concubine for twenty taels of silver and the promise that the buyer would take care of his children and his funeral after his death. Four years later, the *lai* patient is murdered by the buyer of the wife following a dispute over the price and the arrangement of the original deal. The wife confesses during the interrogations, "I was married to Zhao Ying for sixteen to seventeen years and lived in Lerong, and we had never had any scandal. . . . In 1732, my husband contracted *lai* and could not be cured. He was no longer able to work in the fields and the days were difficult. My husband said, 'If you do not leave me, you will also be contaminated by *lai,* and our two boys will also die.' He then spread the word that he would sell me afar. I said I would rather die and was unwilling to go. Later Chen Wenzhang [the buyer] sent a matchmaker, saying that he was willing to support my husband and the two boys on the condition that I became his concubine. I finally accepted, thinking that Chen was nearby, and I was also allowed to take my sons with me." After the murder, besides the punishment—decapitation—of the murderer, the bureaucrats also decide that the selling of the wife was illegal, as it was not a proper divorce, and immoral, as the woman willingly became the concubine of another man. She is consequently sentenced to thirty-five strokes.[21] Clearly the case shows that leaving a critically sick husband in order to marry another was the only chance for an ordinary woman and her children to survive, thus explaining the rationality of the law. However, it also shows the difficulty for peasant women in the late imperial period in obtaining a proper divorce in such a case, not to mention in being officially honored as virtuous women.

Not only material necessities made it difficult for ordinary women to remain virtuous in case their husbands became ill, social tolerance of *li/lai* patients was in general so low that, in many cases, families and communities abandoned their relatives and neighbors, and often with legal consent. The social tolerance of *li/lai* and *mafeng* patients seemed to be diminishing so significantly in the late imperial period that, in certain regions, people resorted to legal actions to expel their afflicted neighbors or relatives from the community. As imperial law did not specify how *mafeng lai* patients should be treated in a community, such legal actions were bound to be ad hoc and sporadic. Their occurrence in the eighteenth century, however, clearly shows the deteriorating social situation of *mafeng* patients. In 1741, in Fengshun district, Chaozhou prefecture, Guangdong province, a certain Hu Zuoting was found to have *mafeng*, and the "clans and people of the community feared contamination by him, and made a public and collective [*gong tong*] decision to expel him." Consequently, Hu was forced to live in a makeshift shed behind the village hills.[22] Another, similar incident occurred in 1749, in Qujiang county, Shaozhou prefecture, also in Guangdong province. A woman married to a villager was found to have *mafeng*. "Neighbors of the village were disgusted, and feared being contaminated. On the eighteenth day of the eighth month of the fourteenth year of the Qianlong reign [1749], her father-in-law, Deng Shining, and his cousin Deng Shizhang went to report the case to the county magistrate. They obtained an order [from the county government] to build a place for her to live outside the village."[23]Contrary to cases of virtuous women who relinquished their legal rights to accept a tragic fate, these neighbors and relatives in rural China made efforts, usually with collective consent, to obtain new, local rulings to expel *mafeng* patients, who otherwise were legal residents in their communities. The late imperial legal system seemed to support such a practice. It is unclear if patients of other chronic diseases were also expelled in this way from their homes and communities, but such rather unprecedented legal actions against *mafeng* sufferers seem to have been common in the late imperial period, at least in the southern provinces. As we shall see in chapter 3, from the sixteenth century onward, because of the fear of contagion, local authorities in the southern provinces of Fujian, Guangdong, and Jiangxi established a network of institutions to isolate these patients.

Such unusual social practices against the victims of *li*/*lai* in the late imperial period certainly had deep historical roots. We see traces of early religious attitudes toward the ailment in archaeological materials, and what follows is an account of Buddhist, Daoist, and Confucian attitudes toward the disease from the early medieval period onward. We shall see that there were continuities in the religious attitudes toward *li*/*lai* victims from the early to the late imperial period, with new elements created by various religious systems in medieval China that sometimes reemerged in the late imperial or even modern period.

THE *LI*/*LAI* VICTIM IN RELIGIOUS TRADITIONS: CURSED BUT REDEEMABLE

While one of the three meanings of the ideogram *li* in ancient texts—that of a ghastly spirit—was fully taken into account in early legal treatment of *li* patients, as we have seen in the previous section, the meaning of moral vileness was still unclear. This aspect of *li*, especially the meaning of an ailment embodying moral corruption, fully developed only in the medieval period in Buddhist and Daoist thinking. In this tradition, *lai* was the most serious of all ailments caused by retribution for the most serious of sins committed in this or a former life, or by one's relatives or ancestors. The typical manifestation of the ailment, consisting of the decomposition of the flesh and bones, stinking ugly lesions, and sores, was considered an exact reflection of the inner moral corruption of the patient.[24] In the Buddhist tradition, serious moral transgressions included blasphemy or disrespect to the Buddha or to the church, such as damaging Buddhist edifices or sutras, insulting monks and sages, and disregard of Buddhist teachings. Other equally unforgivable sins consisted of the transgression of general moral principles, including unfilial acts, insolent behavior toward one's teachers and mentors, and excessive arrogance toward others. All were punishable by contracting *lai*. These ideas were translated from Sanskrit into Chinese as early as the second century.[25] Examples of such retribution are numerous in historical and Buddhist texts of the medieval period. Sins like the assassination of the emperor,[26] the reckless killing of surrendered soldiers,[27] or wanton cruelty to other human beings[28] and to animals[29] were said to cause perpetrators to contract *lai*. We shall see a few concrete examples later.

Early Daoist texts, on the other hand, rarely mentioned the specific worldly circumstances under which victims contracted *li/lai.* Apocalyptic texts of the medieval period, however, confirmed that sinners and nonbelievers would be attacked by disease demons that caused horrifying external symptoms such as malignant sores, *lai* with *chong,* rotten and stinking blood, scabies, and ringworm.[30] However, pathogenic sins or transgressions were not limited to those committed by the victim himself, as "misdeeds could more frequently be traced back to one of the patient's forebears in that miasmic swamp of ill omen, the world of the dead."[31] Daoist texts in general were more interested in the healing process of *li/lai* victims, as we shall also see later.

More important still, ailments caused by moral corruption could be passed from one individual to another. In early Daoist and Buddhist texts, passages on diseases contracted by sinners were often associated with *gu* and *chong,* implying that they could be transmitted to others.[32] Among Buddhist examples, the story of Du Tongda, of the mid-seventh century, most fully shows this. Du Tongda killed a monk in order to steal the silk inside a box containing sutras. Before he died, the monk recited several incantations, and a fly flew into Du's nose. His nose and eyes soon became paralyzed and he lost his eyebrows and hair, and later, his senses. Before long he contracted *eji* and died in less than a year. When he was dying, the fly flew out from him and into his wife's nose. She became sick and died in about a year.[33] In this story, the sin of the thief, the magical power of the monk, and transmission of the ailment by *zhu,* the *chong* flying in and out of a body and contaminating his close relative when dying, formed a complete picture of an occurrence of *eji,* exposing the moral nature of the cause and the danger of transmission. The threat of transmission by *zhu,* so vividly described in this story, was fully incorporated into Chao Yuanfang's medical classic of the seventh century, as discussed in chapter 1. The idea was clearly both religious and medical, as the two realms were inseparable in this period.

Considered as a cursed disease, *li/lai/mafeng* was nonetheless, or precisely because of its horrible nature, redeemable, redemption here meaning the physical recovery of the sufferer, or the physical or spiritual deliverance, from his or her presumed suffering. In the medieval period, roughly from the fourth to the thirteenth centuries, stories of redemption of *li/lai/dafeng* were mostly narrations in the Buddhist or Daoist traditions. In these stories, miraculous healing was normally performed by morally superior men, particularly in the Buddhist tradition. In the Daoist tradition, on the other hand, sufferers sometimes redeemed themselves by means of ascetic practices. Both healers and sufferers in these two traditions were, in the main, male figures. The body to be redeemed or exorcised in particular was typically male. This is especially conspicuous in the Daoist tradition, where recovering from the horrible disease required such physical and spiritual discipline as the "giving up of one's wife and concubines," and the abandonment of all worldly affairs. In the Buddhist tradition, both sufferers of the disease, often depicted as sinful and power-hungry men in the political realm, and their healers, mostly selfless and saintly monks, were also male. Women entered the scene only when the cult of female virtue became increasingly widespread after the fourteenth century and when it was seen as an effective moral performance to redeem a *li/lai* sufferer. However, in most of the stories of female virtue, women are usually not the sufferers but self-denying figures whose filial performance brings about healing miracles that save a sick father or husband.

The understanding that *li/lai* was a particularly monstrous disease caused by moral transgression was a prerequisite for its redemption through religious faith. There are similarities in this between Chinese traditional religions such as Buddhism and Daoism and Western Christianity.[34] In miracle stories in the major religious traditions, illness (punishment) and healing (grace) are often found one alongside the other.[35] We have seen how divine punishment for blasphemy, disrespect to religious figures, and immoral behavior in general was manifested in sinners' contraction of *li/lai,* in both the Buddhist and Daoist traditions. The related question is how redemption or miraculous healing was achieved according to the Chinese Buddhist, Daoist, and Confucian traditions. In a way, there are common points in the miraculous healing of *li/lai* in the three traditions: the condition of having contracted the *li/lai* illness is presented as a particularly effective test for the moral strength of believers, and healing can be achieved through a demonstration of extraordinary faith or piety. However, miracle healing in the three traditions involved different players. In Buddhist miracles, the focus was usually not on the sufferers of the disease but on the monks whose religious faith, charity, and self-sacrifice made healing possible. The stories highlight the superior religious or moral status of the healer-monks. In the Daoist tradition, on the other hand, both healers, in the form of immortals, and sufferers were placed at center stage. Moreover, the boundary between healers and sufferers was particularly blurred, as the latter had the potential of becoming immortals. The idea of self-healing by means of religious bodily techniques was strongest in the Daoist tradition. In the Confucian tradition, there were no extraordinary healers, no holy men with magical healing powers. Miracles were usually achieved by heroically virtuous acts carried out by worldly beings such as close friends or family members, or by the sufferer himself. In this case, the moral superiority of the performer of the virtuous act corresponded to the larger cosmic order producing the miraculous result.

Buddhist Redemption

In Buddhist thought, even though illness was a normal state of the body,[36] serious ailments were the results of retribution for sins committed in this or a former life. Patients of five particular ailments, including *lai,* white *lai,* ulcers and carbuncles, consumption, and insanity were forbidden to be ordained.[37] In this respect, there are similarities between the Chinese Buddhist and Hindu *śāstric* traditions, in which lepers, the blind, insane, and mentally deranged were outcasts and deprived of their inheritance rights.[38] However, precisely due to the seriousness and polluting nature of these diseases, the Buddhist church of the medieval period considered them to be the test par excellence of the power of purification in transforming such polluting conditions into something of the sacred Buddha realm. "Monks and monastic centers become transformative agents able to purify any defilement."[39] Redeeming, purifying, or exorcising these diseases became important tests of the depth of religious conviction, usually not that of the patients but of Buddhist practitioners, mostly monks who cared for the sick. In other words, the religious nature of the causes or characteristics of such ailments necessitated healing or curing only by religious means.

As has been mentioned, *li/lai,* meaning ailments with monstrous skin symptoms such as sores and lesions, including probably some forms of leprosy, was thought to be caused by serious moral transgressions related either to religious faith or to general social behavior. The teachings that such illnesses were caused by bad karma or immoral acts or thoughts were especially pronounced during a period when competition between Buddhism and Daoism was keen, from the fourth to the seventh centuries.[40] Stories of such "punishment," in particular for blasphemies by emperors and high officials, are abundant especially in Buddhist texts.

Cui Hao, a trusted high-ranking official of the Northern Wei (386–534) and his ally, the Daoist Kou Qianzhi, were probably the most frequently quoted examples in Buddhist texts. Both were confidants of Emperor Taiwu (424–451), who was thus converted to Daoism and persecuted Buddhist monks. In the Buddhist tradition, the "sacrilegious" emperor was thus "punished" in contracting *lai,* and was later assassinated, after he executed Cui Hao, who had already contracted *lai,* and his clan.[41] As for Kou Qianzhi, who was said to have built a tall Daoist tower to reach the gods and heavens, he was said to have consequently died also of *eji.*[42] While the killing of Cui and the assassination of the emperor were recorded in official histories, the contraction of *lai* by the blasphemous Daoists was recorded only in later Buddhist texts. Similarly, the Daoist Wei Yuansong, of the Northern Zhou, was said to have presented a memorial to Emperor Wenxuan

(550–559) of the Northern Qi suggesting a reduction in the number of Buddhist monks, as he considered them lazy and greedy. Wei was said to have later died of *eji*.[43] Other frequently quoted examples include that of Prince Wei of the Liang dynasty (502–557), who was said to have contracted *eji* after he destroyed bronze statues of Buddha in a monastery in Xiangyang in order to mint coins for financing the army.[44] Likewise, Xie Hui (ca. 426), a minister of the Southern Song dynasty (420–479), was said to have ordered the destruction of a Buddhist pagoda with its relics. Shortly after having forced soldiers to destroy Buddhist statues, it was said he caught *eji* and had sores (*lai chuang*) all over his body.[45] Other, seemingly lesser crimes, like stealing donations given to monasteries, selling stolen property from monasteries, jeering at monks (an oral sin), could also result in contracting the *lai* ailment.[46] Indeed, such examples are numerous in Buddhist texts and need not be enumerated here.[47] Absent from the official histories, these stories clearly demonstrate the unique position of *lai* in medieval Buddhist moral teachings.

Although sufferers of *li*/*lai* were deprived of such basic religious rights as ordination, their sinful, polluted bodies became important vehicles for the Buddhist church to teach redemption by faith, charity, and sacrifice. Much of the power of the Buddhist religion lay in its claimed capacity to cure impossible ailments by performances of sacrifice and purification rituals.[48] It was in this religious tradition that the famous "quarters for *li* patients" (*liren fang*), of the sixth and seventh centuries, were organized, often associated with Buddhist monasteries, though not always in clear ways. These institutions were not, however, the earliest segregated institutions for lepers, as many Chinese historians of medicine have thought. Isolating the sick from the healthy for fear of contagion was not their main purpose or function. Instead, these institutions were definitely showcases of Buddhist faith and charity, and the place for ritual purification. The more famous examples of such quarters were recorded during the Northern Qi dynasty (550–577). Two asylums for *li* patients, one for men and the other for women, were said to have been built near the capital Ye (near Linzhang, in Hebei) by an Indian monk around 556, when he was received by Emperor Wenxuan of the Northern Qi, an emperor famous for his charity.[49]

The typical ways in which monks treated *li* sufferers clearly reveal the importance of religious rituals and not of "public health." In a mountainous region in Zezhou around 581, for instance, the monk Daoxun was said to preach and provide medical services to villages inhabited by *li* sufferers, and to receive offerings from *li* patients. "Whenever he saw pus flowing out of corrupted sores, he did not have any second thought and cleaned them with his mouth. He washed their clothes, and purified the sins of their hearts."[50] Another example is the monk Seng Chou, active during the reign of Emperor Xiaoming (516–528) of the Northern Wei, who "did not mind the filth and stinking smell [of the patients of *li*]" and mingled with them and enjoyed being served by them.[51]

Indeed, the isolation of patients is not the major concern in Buddhist texts, but the ways patients were cared for and cleansed by the monks, and how the latter achieved sainthood through these selfless and charitable acts. In the Sichuan region, in the area of Fucheng Monastery, in Yizhou, for example, there were victims of *li* with corrupted skin, "their smell was ubiquitous and strong. Everyone would pinch their nose with their fingers, but Monk Daoji provided them with what they needed. His mind and body were totally devoted [to them]. He shared their eating utensils and washed and mended their clothes."[52] Another, more obvious example is one recorded in seventh century, during the Tang. In Shitou, a town near Nanjing, the *li* quarters were visited by the monk Zhiyan around 643. "He preached to the victims, sucked the pus and blood of their sores, and washed them." In 654, he died in the *li* quarters, "his color unchanged, his body nimble, and the room [where his body was laid] had a perfume that lasted more than two weeks."[53]

Monks made such sacrifices in the conviction they were in fact serving Buddha and testing their religious faith. The story of the monk Zhihui, a favorite repeated in many subsequent Buddhist texts, is most typical. Zhihui was said to have cared for a fellow monk, a patient of white *lai,* much dreaded by all others. Master Zhihui fed, bathed, and massaged him. Soon a spiritual light and a strange perfume emanated from the sick body. The *lai*-stricken monk then bid farewell and disappeared. The scabs he left behind emitted an increasingly strong perfume, and a statue of Guanyin was made out of the scabs collected.[54] Some, not unlike Christian missionaries of the modern period or Christian saints of the medieval period, attracted followers and disciples by devoting themselves to the care of *li* patients. During the Northern Qi, the monk Fahe, it was told, cured patients of the malignant ailment on Mount Badie with herbs. Patients usually took the remedy he provided no more than three times and were cured. Many of them thus became his disciples.[55] These examples show that the focus of Buddhist healing was not on the patients, except as Buddhas in the disguise of sufferers, but on the monks and their performance of purification rituals. Emphasis was not on the segregation of patients from society but on the severe test they provided of the monks' religious faith.

One of the most commonly used methods of treating *li* patients inside Buddhist institutions was sutra incantation. There were particular passages in certain sutras that were considered to be effective for healing *lai,* especially the Diamond Sutra and the Lotus Sutra.[56] As mentioned in chapter 1, etiological explanations and therapeutics in the medical tradition were inseparable from religious beliefs and practices. It is very likely that the sutra incantations were gradually incorporated into medical texts as therapeutic methods. In fact, Buddhist chants or incantations were recorded as recipes in some Song medical texts as preventive measures against diseases caused by *zhu* (the pouring on of *chong*) or *gu* magic.[57] The reciting of sutras as a purification ritual, besides its magical healing effect, was probably also an incitation for repenting of former sins of the sufferer.

Indeed, repentance was considered the main method of cure of serious illnesses. We saw in chapter 1 that medieval doctors recommended moral reforms like abstinence and self-imposed exile as treatments for *dafeng lai*. In Buddhist texts, sufferers of malignant ailments were urged to make amends for past crimes. A good example is that of Jiang Tengsheng, of the early seventh century, who suddenly fell victim to *eji*. "His body was erupted into sores and lesions, and the extremities of his limbs fell off." In a dream he saw a white stone statue telling him that if he added a hand to it, he would be cured. In the morning he suddenly remembered that, some years prior, he had hit a white Buddhist statue in his village temple, causing its right hand to fall off. What he saw in the dream was exactly the same as the memory of this incident. He thus went to worship in front of the statue with a sincere, repentant heart. He paid an artisan to repair the statue's hand, had forty chapters (*juan*) of sutra copied, and a Buddhist study built. Consequently his illness was cured within one year.[58]

Buddhist influences on the conceptualization of the cause and cure of *li/lai/mafeng* were profound. The idea that the main cause of the illness was retribution for a particular and serious former sin remained strong in the popular mentality and persisted into late imperial medical texts. Buddhism also provided escape from the otherwise fatalistic view of the ailment. Any serious sin or transgression responsible for the ailment could be redeemed by purification rituals, charitable acts, and self-denial performed by the healer-monk, or occasionally by repentance and good deeds of the sufferers themselves. In Buddhism, as in many religions, caring for the sick by providing shelter and medical care was an important social function that attracted believers, and curing by miracles an otherwise incurable disease was an effective demonstration of the superiority of the religion. The abundance of such examples of healing in Buddhist texts of the early medieval period reveal the Buddhist institution's great political and social influence. However, after the ninth century, with the political decline of the Buddhist church as the result of a series of persecutions by the court,[59] the overwhelming social and political influence of Buddhism declined, never again to claim its former status. Despite the persistence of the Buddhist idea of curse and redemption in relation to *lai*, these colorful stories of notorious sinners, often prominent political figures, and the miracle healing of *li/lai* sufferers by famous monks became rare in the later periods.[60]

Daoist Redemption

The Daoist interest in the redemption of *li/lai* was less concerned with sin and transgression as the cause of the ailment and more with the therapeutic process, either by means of rituals carried out by high priests or self-healing through ascetic bodily disciplines. Both ways were described in early Daoist texts from at least the third century. Rarely, however, were specific earthly crimes committed by *li/lai* sufferers enumerated in any detail in the Daoist tradition. On the other hand, the number and names of disease demons affecting humans, especially those causing *wen* epidemics, ailments involving *gu* and *chong*, those that caused ugly skin symptoms, and so on, and details of the associated therapeutic rituals were greatly elaborated in Daoist texts.

Some classic healing stories in the Daoist tradition are similar to the Buddhist stories in their emphasis on the therapeutic effects of participating in the religion's particular practices. Yu Ji (?–ca. 200), a disciple of Bo He, had the *li/lai* disease and was dying. Bo He told him that, in order to be cured, he should transmit the authentic Taiping classic, the Daoist canon, in manuscript. He was told to edit the text into 170 *juan* and 360 sections and promulgate it throughout the entire empire. Yu Ji, after having obediently followed his master's suggestions, was cured.[61] We can find similar stories in later Daoist texts such as the *Yunji qiqian* (*Bookcase of the Clouds with the Seven Labels* [ca. 1017–1021]), of the Song, in which a man having contracted *lai* was cured after he began to restore the temple housing the Daoist goddess Xi Wang Mu (Queen Mother of the West), which had been destroyed by a fire.[62] Another popular Song story is of a pious Daoist practitioner named Wang Wen, who was said to have bathed with self-made wine two immortals disguised as *lai* patients. The two were cured and turned into handsome young men after three days, and the wine filled the house with a sweet smell. After drinking the wine, all the family, including his dogs and chickens, became immortals.[63] Another Daoist healing story reminiscent of the Buddhist tradition is that of Zheng Rong, of the Song, early eleventh century. He was said to have been endowed with extraordinary healing powers by an immortal, and to have remedies for *dafeng*. Many sufferers asked him for help, and he healed them by giving them bread soaked in blood obtained from his arms.[64] This story is probably the closest, though not quite identical, to the Buddhist tradition of self-denial as a healing method. Such narratives of miraculous healing did not, however, seem to occupy a central position in Daoist teachings.

The more spectacular characteristic of the early Daoist tradition regarding the redemption of *li*/*lai* victims lies in the process of self-healing, consisting of both bodily and spiritual discipline: one had to abandon all worldly desires and pleasures, and to nurture a "repentant heart," not necessarily for any specific sin but for a general lack of kindness. Self-healing was also closely related to alchemy in the early period.[65] Sun Simiao, the Tang Daoist doctor, said explicitly that there were two sides to the malignant *dafeng* disease: "There is an auspicious [*ji*] and an inauspicious [*xiong*] meaning to this illness. If the sufferer of the disease cultivates good, he will have an auspicious end. If he maintains the same habits as other worldly beings, he will certainly have an inauspicious end."[66] Contracting the ailment was like getting a wake-up call about a corrupting lifestyle. The sufferer could either benefit tremendously from the warning by radically changing his way of life, or die from ignoring the warning. In other words, redemption was attained by moral improvement, asceticism, and special bodily techniques with the use of alchemical medicines.[67] Such practices were precisely those required of all believers aiming to achieve immortality and sainthood. The monstrously decomposing and dying body of the *li*/*lai* sufferer being transformed into the immortal body or a body close to immortality represented the gist of Daoist ideas of bodily and spiritual cultivation. Stories of such transformations were abundant in the early medieval period.

A frequently quoted story concerns an event of the Tang period. A victim of *lai,* abandoned by his parents in the mountains, cried and lamented for three days before a man appeared and took care of him. He was taught to do physical exercises and practice *qi* cultivation. Several years later, he was cured. The man told him that he had good karma and would not die of the ailment. He should now return to the human world, however, where he could make a living by palm reading as taught by the healer. He was also warned not to accumulate wealth even if his business went well, otherwise the disease would recur.[68] This story clearly illustrates that Daoist healing involved bodily self-cultivation, moral discipline, and a certain disdain for worldly comfort. A late-Tang Daoist text of the tenth century on immortals mentions a similar story, in which a bureaucrat suffering from *lai* for more than ten years was cured by a Daoist who convinced him to quit his position and serve as his servant. The sick man was given special medicines and books to read. He was said to have the youthfulness of a child when he was 190 years old; he later disappeared into the western mountains.[69]

An even more famous story is one attributed to Ge Hong, the prominent Daoist of the fourth century. In the extant text of the biographies of Daoist immortals, the *Shenxian zhuan,* attributed to Ge Hong, Zhao Qu is said to have had the *lai* disease for years and was unable to get cured. When he thought he was dying, he asked his family to abandon him in the mountains to avoid his dying at home, as "sons and grandsons for generations to come would have transmitted the ailment by *zhu*."[70] Once left alone in the mountains, he cried pitifully and incessantly inside a cave, where food and clothing were left for his use until his death. Some hundred days later, three beings appeared in front of the cave and suggested that he take medicine, consisting of pine nuts and resin.[71] Before exhausting his rations, Zhao was healed, his strength and health restored. He returned home and continued to take the medicine given him. Two years later, he regained his color and his skin turned smooth and clear, his movements became brisk like those of a bird. It was said that, when he was in his seventies, he could still consume an entire rabbit or pheasant, including the bones, and carry heavy things without tiring. He was said to have lived for more than 300 years before he disappeared into the mountains again. There are similar stories in other Daoist texts.[72] As pointed out in chapter 1, pine resin as a common remedy for *dafeng*/*li*/*lai* in Chinese medieval medical texts reflects early Daoist influence, notwithstanding its use as a remedy for leprosy in other ancient cultures.[73] This is yet another example showing the complexity of the Chinese medical tradition.[74]

While records of miraculous self-healing of *li*/*lai* patients through repentance and physical discipline in the Daoist tradition seem to have significantly diminished after the Song, the practice of therapeutic rituals by Daoist priests entered a new age at the same time.[75] This change reflects some profound developments in Daoism in the late medieval period. Although Daoist teachings had emphasized therapeutic or exorcistic rituals since the early period (roughly the third century)—there is at least one collection of talismans in the bibliographical list of the official history of the Sui dynasty that appears to have been applied to *li*/*lai* ailments[76]—it was during the Song that such rituals attained new dimensions. The Daoist therapeutic and exorcistic tradition flourished both locally and at court from the late Northern Song period (roughly the tenth century) onward and enjoyed the sponsorship of the court. Emperor Huizong's reign (1101–1125) was "one of the most fervent Daoist periods in Chinese history."[77] Besides imperial support, Daoism absorbed many local exorcistic rituals and cults into its mainstream, many of which were written down for the first time during the Song. More important, Song therapeutic ritual texts reveal that "the fault for illness . . . has been placed entirely at the feet of the demons and of lesser spirits whose job it is to keep these demons away. The medieval link between illness and morality has been severed."[78] It is thus not an accident that stories of self-healing of *li*/*lai* victims through repentance and spiritual discipline gradually disappeared in later Daoist texts.

Li/*lai* victims thereafter were more likely to search for redemption in ritual exorcism by professional Daoist priests. Michel Strickmann's posthumous work on magic medicine provides a most informative account of therapeutic rituals. As he so vividly put it, these theatrical rituals were comparable to worldly trials: "It was the Taoist priest's task to fight the charges [against the patient or his family in the world of the dead], dispute the allegations, and, if possible, file a countersuit against the plaintiffs."[79] Seals and talismans were commonly used in such rituals to subordinate the demons causing the ailments of the "plaintiffs." As mentioned previously in this chapter, many of the diseases caused by such demons involved *gu* and *chong*. *Lai* is also one of the frequently mentioned ailments in Daoist texts. However, *li*/*lai* did not occupy a special position in the therapeutic system of early Daoism. It was dealt with in the ritual structure as one of the many ailments caused by demons.

For Strickmann, "[Daoist] priests [of the Song] were medical missionaries who went throughout South China, bearing their healing rituals directly into the homes of Chinese and non-Chinese alike."[80] Important illustrations of this trend include the *Tianxin zhengfa* (*Correct Method of the Heart of Heaven*)[81] and the *Yutang dafa* (*Great Method of the Jade Hall*) rituals developed during the Song period. The latter was elaborated by the Daoist Lu Shizhong (ca. 1158). His exorcistic text the *Wushang xuanyuan santian yutang dafa* (*Great Method of the Jade Hall of the Three Heavens, of the Supreme Mysterious Origin*) contains methods for expelling demons that cause *gu* poison and transmission by *chong* emerging from corpses. More important, talismans and rituals to stop transmission of disease in the house through bedding, clothing, and food were carefully described.[82] This exorcistic text was thus more than a description of rituals and could be read as a medical text. Indeed, there was, by this time, "no rigid barrier [that] separated the preserve of the literary medicus or therapeutically concerned official from the world of the ritual healer."[83] In this late medieval period, apparently exorcistic rituals carried out by professional priests became increasingly important in the therapeutic processes and overshadowed the ascetic disciplines emphasized in the Sui-Tang periods. In a way, it was an allegory of the "exorcistic" capital punishment of *li* patients seen in early archaeological documents mentioned at the beginning of this chapter. While the legal execution of a *li* patient in early China for the suppression of the evil spirit was in fact a ritual, the subordination of the disease demon that possessed a patient through a Daoist ritual in the Song was accomplished in the form of a legal trial.

Despite all their differences, in both the Buddhist and Daoist traditions, there was a common and interesting shift from the early to the late medieval period in the stories of *li*/*lai* patients: whereas *li*/*lai* victims recorded in the early period were usually important political or religious characters, the patients mentioned in the Song period were anonymous; it is now the Buddhist monks or Daoist priests involved in healing who are mentioned, while the profiles of the patients are no more. On the other hand, there is an increasing number of vivid accounts of ordinary *li/lai/mafeng* patients experiencing miraculous healing by means of the spectacular performance of typical Confucian virtues such as filial piety, female chastity, or loyalty to masters and rulers.

Redemption Through Acts of Confucian Virtue

The essential difference between redemption in the Confucian tradition and that in the Buddhist and Daoist traditions is that Confucian acts of virtue were performed within the mundane social order, often in the context of the clan or family. Miracles in the Confucian tradition were necessarily of this world, whereas Buddhist and Daoist traditions emphasized the deliberate rejection of worldly values.

In the late imperial period, stories of achieving moral merit by caring for *mafeng*-afflicted family members became markedly more abundant. These stories conspicuously extol Confucian virtues, especially filial piety, female chastity, and loyalty to friends. The specific kinship or friendship bond between the caregiver and the sufferer was key to the redemption process. These stories are recorded in the typical Ming-Qing sources such as official histories, local gazetteers, and writings by literati. Some of these supposedly true stories were used as the basis for popular novels and operas, thus revealing the dramatic appeal of the theme of healing by virtue of moral uprightness.

On loyalty to friends, there is the story of Chen Guang, a "poor orphan from a Confucian family" afflicted by the *feng* ailment living in Wuxi district, Jiangsu province, probably in the early Qing. He was generously cared for by a certain Yan, whose family had a long and deep friendship with his own. The Yan family, however, had an enemy in the region who hated Yan so much that he planned to kill him by bribing a family servant girl to put poison into cakes served to her master. Guang somehow heard about the plot and decided to sacrifice himself. When the poisoned cakes were served, he grabbed and ate them all. The astounded and bewildered household then saw him vomiting numerous small creeping bugs (*chong*). They pressed him for an explanation, but he remained silent. During the night, the servant girl fled, and the family gradually came to understand what had happened. Meanwhile, unexpectedly Guang's health gradually improved and he finally recovered completely and lived into his nineties.[84] In this story, the extraordinary loyalty of Guang to the Yan family and his great moral integrity not only cured him but also turned him into a local hero, earning him a brief official record of the virtuous act in the local gazetteer. The story also reveals a recurrent motif of the miraculous healing of a *li* patient: determined sufferers who attempt suicide for a moral cause by swallowing poison are usually unexpectedly cured. In addition to the power of such moral determination, the popular belief in the therapeutic efficacy of strong, toxic drugs in the case of *li*/*lai mafeng* was behind such a motif, even though toxic drugs had by this time fallen out of fashion in the medical mainstream, as discussed in chapter 1.

Filial piety was a virtue considered of primary importance for sons and daughters.[85] It was reported as a means of healing parents suffering from *li*/*lai mafeng*. During the Yuan, the daughter of a family named Sun took care of her father, who was infected with *lai*, for ten years. During all those years, she prayed to heaven that she should replace her father in his suffering. She began to suck the pus and blood from her father's sores, exactly as medieval Buddhist monks had done for *lai* patients. One month after she began doing this, her father was cured.[86] The healing method described in this story shows the Buddhist influence on Confucian ethical behavior, which persisted throughout the later imperial period. Another example of triumphant filial piety is the story of a man living during the reign of Yingzong of the Ming (1457–1464). He traveled from his hometown in Yongnian district to the Guangyang mountains, more than 400 kilometers away, to collect springwater, which he carted all the way back home in order to bathe his *lai*-infected father. Needless to say, the filial son's extraordinary effort brought about the father's complete recovery.[87] Just as the self-sacrifice of filial sons and daughters was the key to a miraculous healing of a father, the sacrifice of a wife was essential in the curing of a husband, as the following stories illustrate.

Unlike the stories, mentioned earlier in this chapter, of virtuous women who gave up their legal rights to divorce their sick fiancés or husbands and insisted on staying with them, the miracle stories could have a happier ending. The famous early-nineteenth-century Fujian scholar Liang Gongchen (b. 1815) recorded the story of a virtuous Cantonese woman of Nanhai district who insisted on marrying her fiancé, who was afflicted with *mafeng*. She told her protesting parents, probably imitating the famous virtuous fiancée in the classic *Lienü zhuan*, "This is my fate. You should know that following one man in one's life is the way for a woman. My duty forbids me to marry another." After their marriage, the couple, following the local custom, lived by themselves in an isolated lodge in the mountains in order to avoid contaminating their families. Soon, the woman also got the ailment. One night, lamenting their miserable fate beside a stream, the sick couple saw something strange swimming in the water then disappearing into the ground. The woman marked the spot where it had disappeared with her hairpin and dug it up the next morning, when she discovered a 1,000-year-old *Poria* fungus (*fuling*). The couple ate the dried fungus and were cured of their ailment. They happily returned home, and everyone agreed that the virtue of the woman led to the miracle. Liang, at the end of the story, recorded before 1848 and published in 1866, assures readers that the account was told to him by an eyewitness, Xie Lipu (aka Lansheng [1760–1831]), a famous scholar from Nanhai district.[88]

A more famous and earlier story, of the Ming and narrated by the literatus Xu Hao (fl. 1484–1488), who also claimed that the story had a reliable source (a man called Li Han). This story is more interesting because it concerns not only a virtuous wife but also an exceptionally honorable husband. Chen Shou was engaged to a certain woman, but, before the wedding, the unfortunate man fell victim to *lai*. His father consequently asked the matchmaker to annul the marriage agreement, but the fiancée firmly refused, as she considered that a virtuous woman should honor her engagement under all circumstances. Chen, however, did not go near his wife during the first three years of their marriage as he knew his was a monstrous and contagious ailment, whereas his wife took care of him assiduously without any regret. Deeply moved by his wife's devotion, Chen attempted suicide, believing it would free his wife from her terrible ordeal. He secretly bought arsenic and took it. When his wife discovered this, she took the rest of the poison, hoping to die with him. However, after taking the poison, Chen vomited profusely, and his *lai* was cured at once. The wife vomited as well and did not die. The couple lived happily ever after and produced two sons, and the family grew all the more prosperous. Xu records at the end of the story that people considered the happy ending as the reward of the woman's exceptional virtue.[89] Note again the theme of self-denial evident in the determined suicidal attempt that led ultimately to a cure.

This story was re-created as a popular novel during the later Ming period, due probably to its implicit love theme. The creator of the novel was the famous scholar Feng Menglong (1574–1646), who reworked the tale and included it in one of his compilations, the *Xingshi heng yan* (*Eternal Words to Awaken the World*). The hero is, in Feng's story, called Chen Duoshou (literally, Chen the one who will live very long), and the woman has the family name of Zhu. Entitled "Chen Duoshou shengsi fuqi" (The Predestined Marriage of Chen Duoshou), the novel is one of the best known in the collection.[90] Feng's additions to the tale include an exchange of poems between the young couple during their engagement, numerous vain attempts by doctors to treat Chen's illness, the wife's attentive nursing of her husband, and especially the high morality of the couple. Both are portrayed as willingly abstaining from sexual intercourse during the first three years of their marriage, but with different, yet similarly altruistic reasons. Chen declared, "Since we will not be husband and wife for very long, how can I soil the body of a virgin!" Whereas Zhu demurred, "My husband is so sick, his Blood and *qi* are exhausted—how could he survive the assault of sex with a woman [*nü se*]!" As in the story of Chen Guang, the theme of suicide as a virtuous act resulting in miraculous healing is dominant in this story.

Such Buddhist, Daoist, and Confucian stories of redemption illustrate the complexity of the popular conception of *li/lai/mafeng* inherited by late imperial society. The different but often complementary religious systems of China throughout the imperial period helped construct a complicated and sometimes contradictory image of the *mafeng* patient of the late imperial period. However, the redeemed body of the *mafeng/lai* patient in the three main religious systems of traditional China points to a common feature: the visible and problematic *mafeng/lai* body was typically male, and women took the role of caretaker, victim, or martyr. The sick male body was presented not only as a redeemable one through religious ritual but could also be described as a benign, albeit comic, one in the literary tradition until the twelfth century.

The "Comic," Benign Body of the Afflicted Scholar

A modern medical authority, the Cantonese doctor Wang Jimin (1889–1972), wrote his famous piece "Zhongguo mafeng shi zhong zhi mingren"(Famous People in the Chinese History of Leprosy) in 1941.[91] With it, he aimed to rouse public interest in the subject and to destigmatize the disease by pointing to famous historical figures, especially respected literati, who had suffered from *lai.* Using mostly easily accessible historical but nonreligious texts, Wang, and many of his contemporaries, managed to identify about a dozen personalities, all literary talents, who had been afflicted with *li/lai.* The majority of them were pre-Song figures, with again Ran Boniu, Confucius's disciple, as a "first" figure, as seen in chapter 1.[92] At the end of his article, Wang draws the reader's attention to the fact that, "after the Song, there were no more records of famous personalities with leprosy. . . . The ancients also seemed to be less fearful of the disease than the moderns, and they were kinder to the sufferers."[93] Wang's effort is especially noteworthy in that historians after him rarely surpassed his achievement by identifying more examples of famous literati having leprosy in late imperial history. He was also one of the first to throw light on the contrast between the ancient and modern attitudes toward the disease. Wang in fact points out the important fact that the image of the respectable though pitiable *li/lai* literatus existed in early and medieval China but disappeared after the Song.

What was this early image of the *li*-afflicted literatus? In the famous episode about Ran Boniu in the *Analects,* Confucius went to enquire after Boniu, and "grasping his hand through the window said, it is all over with him! Heaven has so ordained it—But that such a man should have such an illness! That such a man should have such an illness!"[94] Modern historians of medicine often overinterpret the text and insist that the Boniu's illness was certainly leprosy, based on other, contemporary texts that name the ailment *eji,* the malignant ailment. They also assume the illness was contagiousness, which is what kept Confucius outside Boniu's house while only holding his hand through the window. I have already dealt, in chapter 1, with both problems of identifying leprosy in early Chinese texts and the late emergence (after the thirteenth century) of the idea of contagion concerning *li/lai/mafeng.* Interpreting the episode as they do is certainly problematic. The significance of this episode in the *Analects* is not that it is evidence for the identification of leprosy or contagiousness. Rather, it presents an image of the literatus with the malignant ailment that later generations readily equated with *li/lai/mafeng.*[95] Such an image of the pitiable but respectable literatus afflicted with the malignant ailment entered quickly into the collective memory. It is evoked in a similar and famous episode of the Liang dynasty (502–557). Zhou Xingsi, a literary talent, first developed sores on both hands, then suffered the *li* ailment, which blinded his left eye. Emperor Gaozu, according to the chronicler, touched his hand and said, obviously imitating the tone of Confucius talking to his disciple Boniu, "How could such a man have such a disease?" The emperor then proceeded to write a recipe for treating the ailment.[96] Indeed, Boniu's ailment, which the great Song philosopher Zhu Xi (1130–1200) glossed as *lai,* was well registered in the repertoire of literary anecdotes that constitute a fine scholar's general culture. The Qing scholar Lu Yitian (*jinshi,* 1836), in his famous jottings on medical questions published in 1858, begins his discussion of *li* by describing the case of Boniu as presented in the *Analects.* He then refers to earlier glosses of the same passage in other ancient classics, and by the Qing scholar Mao Qiling (1623–1716).[97] Only after invoking all these classical literary references does he go on to mention the sixteenth-century medical book on *mafeng* by the doctor Shen Zhiwen.[98]

The typical reaction toward afflicted literati was thus one of pity, mixed sometimes with faint hope. Fear and disgust are definitely not implied in these records. In Song-dynasty examples, scholars are reported to have poked fun at the crippled body of a colleague, as in the famous example of the important Song scholar and historian Liu Ban (Gongfu [1023–1088]), a good friend of the prominent poet Su Shi (Dongpo [1037–1101]). Liu, known to have a quick mind and a sharp tongue, and a passion for debate, was a lively provocateur even after he contracted the *dafeng* ailment. Su Shi was said to have poked fun at Liu's "eyebrows being blown away by the 'big wind'" and at his "heroic effort in trying to keep his nose intact" in a poem he improvised at a party that made everyone laugh. On another occasion, when the two friends chatted in a Buddhist shelter, Liu joked about Su's getting people into political trouble during his numerous poem exchanges, with Su returning the joke by telling a story using a pun referring to Liu's "collapsing" nose.[99] These stories, often quoted to illustrate the conviviality of the Song scholars, demonstrate how a scholar afflicted with *li*/*lai* could nonetheless mix freely in society in Song times and how his physical handicap could be a subject of lighthearted public joking. Though not necessarily representative of a common phenomenon, these stories do show a certain tolerance of the disease during this period. In a way, scholars probably considered *li*/*lai*/*dafeng* as just another illness that might or might not be curable.

At any rate, during the entire medieval period, *li*/*lai* was likely considered not an unusual disease among scholars from the comfortable social classes. The sentiment of shame did not seem to be associated with the ailment. Sun Simiao, and later Wang Tao, who repeated most of what Sun had discussed about *efeng,* allow the inference that many of the patients they treated were literati. "Among my patients, there are quite a few literati, and even extraordinarily outstanding people. . . . If they could give up all their desires, not only could they be cured but they could even become immortals."[100] At least one of the famous literati with *lai* mentioned by Wang Jimin was a patient of Sun Simiao,[101] suggesting that Sun was indeed the doctor for a number of *li*/*lai* patients of the high literary class of his time. This association of *li*/*lai* with the scholar in the classics and mainstream historical texts, a tradition beginning with the *Analects,* buttressed in particular by the Daoist idea of redemption by means of the reclusive life of the hermit, in a sense the idealized lifestyle for the scholar, partly explains the apparently benign, even comic, nature of the ailment as described in literary texts.

From the early texts to medieval religious classics of various traditions, it is apparent that *li*/*lai* victims consistently provoked a profound social fear and anxiety that was often reflected not only in extreme legal treatment but also in complex processes of redemption. The records relating to such victims clearly show their negative image: they are often portrayed as cruel generals or emperors, political go-getters, greedy thieves, ruthless traitors, nonbelievers, sinners with insatiable desires and unkindly hearts, or simply ordinary people with however sinful ancestors and bad karma. Actual social attitudes toward *li*/*lai* were much more complex, with class and possibly regional variations, as shown by the milder attitudes toward scholars from the pre imperial to the Song periods. Limited available sources do not allow us to reconstruct the full spectrum of social attitudes toward *li*/*lai* during this span of history. It is possible to note, however, that all the victims described in these relatively early texts were men situated in mainstream society. *Li/lai* was apparently seen as a punishment from heaven on educated, wealthy, or powerful men who had committed serious crimes, or as an intrusion of evil spirits into the human world. Religious redemption was their only hope for deliverance from a painful death. Moreover, redemption from terminal *li/lai* cases became showcases of religious faith or efficacy. All players in the grand theater of religious redemption up to the Southern Song contributed to the consolidation of mainstream values: the infected sinners, the monk-healers, the exorcising priests, the dying husband and his loyal wife, and even the comic sick scholar—all helped to buttress the mainstream values of Chinese society up to the Southern Song period.

The theme of deliverance from the disease through magic or moral uprightness underwent radical changes when the sufferer of *li/lai* became typically female. It was only after the Southern Song, of the thirteenth century, and especially during the late imperial period of the Ming-Qing, that the female sufferer of *li/lai* took center stage. And the stage moves to southern China. This part of the story we examine in the next chapter.

The Dangerously Contagious Body

Segregation in Late Imperial China

THREE

The problem of *li*/*lai* in China was perceived very differently in the late imperial period, especially from the sixteenth century onward. Even though the question of the contagiousness of the ailment had already been mentioned in medical and Daoist texts in the thirteenth century, and contemporary local customs in the Fujian region reflected the popular belief that the ailment could be transmitted by sex, it was only after the sixteenth century that the fear of the contagiousness of *li*/*lai* became a widespread social phenomenon. The fear was, moreover, associated with several new developments in the conceptualization of *li*/*lai,* introduced in chapter 1: that it was mostly endemic to the southern, miasmatic region, that it was transmitted sexually, especially by female sufferers, and that it was basically incurable. At the same time, *mafeng*/*lai* victims were increasingly considered by society as the sick or corrupt part of the social body that had to be amputated via a form of collective segregation. It was not only a physically but also a morally corrupt body that threatened to pollute the healthy part of society.

The unprecedented fear of the ailment was behind the establishment of asylums to segregate *li*/*lai* patients beginning in the sixteenth century. *Mafeng* or *lai* was the *only* chronic disease in post-sixteenth-century imperial China necessitating institutional isolation. The institutionalizing of patients, though never thorough or of a truly national scale, definitely rendered *mafeng lai* as the most polluting and horrifying disease, in both medical and social terms. The unprecedented practice of social segregation introduced a new period of stigmatization of *mafeng lai* as a disease of the environmentally flawed, culturally backward region generally known as the "south," or of a stratum of the morally base, socially marginal or of semicivilized, promiscuous women.

Indeed, the contagious female patient was considered the most dangerous of all in this late imperial period. She was believed to be desperately seeking a cure by sleeping with innocent men, to whom the disease was passed on. This *guolai* (passing on of *lai*) custom most perfectly symbolized the horrifying contagiousness of a peculiar female disease of the miasmatic, semicivilized south. *Mafeng/lai* thus became an ailment par excellence of the culturally other.

CONTAGION AND IMMORALITY

As we saw in chapter 1, the *chuanran* notion of contagion in connection with *li/lai* first appeared in Chen Yan's medical classic of the thirteenth century. Chen explicitly wrote that the idea of *chuanran* contagion was different from retribution and bad fate. "One is not [in the case of *chuanran*] accountable for [contracting the disease] as one is only being careless [*bu jin*]. The transmission through *qi* and Blood is not quite the same as retribution for former sins."[1] That contracting a disease was independent of premeditated wrongdoing echoes a similar idea emerging in Daoist exorcistic texts of the same or slightly earlier period.[2] While Daoist priests were explicit in their explanation that the spread of such ugly ailments was caused essentially by specific disease demons, medical doctors remained reticent on the nature of *chuanran* contagion. I have argued that Chen Yan's idea of carelessness implied "careless" sexual activities. The contagiousness of *li/lai* independent of retribution (caused by deliberate sinning) but closely related to promiscuity was vague, however, in Chen's text and was only fully developed by doctors from the sixteenth century onward.

I would argue here that there are two types of immorality related to *li/lai* in two different historical periods. Before the Southern Song period, serious transgressions, often religious but also political and generally social, were associated with *li/lai,* as we have seen in the early Buddhist and Daoist traditions. We even know the names of the sinners and the specific offenses they committed before they contracted the deadly ailment. After the thirteenth century, however, such examples became rare. Human acts causing *li/lai* were by now more related to the lack of bodily care and discipline, including sexual excess. Disease transmission in the early period was described as mostly confined to family members or within the same lineage or clan (from ancestors to descendants) as a punishment for shared guilt (see chap. 1), whereas in the late imperial period *chuanran* contagion through careless behavior had a much wider and more dangerous scope; it spread outside the family and reached all corners of the empire.

Among all types of careless behavior, indulgence in sex appeared to be the most serious. It epitomized the new "immorality" related to *li/lai* of the post-Song period. We saw in chapter 1 how Ming doctors such as Li Shizhen and Chen Sicheng considered debauchery a cause for the spread of Guangdong sores, which historians of medicine identify as syphilis. From there specialists of *li/lai mafeng* like Shen Zhiwen associated *mafeng*, which had similar symptoms, with such "undisciplined" behavior. By then, of course, *mafeng* and Guangdong sores were considered by mainstream doctors as basically diseases originating from the semicivilized populations of the south, imagined to be a region with swampy lowlands and steamy mountains, constantly under great heat and dampness, where nonhibernating vipers and vermin thrived. It was seen as a place with accumulated filth generating poisonous *qi* and malignant ailments. There was an unstated but understood relation between such an untamed setting and the semicivilized behavior of the natives, both in the medical texts and other literati texts from the Southern Song onward, and especially after the sixteenth century. From then on, ailments thought to have originated in these hot, damp, polluted regions were considered to be highly and widely contagious. The words of Li Shizhen, of the late sixteenth century, writing on Guangdong sores, can serve as a reminder: "The noxious sores . . . are mutually contagious among people [and spread] from the south to the north, so that the disease is now everywhere. But then all those who fall victim are lascivious people."[3] The relation between sexual corruption and contagion was clear.[4]

Contagion was no longer thought to be limited to the same household or individuals related to a patient by blood but was seen to spread from one region to another, from one population to another. It was an anonymous, collective, and thus extremely dangerous and horrifying phenomenon. Even though *mafeng* did not spread quickly, as did *wen* epidemics (those caused by the Warm factor), its contagiousness was equally dreaded. At the same time, the associated lack of discipline, civility, and decency that led to debauchery, aggression, irascibility, and craftiness were seen as highly immoral.[5] What follows is an account of popular accusations against victims of *mafeng/lai* based largely on records of eighteenth-century judicial cases involving murder and capital punishment.[6]

Undisciplined Polluters

Mafeng patients were, first of all, described as thieves, as polluters in the community. In a village in Leping county, Jiangxi province, around 1742, a group of villagers with *mafeng* living together in two huts outside the village were accused of accommodating outside *mafeng* beggars, stealing vegetables and poultry from villagers, and of bathing in the village's pond, thus polluting the community's main source of water. Several villagers decided one night to burn down their sheds while they were sleeping in order to eliminate what they considered as a major threat to the village. One of them confessed during the interrogations, "These *mafeng* people drink the water and wash themselves in our pond. Sooner or later they will pass the disease to us and our lives will be in danger. We asked them to move somewhere else and they refused. . . . The solution was to burn down their sheds while they were asleep. In so doing, we eliminate this evil [*hai*] from our place and people will now not be contaminated [*chuanran*]. . . . [One of the accomplices said that] even if we burn these *mafeng* people to death, I don't think we will be in deep trouble, as we do this to eliminate an evil for the community." Two of the most crippled *mafeng* villagers, unable to run for their lives, were burnt to death, and the culprits were sentenced to decapitation and hanging.[7] It is interesting to note how these villagers perceived the legal consequences of killing *mafeng* patients. The latter were seen as such a social evil that the villagers sincerely thought that there would be no serious punishment for their crime.

Mafeng patients were also described as violent, suspicious, jealous, greedy, and self-centered. Their emotional indulgence provoked serious domestic or communitarian conflicts that often resulted in tragic deaths. In Zhennan county, Yunnan, in 1740, after the funeral of the mother of a *mafeng* patient, there was a big fight between the son and his cousin, who had come to organize the ceremony. The sick son was described as having gotten drunk and cursing everyone who came to the funeral. The cousin admitted during interrogations that he had also used strong words in the exchange: "I said, 'You could not support your mother when she was alive and are unable to bury her now that she is dead. I come to give you a hand and bury your mother and prepare a meal for the guests, and all you do is ruin the whole thing by cursing everyone. And now you curse me. What kind of a man are you?' On hearing this, he started to curse my parents." In his rage, and encouraged by the sister of the sick son, the cousin put a rope around the son's neck with the intention of dragging him out of the house and back to where he lived, outside the town, killing him in the action.[8]

Self-centeredness was also the cause of conflict between a tenant and landlord, resulting in the death of the landlord, who had *mafeng*. In 1739, in a village in Laiyang county, Shandong province, a set of houses were rented out by the brother of a *mafeng* patient for three years. Soon the sick brother found having a neighbor inconvenient and tried to force the tenant to leave. In a violent dispute, the sick landlord hit his tenant in the face, receiving in return a strike that killed him instantly.[9]

If male *mafeng* patients were often seen as egotistic, violent, and perverse, female patients were often described as gross and improper. In 1738 in Nanfeng district, Jiangxi province, an elderly woman of fifty years of age, a sufferer of *mafeng,* provoked disgust in both her husband and mother-in-law, being accused of "paying too frequent visits to neighbors and relatives." Her mother-in-law confessed that, when she tried to stop her from doing so, as people probably abhorred her visits, she only answered back rudely. One day, the husband, in a rage, strangled her after hitting her with a wooden hammer. He confessed, "It is true that I was disgusted by her poisonous *mafeng* sores, but if my mother had liked her better, I wouldn't have killed her."[10]

More typical still, *mafeng* sufferers were also perceived to exhibit excessive sexual drive and violent behavior, not unlike their counterparts in early medieval Europe.[11] A late Ming magistrate of Boluo county, Guangdong province, Deng Yigao, was infuriated by the 300 *mafeng* patients dwelling in a nearby mountainous area, where they were said to systematically rob men and rape women passing by. Deng consequently rounded them up and drowned all of them, so that "the *lai* problem disappeared in a single day."[12] Wang Zhi (*jinshi,* 1721), magistrate of another Guangdong county, Luoding, reported around 1730 a case in which a peasant woman, Huang, while cutting grass in the hills, was stripped of her clothes and gang-raped by three outside *mafeng* patients. Afterward, Huang ran naked to the magistrate's office for help. A runner was sent immediately to arrest the rapists but was deterred by the three threatening him with a sickle. When Huang's fellow villagers heard the news, they all rushed to the spot and rounded up the three. The rapists defended themselves, saying, "We did this not for pleasure but for curing our ailment." The enraged crowd picked up stones from the ground and stoned the three to death. The magistrate decided not to prosecute the villagers who had killed the three, as he considered that the rape had caused the victim to be subjected to "excessive poison" in the first place, and, second, resistance to arrest was a serious crime punishable by death. His decision was approved by his superior.[13] This incident shows the popularity of the belief of passing the ailment onto a sexual partner in order to get cured, not only from women to men but also men to women. It also illustrates the extremely negative image of lepers in southern China as lascivious and violent antisocial beings and the dread and hatred they provoked. Stoning the rapists to death, a relatively rare act in China, probably reflects the villagers' determination to kill the lepers without touching them, for fear of contagion.

Mafeng patients were feared and hated not only by society at large but also within the family. Husbands suffering from the disease, depicted as having excessive sexual drive, were recorded as killing their innocent wives out of jealousy and suspicion, and in extremely violent and deliberate ways. In a village in Zengcheng county, Guangdong province, in 1736, a young wife refused to share her bed with her husband of six years, as he had been found to have *mafeng* one year earlier. In the evening of the tenth day of the first month, the husband threatened his wife with a knife, finally killing her when she again refused him, saying that he was "useless." The husband confessed that his wife had refused to sleep with him "even when my limbs were not yet rotten."[14] In 1738, in another village, in Chongren county, Jiangxi province, a young husband infected with *mafeng* became suspicious of his pregnant wife, who had refused to share her bed with him. He also developed a grudge against his brother, who refused to share clothes and meals with him. In the end, he was convinced that the two had had an affair. In his confession he admitted that he had planned to spare his wife if she had given birth to a boy. As the unfortunate woman gave birth to a girl, on the twenty-ninth day of the seventh month in 1739, the frustrated and angry husband took a knife and killed his brother and his wife in their sleep. The murderer's mother strongly defended the virtue of her daughter-in-law: "She spent every night with Zhangzhen [the husband], and during the daytime, she never left my eyesight or that of her husband," whereas her sick son "sat idly all day at home since contracting the ailment," and "it is just normal that his wife and his brother would not want to be close to him after he got sick."[15]

Sitting idly at home after getting the disease was indeed yet another cause of serious domestic conflict. In a village in Anyi county, Jiangxi province, an exhausted peasant went home for lunch one day in 1741, only to find his thirty-two-year-old cousin, a sufferer of *mafeng,* asleep next to the dining table. In a rage, he shook him awake and ordered him to get to work in the fields. The sick cousin replied by saying he was sick. The angry cousin then accused him of laziness and began to hit him. Hitting back with his crippled hand, with its crooked fingers, the patient killed his cousin. In the confession, the sick man said, "[My cousin] always accused me of laziness, but I couldn't work because of my ailment. He then asked me to go begging. Not only did he not find a doctor to treat me, he even asked me to work." When asked if his ailment could be cured, he replied, "I have had the ailment of *mafeng* for seven years, I will not be cured."[16]

Fear of Contagion

Indeed, murderers of *mafeng* patients, relatives of those they murdered, witnesses of murders, or bureaucrats who signed the written records of these cases tended to describe the sick as people with serious character flaws. It is unclear if these moral weaknesses were considered as underlying causes of their ailment or its consequence. These perceived weaknesses were clearly causes for serious domestic or communitarian disputes, leading to violent deaths. Yet, one underlying thread was woven through almost all the cases: the dread of contagion. A large part of the perceived moral weaknesses of the patients was in fact a reaction to such a fear in their closest relatives and neighbors. The fear dramatically changed relations between them and brought out what were considered as the patients' moral flaws. Some sufferers reacted with excessive aggression and violence toward others, others with extreme indulgence in self-pity. These responses were probably the result of the reluctance in accepting a tragic fate increasingly considered unredeemable and cruelly reflected in the barefaced rejection by their closest relatives and friends on the grounds of the danger of contagion. The fear was often the immediate cause of the murders involving these condemned bodies. Most of the mentioned cases reveal how this fear bred distrust, jealousy, and hatred within the household or village community. It clearly was the main reason for which the *mafeng*-afflicted inhabitants of the village in Leping county were burnt to death in 1742.

There were other, similar cases showing the tragic consequences of this fear. In a village in Huichang county, Jiangxi province, a woman, Xiao, who had married into the Zhong family, contracted *mafeng*, provoking increasing protest from her disgusted neighbors. Xiao decided to move out and asked her son to build her a house on the public land (*gong di*) on the opposite bank of the river. The son, Zhong Xuanwen, started building the wall in the fourth month of the sixth year of the Qianlong reign (1741); this action brought a protest from the family of his cousin, Zhong Hongliang, who lived nearby. Hongliang's family claimed that the land on which Xuanwen was building the house belonged to them and it was also too close to where they lived. Fearing contagion, they pulled down the wall. The two sides then came to an agreement whereby Hongliang would reimburse Xuanwen for the initial building fees, in return for which Xuanwen was to stop all construction and Xiao remain in her home. Since Hongliang did not pay the fees, Xuanwen continued construction, leading to a fight between Hongliang and Xiaosi, Xuanwen's cousin, in which Hongliang was killed. Xiaosi was sentenced to hanging, and those who were responsible for starting the fight were sentenced to eighty strokes. The magistrate, following the original agreement reached in the presence of the local constable (*baozheng*) and senior members of the Zhong clan, ordered Xiao to remain in her original place, and no house was to be built on the riverbank.[17] The magistrate obviously did not want to get involved in the local fear of contagion, and we do not know how Xiao's family resolved the original problem of the protest from their neighbors.

In other cases, the magistrate showed more concern for the problem of *mafeng* contagion. In a village in Fengshun county, Guangdong province, Hu Zuoting, forty-three years of age, was expelled from his village by a collective decision in 1740, slightly more than a year after he had been diagnosed with *mafeng*. He left the village to live in a shed on the other side of the mountain in the sixth month of that year. Two months later, as food ran out, he returned home to get some rice. Two former neighbors, who were brothers, saw him in his old home and accused him of breaking the collective agreement. This led to a violent fight between Zuoting's brother, Zuoxian, who lived nearby, and the two neighbors, in which the brother killed one of them with his carrying pole. Later, the victim's brother confessed, "Zuoting had contracted *mafeng*, and in the sixth month of the fifth year of Qianlong [1740], the entire village, fearing contagion, made a public and collective decision to expel him to live in a shed on the other side of the mountain. He was no longer allowed to live in the village. On the thirteenth day of the eighth month, in the afternoon, my brother and I returned home after cutting grass. While passing by Zuoting's old home, we saw him inside. We reproached him, saying 'You were expelled by the villagers because you have *mafeng*, how come you are back?' We then began to dispute." Zuoxian's confession, on the other hand, fully articulated the feeling of injustice he felt for his brother. He heard his brother crying out for help and ran out with his carrying pole: "I knew that my brother had contracted this malignant disease and had been expelled by the villagers, who would not allow him to live at home. That day he just happened to make a visit home and was beaten up. He was beaten to the ground, and even then they didn't stop. I was afraid that he would be beaten to death [and thus he hit one of them with his pole]." The magistrate sentenced Zuoxian to hanging, and forty strokes to the neighbor who started the fight. More important, not forgetting the immediate cause of the fight, Zuoting's ailment, he noted, "Hu Zuoting's malignant ailment of *mafeng* is the most contagious [*zui yi chuanran*]. I made an investigation and found that there is no asylum for *mafeng* patients [*feng yuan*] in the newly established county of Fengshun, so he could not be accommodated [there]. He should from now on live in a shed built in a remote and uninhabited place, and should not be allowed to dwell furtively in the village."[18]

In another case, in Qujiang county, Guangdong province, in 1749, a murder was caused by a dispute over expelling a *mafeng* patient, in this case, from her family. A woman by the name of Yang married into the Deng family in 1738. She later contracted *mafeng* and gradually came to live separately from her husband. In 1749, according to the Deng family, their neighbors had grown so disgusted with her presence and so feared contagion that they wanted her to leave. Upon her refusal, her father-in-law and his cousin brought the case to the district magistrate and obtained an order to expel her from the village. When the woman's father heard this, he came with his own brother to the Deng house to protest against such treatment of his daughter. He accused them of improperly bringing the case to the district magistrate and insisted the Dengs build a house for her nearby, not outside the village. The dispute ended in a deadly fight in which a grand uncle of the Deng family died after being pushed to the ground. The father-in-law confessed during the interrogation, "In the fourteenth year of Qianlong, [Yang's] *mafeng* was getting more serious, the neighbors of the village were all disgusted by her, and they feared being contaminated. . . . Now, my daughter-in-law's limbs have all decomposed and she cannot move. I have already built a hut for her in which to live." Yang's uncle, who had pushed old Deng to the ground, was sentenced to hanging; her father, who had started the dispute, was sentenced to twenty-five strokes. Yang was ordered to remain in the shed built by her father-in-law, presumably outside the village.[19]

Revenge of the Contagious Corpse

It is well known that in southern China of the Ming-Qing, the dead bodies of *mafeng* patients were considered extremely dangerous, as *chong* (poisonous bugs) were believed to fly out from the orifices of the corpse and into the bodies of healthy people nearby, thus causing the same ailment in them. We saw descriptions of this process of transmission in medical texts in chapter 1. Due to this fear, the bodies of *mafeng* patients, dead or dying, were often treated with cruelty and violence. Such treatment was undertaken sometimes as a ritual of exorcism, or as a means of preventing contagion, especially through flying *chong*. The story of the gruesome murder of a *mafeng*-afflicted peasant in rural Sichuan province in 1744 clearly reveals the popularity of such beliefs and how they ironically avenged the cruelly murdered victim.[20]

In the second month of the tenth year of the reign of Qianlong (early winter of 1745), an inhabitant of a village in Ya'an county, Sichuan province, was walking along a riverbank, some twenty *li* from the county center, when he noticed a bad smell. He followed the source of the smell and discovered a body washed up on the sandy bank. Not recognizing the dead person, he reported it to the magistrate, Tao. Tao arrived immediately on the scene, accompanied by only a few necessary specialists, including the coroner. The latter reported in a loud voice on the spot on the conditions of the body:

> The dead body is that of an unnamed male of about forty years of age. He was about five *chi* and three *cun* tall. His head and face have decomposed. His hair, pigtail, and beard have fallen out. His eyes are missing. There is a fatal cut on the top of his head. The wound is one *cun* long and one *fen* wide, two *fen* deep. The skin has been torn and the bone damaged. There are two other wounds on the left and on the right [of the fatal wound]. . . . He was stabbed to death by a knife. . . . There is a round wound on the right side of the back . . . of a blackish purple color, and one on his right buttock . . . of a reddish purple color, and two other round, reddish purple wounds near the anus. These are bedsores developed while he was alive. The flesh and skin of the entire body are swollen. It seems that he had suffered from *mafeng*. There are no other particularities. He was killed and the body thrown down the river.

As the villagers in Ya'an did not know the dead man, the magistrate launched an investigation in the villages along the river. They had a breakthrough finally when officer Hu of a postal relay station in neighboring Mingshan county reported that something unusual had happened on the night of the eighth day of the twelfth month of the preceding year. He reported that on that night, "Around the time of the fourth *geng* (about one in the morning), someone knocked at the door and wanted to buy a torch. I went out and saw four people, two of whom were carrying something with a bamboo pole. I asked them where they were from, and they answered they were from Zhu village, on their way to bury a relative who had just died. I sold them a torch and they left. I did not think about this anymore." Hu told the interrogators that he did not know the people but could still remember their faces and could identify them in the village. Hu thus went, on the twenty-fifth day of the second month, to Zhu village and identified four villagers: Liao Fuxian, Liao Shourong, Tang Zijie, and Gao Qixue. Tao then ceded the case to Cai, the magistrate of Mingshan county, as it was now obvious that the murder should be investigated and tried in Cai's jurisdiction. Under interrogation, the four told what had happened that winter night.[21]

Fuxian, the brother of a woman by the name of Liao, of Zhu village, paid a visit to his sister on the seventh day of the month. Liao told him that his brother-in-law, Liao Zonglin, had died two days ago, on the fifth. The death was somewhat expected. Zonglin, suffering from *mafeng* for years, had also contracted an ailment caused by the cold in the twelfth month. Fuxian did not see, however, the dead body of Zonglin, as it was already entirely wrapped in cloth and put in the sitting room. And there was no coffin. His sister told him, "He died of *mafeng*. And there will be poisonous *chong* flying out from the body to contaminate [*chuanran*] healthy people. We should not bury him nearby." She asked Fuxian to carry the body with Shourong, his cousin, and Tang Zijie, Liao's son-in-law, and Gao Qixue, Tang's nephew, to the river and throw it in. As the mountainous road between the village and the river was long, it took the four of them almost one whole day to do the job. They set out early in the morning of the eighth, and after midnight they were still on the road and out of light, which explained their stopping at the relay station to buy a torch. The other three, Shourong, Tang, and Gao, all gave the same version under interrogation. None of them dared to open the wrapping for fear of being contaminated by poisonous *chong* flying out of the *mafeng*-infected body. Shourong, however, provided some interesting information to the interrogators: "Liao Fufeng is my father, the woman Liao is my aunt of the same lineage [meaning a cousin of his father's]. She often comes to our house. On the seventh of the twelfth month of last year, my aunt sent her daughter to fetch me. When I got to her place, father was already there. My aunt said that my uncle had died of illness. . . ."

All evidence was against the woman Liao, forty-four years of age, who finally made her confession under interrogation on the eighth day of the third month of the tenth year of Qianlong:

> My husband, Liao Zonglin, had originally the family name of Wang. His grandfather married into our family and changed his name to Liao.[22] Zonglin and I have been married for years, and we have one daughter and two sons. My daughter's husband is Tang Zijie, who also married into the family and lives with us. Our sons are still young. Liao Fufeng and I belong to the same clan, but we are not directly related cousins. In the ninth month of the ninth year of Qianlong, I went to his house to sort seeds, and I spent the night there, as I could not go home due to the rain. Fufeng [a widower of fifty-five years of age] flirted with me and we committed adultery. In the eleventh month, I again went to his place and we did it again. My husband was suffering from *mafeng* and Fufeng asked me to kill him, as he was an eyesore. But I refused. Then Zonglin caught this cold disease and was bedridden in the twelfth month. On the fifth day, my daughter and son-in-law left home for various errands, Liao Fufeng came and sent away my sons. We committed adultery again in the kitchen and drank wine sitting next to the stove. . . . He said, "His illness is incurable. It's better to kill him now as people wouldn't be suspicious of his death." He asked me to do it first and he would finish him off.

Under the influence of passion and alcohol, Liao took a knife and struck the head of the husband three times while Fufeng held him down. Fufeng finished him off with the last fatal stroke. Since the patient had been ill for a long time and had almost completely lost his voice, he could not even cry out for help. And even if he had, there were no close neighbors nearby who could have heard him. The bedsores on his back and buttock also showed that he had been immobilized by *mafeng* for a long time. The two murderers wiped the blood off the bed with the dead man's clothes and cleaned the wounds that they then covered with mugwort herbs before putting a robe on him and wrapping him up entirely with layers of quilts. They then burnt the dead man's blood-soaked clothes. The rest of the story was told by the four unknowing carriers of the dead body.

When the knife and the bloodstained lined winter coat of Fufeng were found, the crime of the two murderers was confirmed. Liao Fufeng was sentenced to death by immediate decapitation, and the woman Liao was given the heaviest possible punishment, death by slow dismemberment (*lingchi*), a standard punishment for adulterous women who murdered their husbands. The four carriers of the body were also punished with beatings and exile, as abandoning dead bodies was also an offense.

The magistrate Cai of Mingshan county did not interrogate (or he did not put it in the detailed report) the true motive of Liao and her lover in treating the dead body the way they had—wrapping it up entirely before having it thrown into the river, a day's walk from the village. They might have considered this way of disposing of the body the perfect way to cover up their crime. At the same time, they might also have truly believed that this was the proper way of treating a *mafeng*-afflicted corpse. Indeed, the reason they gave to their relatives—that poisonous *chong* would fly out from the dead body and infect the healthy was sufficient to convince them not to bury it in a coffin nearby, as convention would have required. That the body was to be thrown into the river was probably also a customary way to treat the dead bodies of *mafeng* patients, as water and fire were considered equally effective in preventing postmortem contagion. The popular fear of contagion also discouraged the carriers from opening the wrapping on their way. One might speculate that had the murdered husband suffered an ailment other than *mafeng*, the adulterers might have had him buried in a coffin nearby, hence gotten away with the murder. It was really the beliefs surrounding *mafeng* that sealed the fate of the unfortunate husband, and his adulterous murderers. Such beliefs provided the perfect excuse for the couple to treat the body in this particular way, and precisely due to that treatment, the crime was uncovered. The sick husband was betrayed and savagely murdered because of his ailment. But it was also his *mafeng*-contaminated body that had finally avenged him, totally. This true story provides an interesting allegory of the way society persecuted *mafeng* patients in the late imperial period, only to be victimized by them ultimately.

MING-QING *MAFENG* ASYLUMS

In the eighteenth-century judicial cases examined in the preceding, even though only two mentioned excluding *mafeng* patients from their villages through bureaucratic procedures, most of them mentioned or hinted that the *mafeng* patient involved was expected to live in isolation outside the community. The "disgust" of the neighbors, or even of family members, was frequently mentioned as the cause of their social exclusion. There seemed to be little sympathy for *mafeng* patients in these cases, except for one or two close family members. The patients were depicted as repulsive and unlikable, at best useless, and, above all, contagious. Systematic exclusion of such a group was considered as a necessity. Institutional exclusion of *mafeng* patients had actually begun more than two centuries before these murders occurred, in the early sixteenth century. Probably the existence of such institutions made expelling them from the community the most "reasonable" solution in places where such asylums had not yet been set up. *Mafeng/lai* was, it is worth recalling, the *only* chronic disease necessitating segregation in imperial China, for the reason of preventing contagion.[23] Collective memory of such institutions recorded in local gazetteers, official histories of localities, reveal the communal attitudes toward *mafeng/lai* in the Ming-Qing periods, characterized by a growing fear of contagion. One finds that often such attitudes echo perfectly those seen in the eighteenth-century judicial cases just mentioned. There is, first of all, an interesting geographic coincidence in the two kinds of sources: Ming-Qing gazetteers and other archival materials that recorded the collective exclusion of *mafeng/lai* patients show that such institutions were found mainly in Fujian, Guangdong, Jiangxi, and Sichuan provinces,[24] and among the fourteen judicial cases that I have found related to *mafeng* patients, five took place in Jiangxi, three in Guangdong, three in Yunnan, two in Sichuan, and only one in Shandong. Other than Shandong, all provinces where capital crimes involving *mafeng* patients were recorded were also known to have collective exclusion of patients, with the exception of Yunnan province, where I have not found any record of an institution. These provinces were, moreover, what contemporaries considered as southern provinces in late imperial China in the sixteenth century. The absence of mention of such an institution in Yunnan province is probably a problem of a lacuna in the extant sources. The same might explain the lack of information on other "southern" provinces, such as Guangxi and Guizhou, that more modern sources reveal to have had a similar social fear of contagion from *mafeng* patients. Second, it can also be seen from these sources that *mafeng/lai* patients were excluded not only because they were thought to be filthy and contagious but also because they were considered to be morally undesirable social outcasts.

As far as extant sources show, there were at least fifteen counties in Fujian province, nineteen in Guangdong, four in Jiangxi, one in Zhejiang and Hubei, and an unclear number in Sichuan that had at least one asylum for *mafeng/lai* patients in the Ming-Qing period (for a list of late imperial leprosaria, see the appendix). Some counties, like Chaoyang and Haifeng, in Guangdong and Xincheng, in Jiangxi, had more than one. The first asylum that I have located so far was the one established in 1518 in Minxian county, in northern Fujian province. Most of the institutions in Fujian were set up in Ming times, while those in other provinces were mostly Qing institutions. There was also a clear, general pattern of development of these institutions. Most of them began as a *yangji yuan* (literally, asylum for support and relief), a kind of state asylum for the sick and the homeless elderly that could be dated as far back as the Song dynasty. The great majority of the Ming-Qing *yangji yuan,* theoretically one in each county, however, were initiated in the early Ming upon an order from the first emperor of the dynasty, as a symbol of state benevolence.[25] All state *yangji yuan* were set up inside the city walls of the county capitals, with a fixed quota of people inside receiving a state relief stipend. After the early sixteenth century, however, changes arose in these institutions. Many of them split into two or more branches, with the old one remaining in the administrative center and the new ones outside the city walls. The reason for such a split was often the presence of *mafeng/lai* patients in the institutions, provoking protests from other relief recipients. The new branches of the *yangji yuan,* sometimes retaining the old name, sometimes obtaining a new name, such as *laizi ying* (camp for *lai* people), *fengzi yuan, laimin suo, mafeng yuan, mafeng liao* (asylum or shed for *mafeng* people), or *cunxu yuan* (asylum for preserving pity), were almost without exception located outside the city walls, and often in distant mountains or on islands. New names containing the word *ying* or *liao* (camps, sheds, huts) implied that the asylums were sometimes makeshift constructions. In many cases, these new asylums for *mafeng/lai* patients were in time forced to move further and further away from the county capitals.

Records show that most of them were established by local magistrates, and that they received state funding to cover the living expenses of their inmates. In the Qing, individual asylums might receive land donations from local people. Still, asylums for *li/lai* patients differed from the rest of Ming-Qing charitable institutions, like foundling homes, widows' homes, hospices for the elderly, charitable dispensaries, and so forth, in that they did not usually receive donations nor managerial assistance from local elites. Local notables usually derived prestige from supporting major urban institutions that promoted Confucian virtues like chastity, respect for the elderly, and preserving lives.[26] These philanthropists had no interest, however, in assisting *mafeng/lai* patients, as they were not considered to be among the "deserving poor," and above all, the asylums were usually physically so distant from local political centers that they were, to most local people, invisible. In other words, these asylums remained essentially government-sponsored institutions set up mostly as a result of growing popular anxiety about the contagiousness of a dreaded disease, and concern about social evils linked to these patients thought to be threats to the community.

The earliest leper houses were established in Fujian province. According to the 1737 *General Gazetteer of Fujian,* a leper house had been established in Minxian in 1518 outside the eastern gate of the district, by the regional inspector Zhou Yuan. It was separate from the original poorhouse built in the late fourteenth century.[27] Similarly, in Quanzhou, a leper house was established on the basis of the old *yangji yuan* built in 1374. Its name was changed to *cunxu yuan,* while the original *yangji yuan* was moved to another spot in town. The change probably occurred in the early sixteenth century, as we know that Hu Cheng'an (1490–1572), an assistant administrative commissioner of Fujian sometime after 1527, had resisted the demand of the local rich to expel the *lai* inmates to an island outside the city gate for the purpose of appropriating the land of the institution.[28] The leper house in Zhangzhou, simply called camp for *lai* people (*laizi ying*), was established not later than the first decade of the sixteenth century. It was one of the town's three charitable institutions for the sick and poor, and was furthest from the city gate.[29] Other counties, such as Zhangpu, Changle, Sha, Jianyang, Zhenghe, Jiangle, Shaowu, and Lianchen, either had a *cunxu yuan* or *laizi ying,* or a *yangj iyuan* that explicitly claimed to accommodate *lai* or *mafeng* patients or sick poor with a "malignant ailment" (*eji*).[30] They were most likely established during the sixteenth century, just like those in Quanzhou, Zhangzhou, and Minxian. In peripheral Taiwan prefecture, a *yangji yuan* accommodating some forty *mafeng* patients was built by the magistrate in 1736.[31]

Similar institutions were also set up, after the mid-Ming, in Guangdong province. The one outside the city of Canton was built in the Ming. John Gray (1828–1890), a missionary visiting Canton in the 1870s, saw an inscription on which the date of its establishment, 1380, and restoration, 1573, were marked.[32] According to Qu Dajun (1630–1696), the famous Cantonese literatus who had witnessed the fall of the Ming, this *fafeng yuan* (asylum for patients with declared Wind ailment) had existed in the northern outskirts of the city, but the building was ramshackle and had been abandoned in the early Qing when the local government established a new one. According to early-nineteenth-century witnesses, the renovated asylum was located outside the eastern gate, providing relief for 174 local patients, 134 non-Cantonese patients, and 33 nonresident ones. The same quota seems to have been maintained well into the mid-nineteenth century, when Western observers provided the same information.[33] W. Milne reported that, in Canton, "where leprosy of a most hideous, disgusting, and incurable form has too many victims," there was this leper hospital, where, "in 1832 the number of patients in it was 341, who were supported at an expense of 300 taels per annum or 100 English pounds."[34] Gray reported in 1875 that, in fact, many patients had to live in mud huts constructed outside the asylum, as there was not enough room for them, implying a number of patients larger than the quota.[35] The leper house in Xinhui county seems to have been built in the late sixteenth century, close to the *yangji yuan* inside the city. After *mafeng* patients were accused of robbery by city dwellers, the institution was moved outside the western gate of the city. Most asylums had a similar history.[36] The example of Jingning, Zhejiang province, is revealing. The *yangji yuan,* renovated in 1483, originally accommodated the district's sick and elderly. However, as the number of interned *lai* patients grew and the other sick and poor no longer dared to live there, the institution was eventually turned into a *mafeng* asylum.[37]

An increasing number of such asylums were built or rebuilt during the Qing in the southeastern provinces. A systematic policy to intern *mafeng* patients seems to have been followed during the first years of the Yongzheng reign. We know that the Yongzheng emperor issued an edict to encourage the establishment of poorhouses and foundling homes in every county of the empire in 1724, the second year of his reign.[38] After that date, *mafeng/lai* asylums in Fujian, Jiangxi, and Guangdong provinces were built or rebuilt regularly with a fixed, subsidized quota, and efforts were made to separate patients of *lai* from the other sick and poor, revealing conscious attempts to prevent contagion. In Longxi, Zhangzhou prefecture, the policy of providing relief to the impoverished sick was carried out according to the 1724 edict, at the same time separating *mafeng* patients from the others in two different buildings.[39] Many further reformed or enlarged the original leper asylums during the Yongzheng and Qianlong periods. A number of institutions were moved further away from the county centers (Zhenghe), or simply to isolated spots (Liancheng, Shaowu).[40]

Hospices in Jiangxi province, on the other hand, seem to have been built mainly during the Qing, especially from the eighteenth century onward. Some of the better-known ones include those built in Dayu (1736), a county neighboring Guangdong province, in Wuning (1743), and Fengxin (1774).[41] We have very little information on asylums in other provinces, although we do have a record of one established during the Ming in Jingning, in Zhejiang, as mentioned. An asylum was also built in 1731 in Hanyang district, Hunan. However, both institutions were no longer active by the latter half of the nineteenth century.[42]

The preceding descriptions of leper institutions in the southern provinces, particularly Fujian, Guangdong, and Jiangxi, indicate that many such asylums appeared in the sixteenth century and became common in the Qing, especially after the eighteenth century. By 1800 the existence of such places was well known to scholar-officials outside these provinces, only to increase their fear of the disease. Song Xiangfeng, a scholar from Jiangsu province, and a successful civil examination candidate at the provincial level in 1800, wrote a poem on these asylums: "There is a strange disease south of the Five Ranges, / a fruit of excessive poison in humid swamps . . . / I hear that there are *mafeng* hospices / that have been taking in patients since time immemorial. / But I fear that the disease will not thus be stopped, / but will spread ever more quickly."[43] Scholars of the region, watching the development of such asylums more closely, suggested also that these asylums reflected profound popular fear of the disease. Liang Shaoren (1792–ca. 1837) observed that, in eastern Guangdong province, "There are *mafeng* asylums everywhere." His explanation for the phenomenon was the population's fear of being contaminated: "Once contaminated [by *mafeng*], one is doomed to death,"[44] implying that the asylums were there to prevent such fatal contagion. Indeed, even the most destitute did not want to live with *mafeng* patients. The fact that many asylums were offshoots of former poorhouses and relocated to remote, sparsely populated areas reflects the popular fear of person-to-person contagion, a fear rooted even among the most impoverished.[45] From the Qing onward, these institutions were set up either outside the city gates or far away from the town centers. In Zengcheng, Guangdong province, the *mafeng yuan* established in 1736 was on an isolated spot in the mountains "hardly visited by humans."[46] Often, interned *mafeng* patients were forbidden to enter the city gates.[47] Rules of these institutions seem to indicate that patients were not locked inside the building but were allowed to roam or beg in nearby areas. The institutions provided them with basic room and board and the means for minimum survival.

Unlike medieval Christian leprosaria or asylums visited by Buddhist monks, these late-imperial Chinese institutions did not seem to carry out religious rituals. On the other hand, even though these late institutions segregated the sick, as had medieval European leprosaria, they were not assigned the judicial function of disqualifying the social and political status of the patients, as *mafeng/lai* victims did not suffer from the same religious bias as did lepers in European Christianity. Foucault's conception of medieval leprosaria as an "exclusive model" for the execution of a grand "rite of purification" cannot explain the Chinese asylums

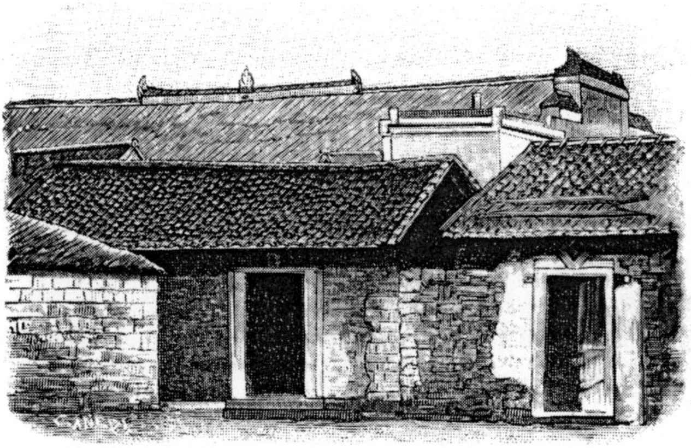

INSTALLATION ANCIENNE DE LA LÉPROSERIE.

Old leprosarium in Raozhou, Jiangxi province, as seen in the 1890s (*Missions catholiques,* no. 29 [1897]; courtesy of Missions Étrangères de Paris).

of the late imperial period. His idea of the "inclusive" quarantine hospital emerging during the plague epidemics of the Renaissance as a model that announced Europe's "modernity," on the other hand, *partially* fits the profile of these Chinese asylums. Both were mainly for the purpose of protecting the healthy population by segregating the contagious sick,[48] while it is questionable whether early medieval European leprosaria and Buddhist asylums for *li*/*lai* victims were instituted for the purpose of preventing contagion.[49] However, whereas the control and surveillance methods employed in the new quarantine institutions of late medieval Europe had the ultimate purpose of healing the sick so that they would eventually return to "normal" society, the Chinese late-imperial asylums did not emphasize healing, as the disease was believed to be incurable. What then was the rationale of the Chinese asylums?

Rationale of Ming-Qing Asylums

The rationality of the Chinese asylums as a model to maximize separation between the contagious sick and the healthy population can be observed in some of their records, especially those of Guangdong province, where they were most widespread in the eighteenth century. The principle of exclusion in this case was not exactly by law or force, but by means of paying *mafeng* patients to stay inside the asylum, and by appointing one among them as a "supervisor," who made sure that they did not loiter in the cities. Qing records clearly show that each asylum had a quota of patients to be assisted regularly by the government. As we have seen, the Canton asylum obtained some 300 taels of silver annually for its 341 residents and nonresidents. The Haiyang hospice in Chaozhou prefecture had obtained, as of around 1744, more than 480 taels of silver a year for its 128 inmates and 519 nonresidents.[50] Similar subsidies were given to registered *mafeng* patients in Jieyang, Huilai, Chenghai, Puning, Haifeng, Shunde, and Zengcheng. Some hospices gave relief in the form of rice, as in Chaoyang and Boluo.[51] In Huilai district, stipends were even classified into three categories corresponding to the different degrees of handicap: the "decomposing" (*kuilan*), with a quota of forty-one, received the most (six *li* of silver [0.006 tael] per day); the "old and infirm" (*pilong*), with a quota of sixty-four, received five *li;* whereas the simple "cripple" (*canji*), with a quota of sixty-six, received only four *li* a day.[52] Even though information on asylums in the other provinces is less complete, it is reasonable to believe that the great majority were financed by the government in similar ways.

On the question of management, the Qing authorities minimized costs and maximized efficiency by appointing one among the inmates as the supervisor to receive and register patients according to the official quota, to distribute stipends, and to oversee their activities. Qu Dajun again gives us one of the earliest descriptions of the organization of the asylums in the mid-seventeenth century: "There was an old *mafeng* asylum north of the city [of Canton]. It became ramshackle after years of existence. The authorities then bought land and undertook to build [a new asylum]. It accommodates as many as possible of male and female *mafeng* patients and supports [their living]. A headman [*shouling* (literally, head collar)] was chosen among the patients to oversee them, to make sure that not one would escape [from the asylum]. And this evil [disease] thus gradually lessened. This is really a beneficence bestowed by kind people that will last for centuries."[53] In certain cases, local constables (*dibao*) were responsible for keeping them off city streets, as in the case of Chenghai.[54] In other districts, the headman was sometimes called the eye among *mafeng* patients (*feng mu*), and the number of patients he had to supervise was officially determined. In Chaoyang, Guangdong province, for instance, one *feng mu* was assigned thirty-six patients in the eastern asylum, one fifty-four patients in the western asylum, one twenty-four in the Heping Weiwai asylum, and one fifty-two in the Xiashan Dongshan asylum.[55] Choosing a leader among the inmates to supervise their movement seems to have been a standard way of managing the asylums.[56] This arrangement had the advantage of minimizing bureaucratic expenses while maintaining efficiency, as such a headman was likely to be best informed not only about his subordinates but also about the local community. He was the ideal link between the bureaucracy, the community, and the marginalized group. More important, he did not fear contagion.

Running an asylum through the intermediary of a selected headman still functioned in the mid-nineteenth century, as recorded by Western missionaries. Wong Foon (Huang Kuan [1829–1878]), the above-mentioned British-trained Cantonese doctor, interviewed a number of headmen to write up his report on leprosy in the Canton area in 1873.[57] Justus Doolittle made perhaps the most detailed account of the asylums in Fuzhou, in 1865: "Each asylum is under the control of a head man, who must reside at the institution, and who is nominally or really one of the lepers. It is the duty of this head man to report at stated times to the district magistrate the number of deaths, accessions, etc., and to manage the general affairs of the asylum. Matters he cannot settle must be promptly reported to the proper magistrate. He has great power over the unfortunates connected with his establishment. The rules are very rigid. . . . These head men have the reputation of being rich, and of having money at interest."[58] Where did the power and wealth of the headman derive? "On entering an asylum, the leper must give to its head man a sum of money, regulated somewhat by the wealth of the individual." And if a wealthy family wanted to keep a patient at home instead of sending him/her to the asylum, again the headman had to be given a large bribe.[59] James Cantlie, who visited what he called a leper village in Canton, made the same observation. He arrived at this asylum in the winter of 1890/1891 with his student Sun Yat-sen, the future "Father of the Chinese Republic." He described its headman thus:

> Perhaps the most interesting feature in the village was the fact that the head man, through whose fingers all the money passes, had been in the asylum in that function twenty-two years, the longest lived leper in the community. He was reputed to be a rich man; he was certainly well dressed in fur and silk. It was January, heavy clothing was requisite. He smoked a wonderfully decorated pipe, he wore faded ornaments,—in fact, gave evidence of being a man well off. His fingers, however, were fewer than they had been, his ears were cropped close, his left eye stared when his right was closed, and his face and neck bore signs of old leprous scars. Still he was fairly strong, and all this after being a leper for a quarter of a century.[60]

The Western observers' fascination with the Chinese headman showed their sensitivity to the Chinese game of local power that most contemporary Chinese writers overlooked, or more often, took for granted. It was taken for granted

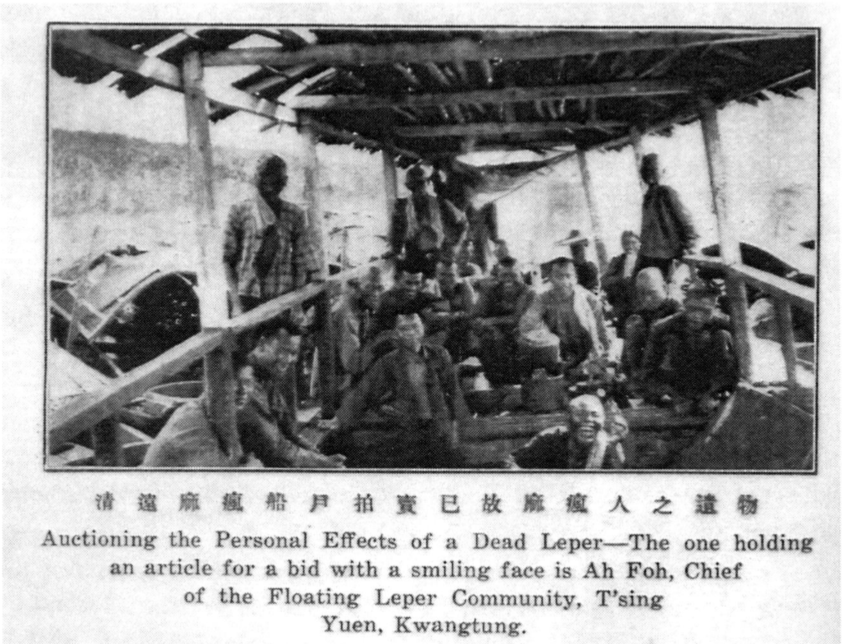
清遠痲瘋船尸拍賣已故痲瘋人之遺物
Auctioning the Personal Effects of a Dead Leper—The one holding an article for a bid with a smiling face is Ah Foh, Chief of the Floating Leper Community, T'sing Yuen, Kwangtung.

Leper boat in Qingyuan, Guangdong province, with the headman auctioning belongings of a dead leper. (Photo originally published in *Leper Quarterly* 6, no. 2 [1932])

and often went unreported because such an arrangement—governing through trusted and well-informed local agents—was inherent in the traditional philosophy of local administration, and the headman was an integral element of the social fabric. Chinese writers were simply oblivious to it as part of the everyday landscape. Such a self-governing system, the product of local power relations and rules of the game unique to China, had little to do with the Foucauldian disciplinary model of the modern European prison or asylum.

The rationality of these institutions resided not only in their financial and managerial organization but was also reflected in their popularity among local populations. These asylums were created, organized, financed, and located in ways local inhabitants wanted them to be. Gazetteers often record, albeit with occasional exaggeration, popular support of such asylums. They were popular essentially because the local populations wanted to be protected from the contagious sick, seen also as socially dangerous and rapidly self-reproducing. The leper house in Xinhui district, built in the mid to late sixteenth century, for example, was, at the beginning, close to the poorhouse inside the city. After inmates were accused of robbery by city dwellers, the institution was moved outside the western gate of the city to pacify local wrath. The moving away of the *mafeng* asylum in Leizhou was, according to the author of the gazetteer, "heartily welcomed by the literati and people."[61] Relevant sources mostly indicate that the incarceration of *mafeng* patients was similarly appreciated by local populations, who considered the patients to be filthy, greedy, malicious, and, even worse, dangerously gregarious and fecund, implying their repulsive promiscuity. In Chenghai, Guangdong, for example, there were sixty-six *mafeng* patients registered in 1752, and, twelve years later, several hundred of them were said to have grouped together in the city. They were accused of organized crimes, including the extortion of money from families having banquets or funerals. Their forced exclusion from the town center was much applauded by the local population.[62] In Shaowu, Fujian province, *mafeng* patients in the poorhouse were said to have grouped together to illegally purchase houses on the main street, causing a general panic. In 1788, the magistrate had to expel them from the city and forbid their reentry into the poorhouse.[63] In Xinhui, the asylum was first relocated, in the mid-sixteenth century, outside the city on a hill along a river because inmates were accused of robbery. Later on, city dwellers began to accuse them of polluting the river that flowed into the town and demanded a second removal. In Fengxin, Jiangxi, city dwellers found the two *mafeng* sheds just outside the northern gate an eyesore and too near to the main avenue. In 1774 money was pooled together to remove them to an isolated spot in the mountains.[64] Like the inhabitants of Leizhou district, those of towns purged of *mafeng* patients must have "felt content and relieved."[65]

From the perspective of the authorities, however, setting up asylums for *mafeng* patients had another important function: to protect the patients from a hostile society. This function was rarely mentioned in the gazetteers, which usually reflected the wider interests of local society. The story told by You Shaoan, magistrate in 1736 of Dayu county, in southeastern Jiangxi province, neighboring Guangdong, illustrates this particular concern. You Shaoan wrote that, when he first traveled in the district in 1734,

> A crowd of beggars knelt on the roadside and I asked them why. They said that they were unfortunate to have contracted *mafeng*, and the inhabitants of the old town forbade them to enter the town to beg. Even the destitute of the poorhouse refused resolutely to share the same roof with them. They were on the verge of being starved to death. Their words thus roused great compassion in my heart. . . . [And I later

learned that] there were twenty-two *mafeng* beggars, half of them local, half from Guangdong province, who had never had a real lodging and shared nine huts on the southern bank of the river, three *li* from the town so that the town is far from the harmful effect . . . . I sighed: they are not only abandoned by heaven, they are also abandoned by men.[66]

He thus negotiated with the provincial authorities to increase by ten the quota of the destitute of the district, and a separate poorhouse was built to accommodate *mafeng* beggars.[67] Similarly, the only leper institution set up in Taiwan during the Qing, the *laibing ying*, built in 1736 in Zhanghua, was apparently initiated by the magistrate out of pity and compassion.[68] In both cases, it appeared that the destitute *mafeng* patients themselves *asked* to be interned and so given relief. In such cases, the state was the only source of legitimate relief and arbitrator between the victims and a hostile society.

The social problems caused by *mafeng* patients caught the attention of the emperor at about the same time. The Qianlong period (1736–1795) was one that I consider marked by bureaucratization in regard to the history of charitable institutions, in the sense that these institutions, mostly initiated by local elites in the seventeenth century, underwent a period of standardization by bureaucrats in the Qianlong period.[69] As *mafeng* asylums were, from the beginning, government institutions, they did not go through the process of bureaucratization, even though there was increasing and systematic governmental resources granted them in the same period. A memorandum from a high official in Sichuan province in 1742 clearly shows the serious social problems caused by *mafeng* patients in the province, and the imperial attitude toward such problems. Li Rulan, the surveillance commissioner (*anchashi*) of Sichuan province, provided the following report on the situation of *mafeng* patients in 1742:

I have always heard that *lai* or *mafeng* is rampant in Guangdong and Fujian provinces. Now the situation in Sichuan is even worse. Probably it is due to the humidity of the earthly *qi*, and immigrants and visitors from Guangdong and Fujian causing contagion [*chuanran*]. Since there is no healing formula . . . even though patients take a long time to die, the harm done has been tremendous. There are cases where patients are abandoned by relatives; some escape into the mountains for fear of passing the ailment to their children; others commit suicide by drowning or hanging. Some parents burn their sick children to death or drown them alive. Because people fear that the *chong* of the *lai* ailment will fly out from the dead body of a patient, the ways patients are killed are particularly cruel. And there are cases of revenge involving death because of contagion.

And of course, the behavior of the *mafeng* patients themselves was also a source of social violence: "Beggars with *lai* are often excessive in their extortions and they harm local businesses. They often get killed for such behavior. The administration has issued numerous orders to prohibit such behavior. Yet these customs have been going on for so long that it is difficult for them to be abolished overnight." There were other, unforeseen administrative problems caused by *mafeng* patients: "Sometimes criminals with *lai* are sentenced to imprisonment, yet other prisoners refuse to share the cell with them. [For the same reason] Poorhouses such as *yangji yuan* and *puji tang* also refuse to accommodate them."

All these problems pointed to the obvious solution that a special place had to be constructed to isolate *mafeng* patients. Li thus petitioned the emperor for the setting up of asylums initiated and financed by the government on a provincial scale. In uninhabited places outside of towns, "houses from several dozen to over one hundred units should be built. A wall should be constructed surrounding these houses, forming a big complex [*da yuan*]. All those who have the *lai* ailment should be sent to live there. An assistant medical official should supervise [the complex]; no one should be allowed in or out, causing unnecessary trouble." He even had a financial plan for the project: 2,000 taels from the surplus (a total of 4,465 taels) in the balance of the provincial prison budget during the several years preceding 1742 could be used to build a provincial network of *mafeng* asylums. Major prefectures were included in his plan.[70] Once incarcerated, inmates would receive regular stipends provided for by part of the "allowance to encourage honesty" (*yanglian yin*) given to bureaucrats above the magistrate level. His objectives for the project were to protect both the sick and the healthy populations: "Such legislation would protect people not having *lai*, and prevent families with *lai* members from hurting each other. If the patients are not allowed out, social disturbances will decrease, and there will be fewer floating corpses." In his eyes, the asylum was something like a charitable prison, and it was only logical that it should be financed from the provincial prison budget. Upon reading the memorandum, the emperor ordered the provincial governor to take charge of the matter, in accordance with available resources.[71]

In other words, the establishment of *mafeng* asylums had, by the eighteenth century, become *the* "solution" to the increasing social and administrative problems that the ailment was causing. It was welcomed by the healthy population, fearful of contagion and bad moral influences, demanded by patients, especially those of the lower classes concerned about sheer survival, and deemed necessary by the authorities themselves for the prevention of many difficult social conflicts and for solving tricky administrative difficulties like incarcerating *mafeng* prisoners.

Besides the widespread state-financed and state-organized *mafeng* asylums, expelling patients from the community by setting them adrift on boats was another common method of segregating them in southern China. Again, Qu Dajun, of the early Qing, provides us with one of the first descriptions of such customs: "Whenever one is found to have *feng*, the family puts him or her into a small boat, with food and clothes, and sets the boat on the river or on the sea."[72] John Gray was an eyewitness of such a custom in Canton in the 1870s: "As the asylum at Canton is not large enough for the numerous lepers who seek admission, several anchorages are set apart on the river for boats in which they are accommodated. . . . They are under the necessity of paddling about the river asking alms from the crews of the junks and boats with which the river is crowded. The leper-boats generally go in fleets of ten or twenty each, and money is almost forced from the sailors. Not infrequently the lepers eke out their scanty subsistence by stripping the dead bodies which are too often found floating on the river. . . . In the silk districts of Guangdong . . . at almost every town, and on almost every creek and river, I found anchorages for leper-boats."He also mentions that, in Guangxi province, "I found a leper residing in almost every one of the small shrines erected at intervals on the banks. . . . Each leper . . .was provided with a rod and alms-bag."[73] Such customs were also reported by other mid-nineteenth-century missionaries in other southern provinces. A missionary living in Fuzhou, Fujian province, wrote, in a report of 1847, "My Chinese teacher tells me that on the river Min . . . are one or two counties in which the unhappy leper is thus treated. He is put into a small boat furnished with a small quantity of rice, wood and some other necessaries, and suffered to float down the river, all other boats avoiding contact with him. A few days generally terminates his wretched existence."[74] The exclusion of *mafeng* patients by means of boats was even used by missionaries in the early twentieth century for evangelical purposes. A "Gospel boat" was said to have been organized on the rivers in Guangdong and Guangxi provinces, "because when a person gets leprosy the people will give him a boat and make him live on the water. . . . We have here about eight Christians . . . who have established a Gospel boat especially for the lepers."[75]

Setting patients adrift on boats is reminiscent of the rituals of the expulsion of pestilence in southern China. The Wangye cult in Taiwan, Marshal Wen cult in Zhejiang, cult of the Five Emperors in Fuzhou (Fujian province) all involved the act of putting the plague demons or deities on a boat that was set off on the water. The boat was either set to drift, paraded, or set on fire. A version of the ritual of expulsion by boat can be found in the Daoist canon as early as the twelfth century.[76] Separation by water or destruction by fire were popularly believed to be effective ways to stop pestilence. The punishment by drowning alive of *li* patients in early Chinese law reveals the early importance of the water element. We have already learned from the eighteenth-century memorandum of Li Rulan that, in Sichuan province, the *mafeng* demon was tamed either by water, fire, or exile. Some missionaries in the mid-nineteenth century and reports of the twentieth century described the custom of lepers being buried alive, echoing another ancient punishment of *li* patients that had ritual meaning.[77] In brief, the ancient idea that a *li* sufferer embodied an evil spirit and the medieval Buddhist notion of his moral corruption seems to have lasted well into the late imperial and modern periods, in addition to the widespread fear of physical contagion, further dramatized by the idea of bewitched *chong* flying out of the corpses of *mafeng* victims. The subjection of such patients to social seclusion or tragic and violent death throughout history reveals something more than a fear of contagion, as it also had deep-rooted religious and ritual significance.[78]

Revenge of the Ostracized Body

Paradoxically, the increasing stigmatization of *mafeng* patients and growing fear of their contagiousness were the very source of their empowerment. Increasing communal hostility toward them greatly restricted their social space, but at the same time lent them a new identity that they could exploit to their advantage, and for their survival. The empowerment came specifically from the fear of contagion, and from the presumption about the promiscuity of *mafeng* patients. As a consequence of the prolonged seclusion outside society, these *mafeng* patients, at least in some parts of southern China, inevitably developed a new group identity, or formed pseudolineages that was reinforced by the growing belief that *mafeng* was a hereditary disease. Although late-imperial written sources do not allow for an in-depth analysis of the nature of such an identity, existing records on their collective activities, sometimes criminal, imply that they were forming permanent groups on the margins of society. In many ways, they were similar to beggar groups. Yet the nature of their particular ailment stigmatized them further and possibly contributed to the forging of a stronger group identity.

In a sense, *mafeng* patients were empowered in ways similar to those of beggars. They acquired their power from the fear society held toward them. Their reputation as dangerous and unscrupulous carved out a specific social space strictly reserved for activities corresponding to their perceived identity. In Guangdong province, *mafeng* patients were often considered the worst of beggars.[79] They were the worst because they were the most dreaded among the socially marginalized. We again turn to Qu Dajun for a first, colorful picture of these often crippled but powerful bodies active in Guangdong province in the mid-seventeenth century. Like beggars, *mafeng* patients extorted money from families having celebrations or funerals. According to Qu, "they were the most harmful," as "they arrive in groups in front of the concerned family, and shout and curse. Unless they are given enough money, things, food, and wine, they refuse to leave. They have a leader called 'A Hu,' who has to be given a big sum of money first. He then distributes the money among [his followers]. Once he has been paid, A Hu hangs a basket in front of the family's door so that his followers will not come again. Among the beggars in Guangdong, those with *mafeng* are the most wicked. Whenever they go out begging, they go in groups of three or five, including women and men. People dare not treat them with a stern voice and countenance."[80] Xu Ke (1869–1928), a literatus, recorded toward the end of the Qing, in the early twentieth century, a similar interaction between *mafeng* beggars and the general public: "[They] often go out and beg, and wander in the marketplace. They usually have swollen faces with sores, fallen-out eyebrows, and crooked hands and feet. Those who see them are greatly appalled and vie to give them money. That is why they often receive much more alms than other, ordinary beggars."[81] Similarly Gray, reporting in the 1870s, describes strategies used by organized lepers: "Lepers of hideous aspect . . . awaiting the arrivals of funerals to exact money from the mourners. Their demands are invariably complied with, as the mourners believe that the souls of their departed relatives would be persecuted by spirits of departed lepers were alms refused." If exorbitant extortion was refused, "the lepers not unfrequently leap into the grave, and resist all the attempts of the undertakers to lower the coffin."[82]

By the same principle, *mafeng* patients in the Ming-Qing period were said to have monopolized several lucrative "trades": they were employed by pirates and gangsters as agents to retrieve ransom from families of kidnapped persons; they were even employed by local bureaucrats to collect overdue taxes in villages and communities. The way they pressed taxpayers to pay their due was particularly telling: "For those families who have not paid all their due taxes, these *mafeng* people would go with their likes to eat and sleep in their houses. Day after day they would burst out unbridled curses, and contaminate [the family] with their filth and poison, with the purpose of infecting them with the vicious ailment. Thus the administration uses these *mafeng* people as its claws and teeth, and gangsters use them as agents. These useless people can thus become so useful!"[83] Indeed, not only the patients themselves realized the power they had over the general population due to the fear and repulsion their sickness generated, others, including local petty bureaucrats, were also fully aware of the nature of their power and thus made maximum use of it.[84] It is thus not surprising that, from at least the eighteenth century onward, we find, in Guangdong province, public condemnation of *mafeng* patients together with beggars and hooligans. Public announcements engraved on public steles forbade them to enter villages, and villagers were authorized to chase them out or turn them in to the magistrate with the help of local constables.[85]

Heredity and Pseudolineages

Such power of *mafeng* patients partially came from their exclusion from society from the sixteenth century onward. Even though stigmatization brought with it a deteriorating image, it also generated a new identity for these sick bodies that was somewhat reinforced by the increasingly influential medical idea that *mafeng* was hereditary. This belief, and the fact that most patients increasingly led a markedly different and separate life from the rest of society, gave birth to the curious notion of them as a peculiar pseudolineage, reminiscent of a tribe, or of a new pariah group.

An early Qing scholar, Wu Zhenfang, recorded in 1705 that patients in the asylum of Chaozhou (Guangdong province) "marry among themselves and produce children like normal people do."[86] The Cantonese scholar Liang Shaoren (1792–?) wrote in 1837, "There are so-called *mafeng* patients in eastern Guangdong province. Once they are contaminated [*ran*], they cannot be cured by medicine. That is why there are *mafeng* asylums everywhere. Inside [these asylums], they are allowed to marry among themselves. After three generations, they are allowed to move out [of the asylums], because the poison [inside them] will have been exhausted."[87] Obviously that *mafeng* sufferers married among themselves was well known in the eighteenth century, and the explanation of the disease's peculiar hereditary nature probably developed at the same time. More details of such a belief are given by another scholar of the same period, Chen Huiyan, who, in 1850, reported, "There are *mafeng* asylums in Canton and Chaozhou districts. Inmates are either of the first or second generation. Headmen arrange marriages among them so that there will be no confusion [of generation], and those born of the third generation no longer bear the poison and can be released from the asylum. That is why one says that the *mafeng* ailment does not exceed three generations."[88] This belief, a mixture of facts (that patients married among themselves) and fiction (that the cured third generation of patients were released) was obviously widespread by the mid-nineteenth century. It was not, however, recorded in any medical text, even though medical doctors from at least the sixteenth century onward wrote that *mafeng* was congenital, that parents passed the poison to the fetus during coitus. That the innate poison would diminish within three generations was purely a popular belief, albeit an influential one. As we will see in chapter 4, even modern Chinese medical doctors with complete Western training in the late nineteenth century still held this to be true. The idea even found its way into medical reports on leprosy in China written by Western leprologists who seemed to accept that the leprosy in China had special hereditary characteristics, different from what they observed in other parts of the world. This very belief, in my opinion, promoted the idea that *mafeng* patients formed their own distinct lineages.

Moreover, the system of asylum, with the management of powerful headmen, also seemed to nurture a separate social and cultural life for patients and reinforce a new identity. Qu Dajun again gives us a hint. After all the descriptions of the horrifying uses made of *mafeng* patients by the administration and gangsters, he suggested that the only way to "eliminate this evil" was to put them all in an asylum and forbid them to get out. He added, "In fact, these *mafeng* people do not desire to get out from there."[89] My reading of his last sentence is that he believed that the patients, once given a secure livelihood in a safe place, would not cause trouble, as they would find contentment inside. His observation was confirmed by John Gray, who visited the same asylum some 200 years later.[90] Doolittle's description of the traditional asylum in nineteenth-century Fuzhou detailed its self-contained nature, an aspect that might explain Qu's optimism: "Different sections of the asylum are allotted to the different sexes. Husbands and wives are, however, allowed to live together. In case of their husbands being taken with the leprosy, and required to live in the asylum some wives prefer to accompany them rather than live at their own houses. These asylums present the appearance of a walled village, having streets, a few small shops, and a school. . . . Lepers at the asylums may marry and raise families."[91] The arrangement would produce a social life totally separate and independent from the rest of society. Moreover, it echoes the belief that the innate poison of *mafeng* would be exhausted in a few generations, so that patients were allowed to get married and have children. This practice also implies that, for generations, these people would intermarry only among themselves and stay within the walls of the asylum. Even the healthy children of patients most likely remained in the community the rest of their lives, as they faced strong social bias outside. Generations of patients and their descendants living in a close community naturally nurtured pseudolineage identities. This identity was discernible in a local custom in Fuzhou county, Fujian province, that was still going strong in the early twentieth century. A Japanese observer noted that whenever a resident of the county was known to have the disease, lepers segregated outside the city walls would visit the family, exerting tremendous pressure on the family to let the patient go so that he or she could join the group. The observer concluded that these patients were attached to each other because they suffered from the same disease.[92]

However, Qu's assumption that segregated patients would stay clear of the healthy section of society proved to be quite wrong, as illustrated by the examples of the social disturbances caused by interned patients in some asylums recorded in the gazetteers. On the other hand, such disturbances did not appear to be random, individual acts but organized by well-structured, large groups. Take, for example, the extraordinary case in eighteenth-century Shaowu, in Fujian, where a large and growing group of interned *mafeng* patients furtively bought up real estate in town, extending their property to the town center, causing a general alarm.[93] The disturbing and rapid agglomeration of *mafeng* patients also became a problem in Chenghai district, Guangdong province. In 1752, the quota for *mafeng* patients in the asylum was sixty-six. Twelve years later, according to a gazetteer, reproduction and agglomeration had resulted in several hundreds of them. This huge group continued their usual business of extorting money, now usually enormous sums, as they were so numerous, from families having celebrations or funerals. They became a pressing social problem for the county due to their sheer number, and necessitated draconian bureaucratic measures to stop them.[94]

In some places, *mafeng* patients had their own religious worship. In Jianyang, Fujian province, inside the asylum there was a Guanyin said to be particularly "efficacious and responsive" (*lingyan*) in curing *lai*. It was said to have cured at least one patient every year in the mid-eighteenth century.[95] In the Suzhou area, at the turn of the nineteenth century, there was a temple for the worship of the god for *lai* patients (*Laipi zushi miao*) on a hill north of Mount Peng: "Prayers of those who have *lai* will be heard and answered there."[96] Wu Zhenfang, mentioned previously, who was one of the first to record the intermarrying among inmates of the asylums, also wrote that there was a special well inside the asylum in Chaozhou. This well, called Phoenix (*fenghuang*), was said to produce water that brought the disease under control. However, should a patient leave the asylum and stop drinking the water, the symptoms would reappear.[97] In other words, myths surrounding *mafeng* asylums by the early eighteenth century suggest that the afflicted inmates had every reason to remain strongly attached to these institutions. Unfortunately, we know too little about the religious life of the majority of *mafeng* patients in the late imperial period. Sporadic pieces of information show that, in some parts of the country, they did have their unique deities or worship or other religious practices. This might also have enhanced their group identity, something that we can, however, conjecture about rather than confirm.

In late imperial China, stigmatized and ostracized *mafeng* patients retaliated through various criminal and antisocial acts, and by grouping together in and outside asylums to form pseudolineages to aggrandize their social influence. In this way, they turned their group identity to their own advantage by deliberately reinforcing the negative image society imposed on them. I have not found any materials, written or otherwise, by patients, so that it is difficult to speculate on their subjective views of their social existence in this period. Not until 1940 did the first Chinese journal created and edited by patients of Hansen's disease appear.[98] Only with the availability of such texts did it become possible to look at the subjectivity and individual identity of educated patients of the disease in the modern period.[99] For earlier periods, we have to be content with an analysis of the recorded actions of those from the most deprived classes, records written by people who usually abhorred or feared them.

SEXUAL TRANSMISSION AS CAUSE AND CURE

As mentioned earlier, by late imperial times, the typical *mafeng/lai* patient portrayed in texts was no longer uniquely male. Now it was the female sufferer who came under the spotlight. Moreover, contrary to her male counterpart in the medieval period, she was said to seek healing by a perverse method: *guolai,* or passing the ailment on to an innocent man with whom she had sexual intercourse when her ailment was still in its incubatory stage. By so doing, she was supposed to be able to get rid of the poison of the disease. With the development of this idea, attention shifted from the male body, a political or religious figure, centrally placed in the power game of the civilized world, to the dangerously beautiful and contagious female body at the fringe of civilization. Moreover, the latter usually victimized the former in the transfer of the *mafeng* poison. This critical shift in the social perception of the *li/lai* body corresponded with the reclassification of the ailment from a Wind-induced disease to a skin ailment belonging to *waike* (external medicine), from an illness with no geographic specificity to one that was increasingly considered as endemic to the south, and from a vaguely transmittable to a highly contagious disease, as we have seen in chapter 1. The disease was now increasingly and popularly perceived as a problematic female physical condition. Such a perception eventually influenced medical doctors' view of *mafeng.*

The emergence of the idea of the polluting southern female body, reflecting an ancient conception of the deep south as a locus of extreme yang favoring the feminine yin power,[100] suggests a changing perception of the boundaries of the Chinese empire or civilization. While the south appears as a rather distant site in the cosmological map in early and medieval texts, it obtained a more concrete, at times disturbing image in the later imperial period, when the cultural and economic center was, in fact, shifting toward the south.[101] The *guolai* custom and the idea of contagion surrounding it reflect a growing anxiety coming from China's political and cultural centers regarding the subversive character of the semicivilized south. From the early Ming onward, the increasing penetration of political and cultural orthodoxy into the southernmost regions of the empire and the increasing cultural contacts with the local populace provoked renewed discourse about the region's cultural peculiarity, characterized partly by the presence of semicivilized ethnic groups with curious customs.[102] In this sense, Ming-Qing writings on the *guolai* custom, as well as those on the specific southern endemic diseases, could be read as indications of anxiety over increasingly ambiguous cultural boundaries between the civilized and the uncivilized in this part of the Chinese empire.

The Female Sufferer and the *Guolai* Custom[103]

The first time the female *li/lai* body became a subject of interest in literary writings was, as briefly mentioned in chapter 1, in the late thirteenth century, by which time the image of the scholar with *dafeng* or that of the healing monk was fading from texts. The female sufferer of *li/lai,* unlike her earlier male counterpart, was anonymous and stereotypical, and she was said to be able to cure herself of the ailment by passing it on to her sexual partner. A first description of the belief is found in a text written by the famous southern Song scholar Zhou Mi (1232–1298), from Huzhou, Zhejiang province:

> There is a [custom] called "passing on of *lai*" [*guolai*] in the Fujian region. This is due to the fact that women [there] often have the ailment. Whenever one sees faces red like peach flowers, one can be sure that these are indications of the symptoms of the disorder. Men who, not knowing this, unite with them are contaminated [*ran*] by their ailment, while the women are cured. The local people are all aware of this, but they play all kinds of tricks to set up visitors to the region. There was a man from Hangzhou [capital of the Southern Song] called Ji Gongjia visiting Putian [in Fujian] and met a very pretty young woman walking alone on the road. He asked her where she was coming from, and she answered that she was driven out by her parents and had no place to go. He then took her to his lodge. When night fell, he united with her. Then the family of the woman claimed that they would sue him for illegal sex. He thus left the region in a hurry to avoid being arrested. After he returned home, he began to suffer from the ailment. He lost his ears, the bridge of

his nose collapsed, the extremities of his limbs fell off, and he died. *Lai* is the same as the *dafeng* ailment.[104]

The significance of this thirteenth-century record is twofold: first, the elaboration of the idea of transmission by sexual intercourse would eventually be appropriated by mainstream medical texts in the later imperial period, and it had a prolonged impact on real social behavior until the early twentieth century. The importance of this passage in the history of medicine was briefly discussed in chapter 1, in connection with the mention of the famous doctor Chen Yan of the same period, who wrote the ambiguous passage on *lai* hinting for the first time in a medical text at its contagiousness. I conjecture that what Chen Yan meant by *chuanran* contagion in this passage probably was transmission by sexual intercourse, and that the idea did not come from any medical theory but from influences of popular beliefs. Zhou Mi's short record of this custom in Fujian is an important indication of the existence of such beliefs in southern China in the Southern Song period. Contemporary Daoist exorcistic texts also contain similar ideas of contagion in the same regions. We also saw in chapter 1 that, after the critique of Chen Yan's idea of *chuanran* by Liu Chun in the early fifteenth century, it was not until the mid-sixteenth century that marginal doctors elaborated on that idea. However, mainstream medical texts, such as those written by palace doctors or sponsored by the court, never discussed the custom of *guolai* in southern China. The custom was mentioned only in texts written by *waike* specialists of the ailment, usually marginal doctors. Shen Zhiwen mentioned it in his mid-sixteenth-century text on *mafeng*, as did Xiao Xiaoting, in the late eighteenth century.

Shen and Xiao both devoted lengthy discussions to the differences between the male and female *mafeng* bodies and clinical treatment of the female sufferer, considered to be more resistant to the disease, a point never raised in earlier medical texts. Shen quoted two cases to illustrate such a difference: a girl born of a *li* father never developed the disease but passed it on to her husband. The wife of a *li* husband also did not manifest the disease but, after the death of her husband, passed it on to her second husband. Shen thus concluded that "women received the poison in their viscera and transferred and poured [the poison] onto a man during intercourse."[105] Shen therefore implied that the female sufferer, often not knowing that she had the disease, could transmit the disease to men through sexual intercourse.

Xiao Xiaoting, of more than a century later, further elaborated on such differences in male and female *mafeng* sufferers: "It is rare for a man to transmit the disease to a woman, and common for a woman to transmit it to a man. The reason is that women can get rid of the poison via their menstrual blood. That is why there are fewer women suffering from the disease." Discussing the *guolai* custom, he continued, "The story that women could sell the *feng* ailment[106] is reasonable and believable. There is also a story that virgins of certain localities [were born with the poison] and necessarily seek to sell the disease so that they will not develop it. Men to whom the *feng* disorder was sold will develop the disease. In this case, virgins with this problem should be treated with medication when their first menstrual period occurs. Drugs for the elimination of Heat in Blood should be used together with those that will rid the Wind that has developed in the hepatic orb."[107]

In other words, by the early nineteenth century, the custom, believed to be widespread first in Fujian, then in Guangdong and other southern provinces such as Jiangxi and Guangxi, not only influenced medical thinking on the transmissibility of the disease but also directly entered formal medical discussions. The importance of this development was reflected in the latter half of the nineteenth and early twentieth centuries in writings of doctors with full Western medical training, such as the mentioned Wong Foon, who held the custom to be true. The peculiar way of contagion through sexual intercourse from women to men was even recorded in all seriousness by Western medical missionaries (see chap. 4). As late as in the 1950s, Chinese doctors "fighting" leprosy still warned against the dangers of the *guolai* custom current in Guangdong. They believed that leprosy could truly be transmitted by sexual intercourse, as they claimed that the bacillus was found in the vagina and penis. For them, what was unscientific, superstitious, and thus dangerous about the custom was the conviction that the sick man or woman could get rid of the disease by passing it on to their sexual partners.[108] The superstitious custom, for these doctors of the early Communist regime, only helped spread the disease by encouraging sufferers of leprosy to have excessive sexual intercourse with innocent victims.[109] In other words, the custom was not only just another strange, exotic custom heard of or imagined by bemused scholars but one, too, that had real impact on medical thinking and social behavior for centuries.

The second significant aspect of this custom recorded in the thirteenth century is the unique and peculiar cultural construct of the disease that produces the effect of subtly differentiating "us" from "others," by creating dividing lines between men and women, center and south, outsiders and insiders, the civilized and the savage that continued into the modern period. The "curing" of the female sufferer consisted of the passing of the disease from the southern, semicivilized region to the other side of the boundary, to the northern civilized male. However, written records on the *guolai* custom somewhat disappear in available extant texts in the immediate aftermath of the fall of the Song in 1279. It reappears again not in literary texts but in the medical text on the disease by Shen Zhiwen, in the mid-sixteenth century. As we have also seen in chapter 1, by this time, *lai* or *mafeng* had been reanalyzed as a contagious disease endemic to China's deep south, then represented by Fujian and Guangdong provinces, and the fear of its contagiousness was enhanced by the confusion with Guangdong sores (syphilis) in the sixteenth century, as witnessed in Shen's discussions of *mafeng* mentioned earlier. Shen mentioned the custom right after he noted that *li*/*lai* was called "Guangdong sores" or "*yangmei* sores" in the south: "One hears that in Fujian and Guangdong, virgin women can 'pass on *li*.' [Those who are affected] will develop *chong* that turn into obnoxious sores having extreme filth and poison."[110] It is interesting to note that, with the emergence of Guangdong sores, the *guolai* custom was described by Shen to be current also in Guangdong, a region further south than Fujian, where the custom was first recorded in the previously mentioned thirteenth-century text.

The literary tradition picked up the custom again in the early seventeenth century, in a short collection of notes on Guangdong province by the late-Ming Jiangsu scholar-official Wang Linheng (1548–1601), who was sent to the southern province to deal with judicial affairs. Among the various descriptions of the landscape and customs of Guangdong, he noted that many of the natives of the province were afflicted with the *feng* ailment: "At the beginning of the illness, there is the symptom of insensitivity between the fingers and toes. When women are afflicted, they pretend to run away from their families or get lost on the road in order to seduce men. Once they have had sexual intercourse, the ailment passes on to the men. The custom is called the 'passing on of *feng*' [*guofeng*]." Due to this peculiar custom, Wang continued, most sufferers of the ailment in Guangdong were men.[111] For Jiangnan scholars, Fujian and Guangdong were similar southern peripheries, forming a culturally different region. Even though Wang mentions the existence of the custom only in Guangdong, late-Ming geographical perception of the custom covered both Fujian and Guangdong, as shown by another obscure but interesting medical text, of the mid-seventeenth century, the *Shouyu shenfang* (*Miraculous Recipes for Achieving Longevity*). In this text of the Chongzheng period (1628–1644), the author writes that "the ailment *lai* originated in Fujian. People of Fujian have the method of 'passing on *lai*.' It is a malignant ailment of barbaric seas and islands. People from the center of the country [*zhongtu ren*], once having the ailment 'passed on,' are hardly curable."[112] Here the author draws a clear line between the barbaric south and the civilized "center" of the empire. Bodies and diseases were different in these two regions.[113]

Problematic Boundaries

The *guolai* custom described by Zhou Mi in the thirteenth century establishes all the main themes related to the ailment further developed in the later periods: a native, beautiful, female sexual body with the disease in its incubatory stage, seduction of an innocent man from the northern political center (Hangzhou, then capital of the Southern Song), passing of the *lai* ailment from the woman to the man through illicit sexual intercourse, the former thus cured and the latter infected with the disease, the woman's family as the main author of the plot, and local society as the accomplice. This view was typically formed *outside* the so-called miasmatic south. In the thirteenth century, the site of the custom was Fujian, which shifted further south, to Guangdong province, in the Ming. Other writers on the custom, including medical doctors of the Ming period, upheld and further developed these themes. This is particularly obvious in the seventeenth-century medical text the *Shouyu shenfang,* quoted previously: the disease and the custom were from a "barbaric" region, and men from "civilized" central China were easy prey to the perverse custom. The "barbaric" nature of the custom was composed of several elements: a disease believed to be endemic to a miasmatic region with extreme climate and topography; a differently constituted southern physical body, especially the female body; a custom diametrically opposite to mainstream Confucian ethics, especially female chastity. Needless to say, scholars who had written on the custom until then were all close to the center of Chinese civilization, that is, from regions north of Fujian and Guangdong provinces.

The outsiders' view of the custom continued to elaborate after the Qing, that is, after the mid-seventeenth century. Negotiation of the boundaries separating the civilized and the uncivilized, the normal and the exotic, continued well into the twentieth century. For outsiders, or rather, scholars from Jiangnan and northern China, the idea that the distinctive climate and landscape of the south would produce particularly severe diseases and epidemics was increasingly persuasive in the later imperial period.[114] Many scholars, even though not medical practitioners themselves, were increasingly tempted to theorize on obnoxious diseases like *mafeng* and Guangdong sores that they believed to be rampant in specific ecological conditions. For instance, under the pseudonym Qingchengzi, an early Qing scholar wrote, "Provinces have different climates. Ailments of the natives are thus different. For instance, *mafeng* is widespread in Guangdong because the *qi* of that locality is hot and humid. This [*qi*] is retained and accumulated [in the soil], then steamed [and spread] with the perverse miamastic *qi*. People fall victim to [the *mafeng* disease] because of this. Many thus become blind, especially women. . . . It is because [women] are yin and when the yang is dissipated [through steaming], pure yin becomes [very strong]. Yin is a sign of darkness. Those [women] who are feeble become blind."[115] Women in Guangdong were therefore considered by some nonnative scholars, amateurs in medicine, as particularly vulnerable to *mafeng,* an ailment caused by perverse miasmatic *qi,* and to blindness, due to the cosmic receptiveness of the female body to its ecological surroundings. In more cautious language, mainstream medical texts expressed similar links between *mafeng* and the southern ecology, as did the influential imperial medical compendium of 1742, the *Golden Mirror of Medical Orthodoxy,* representing the typical central view: "*Lifeng,* today called *da mafeng,* is, first, generated [*sheng*] by local climates and environment [*fengtu*]. In the center of the country [*Zhongguo*], the ailment is rare. It is rampant only in miasmatic [*yanzhang*] regions."[116] The boundary between the miasmatic south and central China was drawn by medical and nonmedical writers, even though the "miasmatic south" was never clearly defined in geographical terms. The difference, in a way, was more cultural than geographical, but provinces such as Fujian, Guangdong, and Guangxi, especially the latter two, were mostly implied as far as the "miasmatic region" was concerned.

This ambiguous boundary was constantly evoked by scholars outside the region. The early-nineteenth-century scholar with the pseudonym Yongna jushi also reminded readers that the main victims of the *guolai* custom were outsiders of Guangdong: "This disease can only be 'sold' to outsiders from the northern side of the river [*waijiang* (literally, the external side of the river)] and cannot be 'sold' to natives. This is the reason why there is the saying 'One [anyone from the civilized center of the empire] should not enter Guangdong when one is young.'"[117] The danger for young men outside Guangdong being contaminated by beautiful but dangerous female barbaric bodies was fully described in another collection of notes written by a Zhejiang scholar, Wu Chichang, of the later nineteenth century. According to Wu, in Guangdong's Chaozhou prefecture

> all young women are born with the poison of *lai.* They have to pass the disease on to men before they become an adult so that they can be married later on. All young girls of fifteen or sixteen, rich or poor, make attempts on the doorstep of their houses to seduce lechers from outside the province to have union with them. The men stay a month in their place. After this, the parents of the women hang lanterns and put out feasts to invite relatives and friends to show that their daughters have gotten rid of *lai* and are now available for marriage. The lechers are also invited to the banquets and given great sums of money from rich families. These men all die of *lai* within one

> year. As they can also pass the disease on to others, even their families dare not come near them. Kind bureaucrats build asylums to accommodate them.

Wu then goes on to record the "true story" of the young brother of the prefect of Chaozhou, who fell in love with a beautiful young woman afflicted with *mafeng*. Even though this young man from Suzhou had been warned of this terrible Cantonese custom, he could not control himself and willingly became a victim.[118] The "innate" poison of *lai*, remotely comparable with that of smallpox, was seen as a product of the specific climate and environment of the south, and at the same time hereditary, as it was congenital in most young girls.

However, a different view of the custom soon emerged in the early Qing: the *insiders'* view from native Confucian scholars of the south. These scholars were understandably sensitive to the center/south, civilized/barbaric boundaries, which they attempted to push toward directions favorable to their own cultural position. Basically, they negotiated by proposing the substitution of a more marked male-female/moral-immoral boundary. Qu Dajun, the famous early Qing scholar from Panyu, Guangdong, comes again to our aid, giving us some supplementary details on the custom. He wrote that women with the incubatory ailment all carry bags embroidered with flowers in which they hold fruit and other food.

> They then invite visitors to dismount from their horse. No matter how old or young these men are, they call them all "friends of my age" [*tongnian*] and flirt with them. . . . Five or six out of ten of these women are sufferers of *feng*. At the beginning of the ailment, before [symptoms appear on] the face, if one looks at the face of the "seller of *feng*" [*mai feng zhe*] under candlelight, one will see a color as red as alizarin beneath the skin. The *feng* of a man cannot be "sold" to a woman, but that of a woman can be sold to a man. Once "sold," the *chong* of the "*feng*" ailment is passed on, and the woman is cured. Along the coast, for six to seven hundred *li*, amid bridges and hotels, there is a lot of promiscuity, with a few copper coins changing hands. This is all very scary and is the custom that is called *guolai*.[119]

There are several interesting differences between the "central view" of Jiangnan scholars and the "insider's view" of Qu. First, unlike the outsiders' view, Qu's descriptions are strongly suggestive of prostitution. The term "selling *feng*" and his evocation of money being paid during the activities imply that many women with the incubatory ailment were prostituting themselves in order to get rid of the disease. This again reminds us of the fact that the ailment Guangdong sores, believed to be syphilis, was confused with *lai*/*mafeng*, even by specialists, in the sixteenth century. Whether these prostitutes were selling *lai* or *Guang chuang* cannot be determined here. They sold the ailment as they were selling their bodies together with all their "poisons" to strangers. What seems probable is that the so-called custom of *guolai* or *mai feng* (selling *feng*), when described by seventeenth-century native Cantonese literati, was closely linked with ordinary prostitution and the disease thus "transferred" in brothels was very likely to be confused with Guangdong sores.

The second difference with outside observers of *guolai* is that Qu was quite oblivious to the regional origin of the male victims. Unlike Zhou Mi and other nonnative scholars, Qu, as a local person, considered these men simply the average clients of brothels and not particularly visitors coming from the cultural center. For Qu, it was not at all a problem of contaminating the civilized by the savage but "careless" men polluted by ordinary prostitutes. Most Cantonese scholars after Qu repeated mostly what Qu had said, notably Fan Duan'ang, a native of Sanshui, in Guangdong, of the Kangxi period (1662–1722), in his famous collections on the province.[120] Liang Tingnan (1796–1861), a native of Shunde and a local leader fighting against the British leading to the Opium War of 1840–1842, also briefly recorded, in the spring of 1841, the custom, by which "young women with *mafeng* went out at night to seduce men in order to get rid of the incubatory poison so that they would eventually be healthy enough for a normal marriage." Even though the main victims of the custom that spring were militia from Hunan ignorant of this local custom, Liang's account was in fact a condemnation of these Hunan soldiers for kidnapping small children, whose flesh they believed to be a cure of the disease, and for killing local soldiers who defended their children.[121] For Liang, these young women were seducing men irrespective of their cultural origin, and the fate of the Hunanese soldiers was simply a consequence of their own barbarity and immorality.[122]

The conflict between the central Chinese view and the native view of the custom is vividly described in a passage in the famous late-Qing novel by the Cantonese writer Wu Jianren (1866–1910), who lived most of his adult life in Shanghai, *Strange Phenomena Observed During the Past Twenty Years* (*Ershi nian mudu zhi guai xianzhuang*). The passage is a dialogue between a native person from Chaozhou, Guangdong province, and the narrator, from Shanghai. The narrator is traveling in Guangdong and meets the Chaozhou native, to whom he lends the mentioned book by the Zhejiang scholar Wu Chichang. The Chaozhou native is described as having a fit of rage after he reads the passage on the *guolai* custom in his native district, and he tears the book into pieces. He says to the Shanghai narrator, after quoting the passage in the book translated in the preceding, "This *mafeng* is something that we Guangdong people have, and we do not need to deny it. But how can this writer tarnish the reputation of the entire population of our prefecture! . . . Not only does he make this groundless allegation, but he even puts it in print. Isn't it a most irritable thing?!" The narrator responds, "It is true that one should not put down in print things that one is not certain of. Especially this concerns the reputation of unmarried virgins. If I were from Chaozhou, I would hate him too."

What is most interesting is the way the narrator from Shanghai goes on to demystify the custom:

> In fact *mafeng* is not unheard of in other provinces. I have met one in Shanghai. However, people of other provinces do not treat this as a taboo, whereas people from Guangdong do. That's, however, a difference that I cannot explain. Maybe because the environment is so hot in Guangdong that sufferers of the disease all go rotten, which is not the case if they get the disease elsewhere. In Guangdong, one who gets the disease is denied even by one's father or son. An asylum has been built to accommodate patients and to prevent contagion. The disease has no visible symptoms after [being transmitted through] three generations, even though the root of the disease is still inherent in the bones. For these, the disease needs to be passed on to others [by sex]. It is easy for men to do that, but women can only seduce passers-by in the countryside [where they will not encounter people they know]. They only need to do it once or twice, and it will be over. . . . This is called "selling *feng*," and this is done outside one's home in hiding. Nobody does it openly in one's place, and it does not take a month to get rid of the disease. There is no feasting about it, not to mention the entire population of the prefecture doing this.[123]

Here, Wu Jianren, a Cantonese who had lived outside the province for a long time, demystifies the native custom by breaking down several boundaries: the male/female boundary, as men also need to "sell off" the disease; the insider/outsider boundary, as victims of the custom are not limited to people outside the province, and the disease was not limited to Guangdong populations. He also attempts to demolish the civilized/uncivilized boundary, as women and their families practicing this were described as having a sense of shame or guilt, and women "only do this once or twice" instead of for "a month." What stubbornly remains is the idea of the peculiarity of the Cantonese environment and the specificity of the Cantonese body type: the *mafeng* poison was innate, incubatory, and contagious in this body. This specificity of the Cantonese body type necessitated the *guolai* custom. In other words, for Wu Jianren, an inside scholar of the late nineteenth century trying to look from the outside, the *guolai* custom was purely a particular medical or biological necessity that unfortunately conflicted with mainstream ethics.

As Rod Edmond has put it eloquently, "Leprosy . . . is a boundary disease par excellence. It can focus and dramatise the risk of trespass, serve as a punishment for such infringements, and help to re-establish the categories and boundaries that define our relation to the world by keeping the clean from the unclean, and thereby rescuing purity from danger."[124] Even though the deep south was always conceived as a miasmatic region, it was a remote and abstract idea in the early empire order. When the so-called Lingnan region was increasingly and concretely visible in the cultural map of the Chinese empire with the political and economic centers shifting increasingly toward the lower Yangzi region in the Song period, scholars considering themselves part of the central plains culture began to feel anxious about the polluting effect of the peoples and customs of this tangible southern, semibarbaric periphery. On the other hand, indigenous Cantonese literati of the late imperial period reset the boundaries originally defined by outside scholars in formulating the *guolai* custom from the thirteenth century. In so doing, they were negotiating a new empire order that would include the south as part of the civilized world. They seemed to accept the ecological center/south divide, however vaguely defined, that maintained the peculiarity of the climate, environment, and body type of the south. This conception somewhat confirmed and enhanced their proper local identity. They, however, attempted to blur the division between male and female bodies (except Qu Dajun), shift the dividing lines between the civilized and uncivilized by including Guangdong within the boundaries of the civilized.[125] These efforts to redefine the empire had been visible and deliberate since the early nineteenth century.

TAMING THE BARBARIAN BODY AND REDEEMING THE NATION

Aggressive *mafeng/lai* beggars involved in organized crime and female patients with their perverse *guolai* custom gave *mafeng* sufferers the reputation of a particularly subversive social group threatening the Confucian social order. While crimes by organized groups of patients could be accepted as not uncommon in late imperial society, the corruption of the healthy and civilized society by contagious female bodies was much more disquieting. Beginning in the early nineteenth century, many Cantonese scholars attempted to modify descriptions of the custom to turn it into something radically different: a custom that could even buttress the Confucian body politic. The Cantonese scholar Liang Shaoren, for instance, recorded an episode in which a scholar from Shunde, a district near Canton, fell in love with a pretty young woman living on the east shore of the Pearl River who was also a virgin with *mafeng*. Despite their vows of love, the woman refused categorically to have intercourse with the scholar because she knew that he was an only son and that she had the disease. She finally revealed her illness to him, and both wept over their fate. Soon after the scholar returned to see her, she committed suicide by drowning herself in the river. The woman's virtue inspired a Cantonese scholar, Huang Yujie, to write a long, touching poem.[126] Clearly in Liang Shaoren's version, the custom did not victimize visitors from the center. It was not a trap southern barbarians set to harm civilized Chinese men from the empire's center. More important, female chastity, a Confucian precept upheld in the civilized world, was now totally compatible with the custom. For the first time, the custom was described as yet another opportunity for virtuous Cantonese virgins to demonstrate their moral superiority. His version shows how the originally barbaric southern female body was finally tamed by Chinese civilization in the early nineteenth century.

Liang's version of the virtuous female *mafeng* virgin was only the beginning of a series of similar attempts toward the end of the imperial regime to transform the originally exotic and erotic custom into a stereotypical Confucian story of redemption of severe sickness by superior moral performance. What is more interesting about this transformation is that, ultimately, in a famous play based on such a virtuous virgin, *Bing yu yuan chuanqi* (*Drama of the Love Story of the Sick Beauty* [preface, 1913]), the redemption of the entire body politic sickened by feudal practices and superstitions, as antipodes to modern Western science, was symbolically realized by the curing of her *mafeng* ailment together with the doing away with the feudal and perverse native custom by replacing it with scientific healing of the disease. This ultimate version of the *guolai* custom perfectly fits the discourse of modernization at the turn of the twentieth century.

First let us briefly trace the building up of the ultimate drama of *Bing yu yuan* after Liang Shaoren. After the emergence of the model of the virtuous *mafeng* virgin in Liang's version, even non-Cantonese writers elaborated on the model of the virtuous *mafeng* virgin. Wu Chichang, the Zhejiang literatus whose version of the *guolai* custom was said to have infuriated Cantonese readers in Wu Jianren's novel, gave another version of a virtuous Cantonese *mafeng* woman. The woman was so beautiful that a young man named Cao from Suzhou, well aware of the custom, chose to be intimate with her despite the terrible consequences. After their union, Cao returned to Suzhou secretly, and the young woman realized that her husband would die of the disease. In tears, she vowed that she would not marry again and would prefer to die with him. She found her way to his home in Suzhou and served him like a virtuous wife. One day, Cao accidentally took alcohol with a drowned viper inside, and was cured of the disease, and the two lived happily ever after. Wu concluded the story by saying that the virtue of the Cantonese young woman was the reason for the miracle.[127] Liang Shaoren's and Wu Chichang's versions of the virtuous Cantonese *mafeng* woman were finally combined in a story by the Anhui scholar Xuan Ding (1832–1880), in a short piece, "Mafeng nü Qiu Liyu chuanqi" (Story of Qiu Liyu, the *Mafeng* Girl [1877]), imitating the very refined classical style of Tang-dynasty short biographies of unusual women. The story maintained many of the original themes of the outsider's version, with an unprecedented final twist. The hero is Chen Qi, from Anhui (the same as the author), traveling in western Guangdong in search of a relative. Destitute, Chen accepts the proposal of a matchmaker to marry into a wealthy local family. Ignorant of the *guolai* custom, he is pleasantly surprised to find that his wife is exceptionally beautiful. The woman, Qiu Liyu, falls in love with the man, whom she does not want to contaminate with her deadly disease. On the wedding night, she tells him about the custom and plans his escape by pretending they have united, which they never did. Chen eventually obtains money from Qiu's family and returns to Anhui. Qiu later inevitably develops the disease and is expelled from her family. She begs her way to Anhui and finds her husband's family, owners of a winery. Even though she is warmly accepted by the family, who are grateful to her for saving the young man's life, she is aware that she has become a burden to her husband and decides to commit suicide. One night she sees a gigantic viper falling into one of the wine pots. Thinking that will be poisonous, she takes the wine, and her disease is miraculously cured. The happy couple return to Guangdong and make viper wine as a drug that cures numerous *mafeng* patients.[128]

Xuan's story of the Guangdong *mafeng* woman Qiu Liyu was eventually made famous as an opera written by a Fujian scholar under the pen name of Modengxianzhai Zhuren (Master of the Nonidling Study), based on the same story. This long piece, in thirty acts, was a popular piece performed frequently in the early twentieth century. The opera is in fact still performed in China today, having featured several actresses famous for playing the role of Qiu Liyu.[129] The libretto, first published in Shanghai in 1907,[130] four years before the fall of the Qing, is a fascinating modernized version of the *guolai* custom, with the heroine transformed from a strange, antiquated, female figure of the not-quite-Chinese culture of the southwest to an active, progressive, and modern social citizen reformer of the local public health system. Qiu is not only completely tamed by Confucian morality, she is even metamorphosed into a modern, national heroine after she is miraculously cured.

The little we know about the author should shed some light on the interest of this play. The real name of Modengxianzhai Zhuren[131] was Chen Tianchi, a native of Fujian. He studied boat engineering in Fujian and had visited England. In 1905 he joined the revolutionary group of Sun Yat-sen, the Tongmeng hui, and created a related group in Fuzhou. At the same time, he was active in producing, translating, and publishing revolutionary literature. After the success of the Republican Revolution in 1911 and the following northern expedition led by Sun, he retired from politics and made his living as a traditional Chinese doctor. Not only did he invent his own pills but he also headed a local traditional Chinese medical institution and edited a medical journal, at the same time as being an amateur in the operatic arts. He wrote this long opera obviously during his period as a revolutionary against the Qing dynasty.[132] In other words, the reader has to be aware of the author's identity as a southerner, someone well versed in traditional medicine, and definitely a modernizer, a nationalist, a revolutionary, a creator of the modern Chinese nation-state. That he picked the problem of leprosy and the *guolai* custom to express in an opera his revolutionary ideals is a most interesting and revealing choice.

The success of the opera lies in its interesting mix of traditional and modern topoi, enhancing the effects of the drama. Many of the traditional themes are deployed to accentuate the tragic features of the old feudal custom of *guolai:* Qiu's selfish family, her physical beauty and virtuous character, her tragic fate of being born with a deadly disease, the cure of the disease by means of viper wine, the miraculous effect of her self-denying suicide attempt, and so forth were all typical traditional topoi. However, the infiltration of new, modernizing themes in the opera differentiates it totally from the earlier versions of the story and clearly marks its period. If the emotions of love, virtue, and family obligations are conventionally conveyed within the framework of traditional Ming-Qing drama, the stark contrast between personal, regional, and national redemption of the illness in a moral and scientific way and the cruel, perverse, barbaric local custom of *guolai* is certainly a new strategy in this modern opera. The sentiment of progress and collective salvation thus expressed was certainly a new one in the form of traditional opera. However, we will see that, similar to many contemporary literary works, the emerging elements of modernity in the opera are full of ambiguities and imbued with traditional ideas, making the opera into a uniquely complex and hybrid piece.

Most of the ideas surrounding *mafeng* since the mid-Ming are expressed in the opera as illustrations of the dark side of traditional society. The main idea that goes through the entire drama is the ecological/cultural specificity, that is, the miasmatic nature of the Guangdong region, which is the underlying cause of the endemic *mafeng.* We have seen how the miasmatic region shifted from

Fujian in the thirteenth century to Guangdong, especially the eastern part of the province, in the seventeenth century. By now, the region considered as most miasmatic was western Guangdong, with its "neighboring [tribes of] Dong and Yao," a "barbaric and remote" region.[133] The association between barbaric culture and miasma was obviously strong in the late imperial period. For the author of the opera, this specific perverse *qi* of the locality accounts for the innate and hereditary poison of *mafeng* found in young virgins in the area and consequently the perverse custom of *guolai.*[134] He writes, "This miasma [*zhangqi*] is called *mafeng.* It is very bizarre as it is only linked with women, and never with men. These women do not show the symptoms when they are young. But once they are sixteen or seventeen, the root of the disease manifests itself."[135] The idea that the disease was highly contagious and sufferers should be segregated in asylums, even though it means the breaking up of families, is also prevalent. The dread of *chong* coming out of the dead bodies of *mafeng* sufferers to contaminate the healthy is also evoked.[136] The non-Cantonese author also emphasized the perversity of the custom, especially the way the natives set up innocent outsiders to be victims of the "passing on of *lai.*" Qiu Liyu tells her innocent husband that the trap "is inextricably set up. Guards and arms are installed everywhere so that [the victim] has no escape," even though he will be handsomely paid once the "passing on" is done.[137]

The negative image of the headman of the asylum for women sufferers also confirms the stereotype of these characters as described in gazetteers, literati writings, and later on by Western missionaries. Even though a sufferer of the disease himself, he was portrayed as having no sympathy for the inmates, as he was greedy, corrupt, and cruel. He was given a large sum by Qiu's family when Qiu entered the asylum, which, however, did not prevent him from treating her cruelly later on when the money ran out.[138] The traditional asylum was described as a dark and horrible prison, "it is a dark world where one does not see the sky nor the sun," even though it began as "a charitable enterprise organized by both officials and local gentry."[139]

The traditional, dark side of this uncivilized backdrop is contrasted with a brighter, changing world symbolized by the virtuous Qiu Liyu. The first impression of Qiu on Chen, her adoring husband, is that she has natural feet. Even though her unbound feet fit in with the "barbaric" background of the south,[140] their real significance here lies in their representing the liberated woman, a strong symbol of China's modernity. Indeed, the hero Chen Qi fell in love immediately with this "beauty of natural feet. If she is not a Guanyin of the southern seas, she must be a woman literatus of Western Europe." In the singing verse, Chen asks whether she is "another Camellia of France,"[141] clearly referring to the heroine of Dumas' novel, then very popular for a reform-minded readership.

On the medical discussions of *mafeng,* on the other hand, the author systematically uses modern medical terms. The benevolent ghost of Chen's uncle who guides Qiu to Anhui asks why she got the disease since she comes from a good family, "You must have thoroughly studied the theories of hygiene [*weisheng xueli*]!"[142] Here the term *weisheng* is used as a modern translation for Western "hygiene," or Western ideas of health, and not as the old, traditional medical word, with its strong Daoist connotation, meaning the "defense of life."[143] Later, when Chen tries to find doctors to heal her disease, he says, "If *mafeng* cannot be cured, then medicine is an incomplete body of learning." He thoroughly searches for famous doctors "in Beijing and Shanghai," then the national centers in China, to treat his beloved wife. Chen finally settles on a "Western doctor" in Shanghai, an "American M.D." The role of the American doctor, however, maintains the traditional characteristic of doctors in popular plays: he is phony and ludicrous, and he also fails to cure Qiu.[144] However, in the foreign doctor's monologue, one clearly sees the growing influence of Western medical vocabulary, representing new, scientific knowledge: "I think that eight or nine out of ten of the cases are caused by contagion. This is all caused by microorganisms [*mei jun wei shengwu*]. But don't you panic. Western medicines are perfectly exact, unlike Chinese drugs, whose therapeutic efficacy does not match their reputation."[145] When his medicines have no effect either, Chen encourages Qiu to stop taking them: "Western medicines are much stronger than Chinese drugs. If the prescription is wrong, then she will really be done in!"[146] When Qiu's case seems totally hopeless, she asks Chen to find her a woman "nurse" [*kan hu fu*], yet another new medical professional under Western influence.[147] It is true that no Western drug in the early twentieth century could effectively cure leprosy. The drama truly reflects the medical situation of leprosy at that time. The author seems to be eager to show his knowledge about Western medicine and ideas of modern public health, which apparently was an attraction to the audience. At the same time, however, he subtly defends Chinese medicine and pokes fun at Western "strong" drugs.

The ultimate solution to the *mafeng* problem for the author is a mixture of traditional therapeutics,and modern, Western pedagogy. Finally, the miracle drug that cures the *mafeng* is traditional viper wine, a remedy discussed in chapter 1, where it is pointed out that its therapeutic efficacy was still held to be reliable as late as the 1930s. However, the author does not dwell at great length on the therapeutic aspects; instead, he is more interested in describing the setting

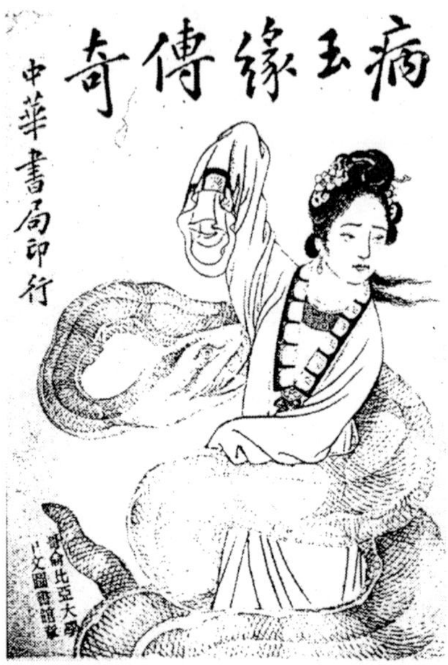

Cover of the play *Bing yu yuan chuanqi* (1932 ed.), showing the leprous heroine Qiu Liyu and the viper.

up of totally new institutions in Guangdong to deal with the problem. Like typical heroes of traditional drama, Chen passes the civil service examination and becomes an important official and is assigned a high position in Guangdong and Guangxi provinces, where he decides to transform the perverse custom. His plan is to "officially ban the custom and give out drugs to heal young girls with the innate disease." He punishes the headman of the old asylum for maltreating inmates by imprisonment. With the wealth of his in-laws, he renovates entirely the shabby building and turns it into a modern, comfortable, and clean hospital, which will be his "*mafeng* hospital." A drug factory is also built inside to make viper wine. To procure enough materials for the drug, he pays people to capture vipers in the mountains. More important, he and Qiu give speeches in the hospital on the necessity of abolishing the perverse *guolai* custom. Local people are encouraged to attend, as free drugs are distributed on such occasions. "Within several months, the two of them have transformed the native bad custom. . . . Isn't it incredible, the power of spoken words!" The happy couple predict that very soon the custom, the disease, and the miasma will disappear completely from the region. When that happens, the hospital and the drug factory "will be turned into a school for boys and a girls in the future."[148] Indeed, China will first be sanitized and made free of ugly diseases before it is completely modernized through mass education.

This modern and long version of the *guolai* custom has clearly broken with the tradition of the creation of the custom and of miraculous healing in literary writings since at least the thirteenth century to the mid-nineteenth century. It has shifted from individual tragedy and redemption to collective and national suffering and salvation. It has slowly moved from the religious realm to become a social and national problem. "The passing on of *lai*" is no longer seen as a curious and exotic custom of the uncivilized south but is presented here as a feudal practice of the old empire, a predicament that obstructs the modernization of China from a corrupt empire into a healthy and moral nation. The miraculous healing no longer stops at the realization of true love for a blessed couple. The curse of *mafeng* can be broken only by an integrated collective social and political reform. The opposition between a backward, immoral, cruel, and superstitious past and a progressive, ethical, and scientific future is constructed through the demolition of the *guolai* custom. Even though the dramatic setting is still the miasmatic south, the real background is undoubtedly the Qing empire. Redeeming the *mafeng* body is, for the author, a redemption of the crippled, weak body politic of China.

FOUR

The Chinese Leper and the Modern World

Even though China was not exactly a colony in the nineteenth and twentieth centuries, the sense of political and cultural crisis was growing rapidly among the elite from the late nineteenth century onward. Modernization was the major task that the Qing government strived to achieve, a task continued to be pursued by the Republican government from 1911 onward. In the midst of such nationalistic endeavors, the Chinese leper came to symbolize what was deplorable in China's past and the obstacle to modernization: physical and moral weakness expressed in repulsive sores and a crippled, incurable body. Even worse, this sick body was seen as contagious. One urgent task of the modernizing Chinese state was to cleanse this corrupting body politic.

In this chapter, I discuss how Chinese in this period perceived the disease in the context of imperialist expansion, and also how Western medical experts considered the same problem. We shall see that, often, the two views reinforced each other. I also show the importance of Chinese agency in the modern construct of the disease, especially in a period when European doctors and scientists were arguing among themselves whether the disease was contagious or hereditary, if it was a miasmatic disease or a problem of bad blood. Chinese society had ready answers to all these questions. Even the Western racial interpretations of the disease had a Chinese version, profoundly rooted in traditional medicine and popular beliefs. These beliefs were so strong that many Western missionaries in China were under their influence.

What made the Chinese leper globally visible was the new international situation in the nineteenth and early twentieth centuries. Increasing labor emigration from China was certainly the main factor. International accusations of China's exporting the disease through infected coolies to the entire world were coming from all directions, and leprosy was soon perceived at home as a shameful national problem. It was no longer seen as merely a regional concern but one of national proportions around the mid-nineteenth century. This development reflected an escalating international alarm over the leprosy problem as Western powers were competing to build their colonial empires.[1] The famous text by H. P. Wright, *Leprosy: An Imperial Danger,* begins: "There are certain burning questions of the highest importance with respect to leprosy. Never before has the disease been so closely and anxiously studied as during the last thirty years; and never before has it excited greater interest (and that interest is daily increasing), not only among medical men, but among the thoughtful, wherever high intelligence and true humanitarianism prevail."[2] Leprosy indeed became a public issue in Britain and its empire in the last decades of the nineteenth century.[3] Even though the situation of leprosy in India had been scrutinized by British colonial medical experts for a much longer time,[4] China occupied a more central position in this perceived world pandemic.

The emigration of Chinese coolies was accompanied by the increasing inflow of Western experts, including missionaries and medical and other professionals in Asia. Westerners residing in China, Japan, India, and other Asian countries soon "rediscovered" the problem of leprosy, something that they readily related to Europe's Dark Ages. The observable leprosy in certain parts of China certainly fit into these experts' perception of China and its people as a backward civilization. China was, like the India described by David Arnold, "understood and represented through science and medicine as an alien territory inhabited by a foreign race."[5] As late as 1935, a Western professor of sociology at the University of Shanghai published a textbook entitled *Social Pathology in China,* in which the section "Health" was introduced by a whole chapter on leprosy.[6] In the eyes of these foreign experts, leprosy was certainly one of, if not the most serious health problem in China.

Western observers' view of the disease inevitably influenced China's own judgment of the epidemic situation. While *lai* was depicted as a mysterious albeit horrifying disease of the miasmatic and exotic south in Ming-Qing texts, *mafeng* leprosy scrutinized by Westerners soon became a most serious *national* public health problem for modern Chinese elites. Wong Foon (Huang Kuan), the

Chinese medical officer, mentioned previously, in the Imperial Maritime Customs, warned in a medical report dated 1873 and based on interviews with Cantonese "leper physicians" and headmen of local traditional asylums, that "leprosy is on the increase compared with what it was ten years ago. The disease is found in all classes of person, rich and poor, in the city and in the country, among artisans, tradesmen, and field labourers."[7] The famous Cantonese scholar Chen Yuan (1880–1971), who had training in Western medicine, also wrote several articles in popular Chinese medical journals at the turn of the twentieth century calling for a more systematic control and study of the disease, which, to him, was spreading dangerously: "*Mafeng* is a terrible contagious disease. How could we let [lepers] roam freely in cities?"[8] At the same time, others began to study the occurrences of the disease in history and to reconstruct the disease's national history in order to rouse public attention to a seemingly disquieting situation. Such writings became even more common in the Republican period (1911–1949).[9]

The situation was not unique to China. The anxiety about the spread of the disease as a sign of some intrinsic weakness of the race was also conspicuous in

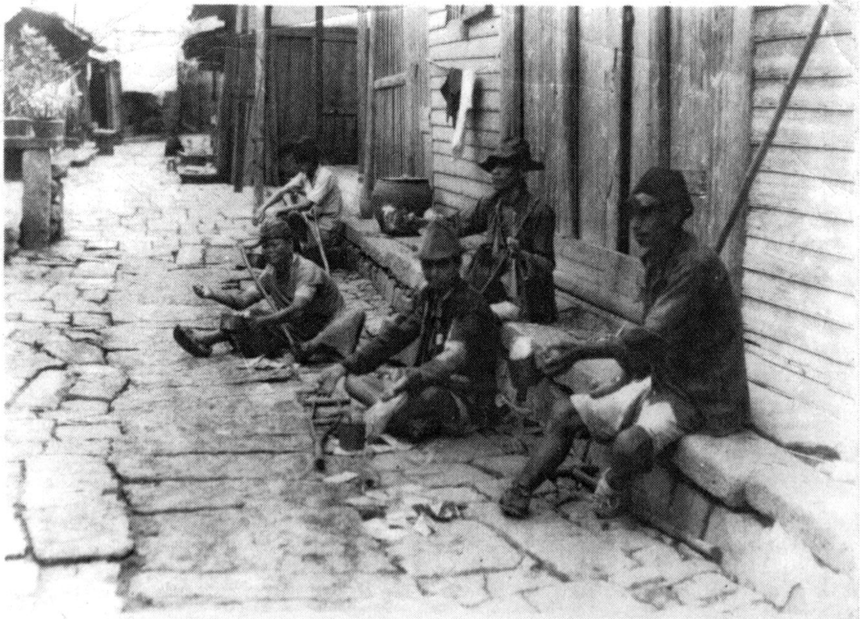

Leprous beggars on a street in a Fujian city, in the early 1940s. (Collection of Dr. Jiang Cheng. First published in Jiang Cheng, ed., *Zhongguo mafeng fangzhi (huace)* [*Pictorial of Leprosy Control in China*] [Taizhou, 1993])

modernizing Japan. In the 1870s, as the Meiji government worked to establish its country "as part of the modern world and to distance it from 'backward' Asian societies such as India and China," the prevalence of leprosy was particularly problematic. Diet member Saitō Toshio submitted, in 1902, a proposal for a leprosy prevention law for the purpose of eradicating this "sign of an uncivilized country."[10] In other words, when leprosy, like syphilis, became associated with the question of degeneration, race, and civilization, an idea brought by Western imperialist powers, both China and Japan began to see the elimination of the disease as an important part of their social and political agenda.

Leprosy control was thus metaphorically linked to China's difficult state-building process in the last two decades of the imperial period and continuing well into the Republican period throughout the first half of the twentieth century. It was an important issue in China's construct of its "hygienic modernity." Neither regime succeeded in dealing with the situation in a way satisfying to Chinese society or to Western observers. It remained a major national public health problem for the Communist regime after 1949. Leprosy became literally a persistent, ugly sore on the body politic of modern China, awaiting amputation when the hope of a complete cure was remote.

THE SHAMEFUL, CONTAGIOUS BODY

From the mid-nineteenth century onward, the Chinese leper embodied two "defects" of the Chinese race: its physical inferiority and the contagiousness of its disease. The racist discourse regarding leprosy in China was not entirely constructed on Western medical theory or imperialist ideology. The Chinese epidemiological view of the disease in the late imperial period unquestionably buttressed such a discourse. *Mafeng* had been redefined since at least the sixteenth century as a disease endemic to the empire's miasmatic south. And southerners, conceived to have a different body type from that of the Chinese at the center of civilization, were believed to be more susceptible to contracting and spreading the disease. At the same time, *mafeng* became increasingly dreaded as a sexually transmitted, highly contagious scourge affecting mostly promiscuous or weak bodies.

Embodiment of the Inferior Race

The progressive and dramatic development of the disease in its victim, especially the monstrous external symptoms, and the persistent cloud of mystery surrounding the channels of its transmission made leprosy one of the most popular and persistent metaphors for degeneration, pollution, and moral flaws, not only for the individual but also for the collectivity.[11] The heavy religious implications of leprosy during the medieval period of the Christian West are well known, and we have seen its other inferences in Buddhist and Daoist religious traditions in premodern China. In the industrial and imperialist era, old metaphors related to leprosy were transfigured to be meaningful in the context of the modern world. Racial degeneration was one idea that was easily represented by leprosy, and embodied by lepers. This was all the more so as modern Western medicine at the turn of the twentieth century had not solved the mysteries surrounding the disease. On the question of the transmission of leprosy, for instance, there was no agreement in European medical circles in the late nineteenth and early twentieth centuries. Heredity and contagion were the two main hypotheses, which did not, however, seem to readily accommodate each other. Underlying the different theories on the transmission of leprosy, however, was the shared belief that the disease was specific to certain races, especially inferior races with darker skin dwelling in hot countries. This idea was naturally in tune with the prevalent obsession of degeneration in Europe in this period. The conviction that the disease was a race-specific one was particularly strong among those who upheld that the disease was hereditary. In a way, it was reassuring for white Westerners to believe that leprosy was limited to colored races that were physically predisposed to contracting the disease.

Two major medical reports that came out of Europe before Hansen's discovery in 1873–1874 upheld that leprosy was essentially hereditary, and definitely not contagious: one was by the Danish doctors D. C. Danielssen and C. W. Boeck (*Traité de la spedalskhed ou des éléphantiasis des Grecs* [Paris, 1848]), and the other was from the Royal College of Physicians in London (*Report on Leprosy* [1867]).[12] The former considered that, pathogenetically, leprosy was a hereditary depraved condition of the blood. Such condition was necessary for the contraction of the disease under certain external circumstances. The latter confirmed this view: "Leprosy is essentially a constitutional disorder, indicative of a cachexia or a depraved condition of the general system." It stated that there was no evidence to show that leprosy was contagious and recommended that ancient leper statutes be repealed.[13] This view, resistant to the contagion theory even after Hansen's discovery, was commonly accepted by medical missionaries working in China in the nineteenth century.[14]

Benjamin Hobson (1816–1873), of the London Missionary Society, the first British Protestant medical missionary to work in China, responsible for introducing Western medicine into China especially in the 1850s,[15] stated, in 1860, that leprosy was a "specific, constitutional, hereditary disease, peculiar to hot countries." He did not "regard it strictly an infectious disease, that is communicable by mere contact; but it is unquestionably an hereditary one." It was, more precisely, "an inter-tropical disease affecting the Chinese, Hindoos, Mohammedans, Africans and other people living within or on the borders of the tropics."[16] Hobson's view in fact predated that of the Royal College of Physicians, of 1867, which also claimed that the disease affected essentially peoples with darker skin living in tropical areas, including Chinese, Indians, and peoples with mixed blood.[17] As late as 1911, James L. Maxwell (1873–1951) , then chairman of the China Medical Missionary Association, and his collaborator, Dr. W. H. Jefferys, observed that "leprosy is more frequent in the coloured than in the white races."[18]

The disease was also seen as specific to races at a certain stage of civilization. The idea was most systematically expressed by Patrick Manson (1844–1922), founder of British tropical medicine, which, in Rod Edmond's words, "can be understood as an attempt to put a fence around Europe, and around the European in the tropics."[19] Manson had done most of his fieldwork in southern China prior to the publication of his classic *Tropical Diseases* in 1898, in which he listed leprosy as a tropical disease and one, moreover, of semicivilization: "Savages are exempt; the highly civilized are exempt; but when the savage begins to wear clothes and lives in houses he becomes subject to the disease."[20] Dr. George Shearer, working in Hankow, also an adherent of the hereditary theory, reflected this view in a report written in 1871 explaining the leprosy situation in different parts of the world: "The disease is said to be on the increase in Jamaica during the last twelve or fifteen years [prior to 1871], because of the retrogression towards barbarism of the bulk of the population. Imperfect tillage, draining and culture of land, furnish conditions for the development of the marsh-poison." Indeed, for him leprosy was contracted by people with a "morbid condition of the blood," a belief reminiscent of the classic humoral theory, and under the influence of "the impure air of certain malarious districts."[21] In other words, leprosy was thought to affect races with a certain hereditary physical predisposition living in a miasmatic environment polluted by "barbaric" ways of living and producing. The Chinese, apparently, were considered one of these degenerated, semicivilized races dwelling mostly in malarial regions, which explained the observed prevalence of leprosy in China.

Both Western missionaries and traditional Chinese doctors agreed that leprosy was rampant in miasmatic regions. Some early missionaries, like Hobson, totally accepted the Chinese view that the disease was rare outside Fujian, Guangdong, and other southern provinces of the so-called Lingnan region. He wrote, in 1842,"The fact seems to be established that the leprosy in China is confined to the southwest provinces."[22] Later on, when leprosy was observed in other parts of

China, the idea of miasma was not abandoned but modified to fit the argument. Dr. Jardine, working in Hankow in 1871, observed the spread of leprosy in his region and concluded that "it is a degeneration which flourishes amidst a variety of climates, of soils, of staple articles of food, and of race." Hankow, for Jardine, was also perfect ground for the spread of leprosy.[23] Miasma was attributed to the spread of leprosy even in northern provinces like Shandong. Dr. A. W. Douthwaite, working in Shandong province in the late nineteenth century, said, in 1892, that he agreed with the natives of his district near Jiaozhou Bay that "leprosy is of miasmatic origin,"[24] seeming to imply that the presence of the disease could define the northern province of Shandong as a miasmatic region. More interesting is the remark of the missionary Joseph Edkins, also working in Shandong in the same period. Quoting the observations of a colleague, Dr. Stephen Hunter, Edkins reported, in 1891, that leprosy was prevalent in that province only in localities where leprosy had been recorded in ancient texts: "Possibly the disease has been where it is now found for more than two thousand years, and in that case *heredity* must have much to do with its presence there now." He then went on to speculate that "probably the climate of China has grown both dryer and cooler than it was, anciently. The result is that leprosy now is differently developed from what it was in the time of Confucius. It seems to be driven to the south by the increasing dryness."[25] Edkins's logic is simple. All of ancient China was warmer, damper, and miasmatic, and leprosy was rampant everywhere. The hereditary nature of the disease, however, explained its lingering prevalence in northern provinces, whereas the continuous miasmatic ecology in the south accounted for the disease's widespread presence in that part of the country.

The famous report by James Cantlie (1851–1926) on leprosy in China prepared in 1894 echoed Edkins's ideas, concluding that the drying and cooling of northern China was that "which was driving the people coastwards; this it is which is sending them abroad over all the tropical lands, and much of the temperate."[26] If Edkins and Cantlie attempted to attenuate geographic differences in China by evoking climatic changes over time, other, less-informed Westerners simply saw China as a highly "uniform" empire, with probably a general pathology all over the country.[27] Indeed, the miasma argument was made to work magic by the end of the nineteenth century in the case of China, asserting that, as leprosy was found in many parts of China, including the north, these regions must be miasmatic, and China, in general, must be a miasmatic, tropical country.

The idea that leprosy was a hereditary disease of specific, inferior races dwelling in miasmatic regions, which should have been distasteful to the Chinese, was, ironically, perfectly in tune with the Chinese traditional idea of the disease in the late imperial period, a notion that lasted until the Republican period. We have seen in the history of the etiology of leprosy how it was reanalysed not later than the sixteenth century as a disease of the miasmatic south, affecting essentially populations not completely civilized by Chinese culture. This idea, nicely echoing the racial assumptions current in the West, was still dominant in the 1920s and 1930s. In March 1929, the Ministry of Public Health, of the Republican government, issued an order to the provincial governments, saying, "At the beginning, leprosy in our country was limited to the provinces of Guangdong and Guangxi. Then from there it was transmitted to Fujian and Zhejiang. Now it gradually penetrates the Yangzi River Basin, and has the tendency to spread to the northern banks of the Yellow River. The degree of harm the disease inflicts and the extent of its spread are the worst of all epidemics." The purpose of the order was to urge the organization of general surveys in the provinces and particularly on existing leprosaria.[28] It is indeed revealing that, as late as 1929, the Chinese political elite still believed in the cliché that leprosy was a disease originating from the southernmost provinces, and cases in other parts of China were caused by the spread of the disease from its region of "origin." This amply shows the weight of traditional beliefs about leprosy in China. This persistent view was in tune with the Western colonial discourse on racial degeneration and partly explains the absence of any challenge to the Western view by Chinese elites.

On the other hand, on the question of heredity, the transmission of the "poison" of the disease to the fetus at the moment of conception, already described in Ming-Qing medical works, was still a strong belief in southern China even in the 1930s. Li Zuwei, a doctor working in Nanning, Guangxi province, wrote, in a 1934 article, that congenital transmission of leprosy was possible, refuting the theory of most Western experts, basing his view on what he thought was evidence of the bacillus found in the wombs of pregnant women, provided by Japanese researchers.[29] More interestingly, as we saw in chapter 3, by the early nineteenth century, the specific belief of hereditary transmission had become well entrenched in southern China. Congenital transmission was believed to be not only systematic but also to diminish over the generations, finally dying out by the fourth generation.[30] The idea, absent in Qing medical texts, appeared to be widespread in southern society by the mid-nineteenth century.

This popular belief on heredity was told to foreigners by none other than the Cantonese doctor Wong Foon. Wong apparently took the belief quite seriously and wrote, in his 1873 report from Canton, "Lepers do not intermarry with the healthy. . . . Nearly all the children of lepers show the disease. As a rule the disease becomes milder in each succeeding generation; in the third, the descendants can only be distinguished from ordinary people by a greater pallor of the face. In the fourth, it is considered safe to marry, although this is not generally done. So long as marriage is confined to lepers there is a tendency to a natural extinction of the disease."[31] Obviously, his Western medical education induced no doubts in him on the validity of the belief and practices in his native place.

In fact, as early as the 1840s, Western medical missionaries working in China were already aware of such a belief. Benjamin Hobson wrote, in an 1842 article reporting on the situation in Macao, that leprosy was "said to become mild in the third generation, and to run itself out in the fourth," a point that he repeated in a later article, published in 1860,[32] without further comment. Wong did more than simply record the belief and practices in Canton: he roused interest in the belief in Western doctors. The French doctor Durand-Fardel translated Wong's report word for word in an 1877 article published in Paris and remarked that "this is an affair of observation," even though he found some of the ideas difficult to accept.[33] Neither he nor Hobson considered the belief outlandish, and both chose to record it with an unspoken reservation. Moreover, the idea was described in the famous 1867 report on leprosy by the Royal College of Physicians. Based on reports sent in by doctors stationed in Hong Kong and Canton, including one by Benjamin Hobson, on the idea of heredity, the authors of the report summarized the survey on the question of heredity by saying, "In China it is said to become mild in the third generation, and to run itself out in the fourth. For this reason, lepers usually intermarry only with those in whom the same grade or degree of the disease exists. . . . Their progeny is then considered free from taint." The British authors were content to synthesize the various observations by concluding that "there is an almost unanimous concurrence of opinion that leprosy is often hereditary."[34]

This attitude probably reflected the Europeans' great uncertainty about the nature of leprosy in the nineteenth century, and their suspicion that it was not a specific disease with universal features. To them, the leprosy they observed in China could have its own specificities, peculiar to the Chinese physical constitution and natural environment.[35] Such uncertainties provided plenty of room for different explanations of the disease, for both the Western observers in China and the Chinese, whose discourse on the disease was not at all subordinated to any dominating Western theory. On the contrary, medical missionaries in the mid to late nineteenth century were attentive to the Chinese interpretations of the disease, which they dutifully recorded with due respect, like naturalists and anthropologists.[36] They were, as we have seen, particularly supportive of the Chinese conviction of the miasmatic origin of the disease, so close to their own. In a way, therefore, both Chinese and Western conceptions of the disease reinforced the idea of leprosy being hereditary and specific to peoples of particular regions and constitutions. For the Chinese, southerners were the main victims; for the Westerners, all Chinese were southerners.

However, the hereditary theory of leprosy did not convince Western medical doctors that the disease would logically remain inside China among only the Chinese race. On the contrary, the idea that the Chinese race was contaminating the world became increasingly persuasive. Even before Hansen's discovery of the bacillus in 1873, providing a strong piece of scientific evidence for the contagion theory, Chinese emigrants were accused of infecting the Pacific region, notably Hawaii, California, and Australia. The belief that leprosy was an inherent condition of the Chinese race was already fixed by the early 1870s, when American public opinion began to accuse Chinese immigrants of bringing leprosy to America. A Cantonese immigrant diagnosed to have the disease in the San Francisco Smallpox Hospital, in 1871, was pinpointed as the beginning of the Chinese leper's "invasion" of the United States in the early 1880s.[37] Even though San Francisco public health officials tried to calm public panic by reiterating the mainstream medical explanation of the time that leprosy was limited to the Chinese and transmitted only hereditarily, the hysteria continued.[38]

The disquieting news of a worsening leprosy epidemic in Hawaii convinced some Americans that Chinese immigrants were turning the United States into a "nation of lepers."[39] Indeed, in Hawaii of the mid-nineteenth century, leprosy was commonly called *ma'i pake*—the Chinese disease, thought to have been unknown in the Sandwich Islands before 1849, when Chinese immigrants began to arrive. A Dr. Hillebrand claimed that he saw his first leper there in 1853. Twenty-five years after this, the percentage of known cases was said to be as high as 3.5 percent.[40] American public opinion had apparently disregarded the cases of leprosy brought into America by Scandinavian, Spanish, English, and French immigrants in various parts of the continent during the earlier phases of European migration into North America.[41] Reports in the late nineteenth century claiming that leprosy existed in Hawaii before the Chinese arrived were also largely ignored.[42] Even the well-documented history of leprosy in Hawaii published by Dr. A. A. Mouritz in 1916, showing that leprosy had already been observed by American missionaries in the 1820s,[43] did not seem to calm the fears of Chinese immigrants as carriers of leprosy.

In Australia, "it is generally agreed that leprosy was brought to northern Australia by Chinese immigrants, and that the first person in the Northern Territory known to have leprosy was a Chinese man whose illness was reported in 1882."[44] Not surprisingly, no research was done on the possibility of an earlier introduction of the disease by European immigrants to the continent before the nineteenth century, as in the Americas. Subsequently, from the 1880s onward, white Australia increasingly associated the Chinese race with the spread of the disease and began to restrict Chinese immigration and set up racial cordons sanitaires.[45]

As mentioned, not only China felt the effects of this international outcry against the spread of leprosy. Japan, the strongest and most modernized Asian nation-state in the nineteenth century, was also a victim of the international panic about the spread of the disease, as the presence of leprosy in the country seemed to indicate that Japan was not quite qualified as a member of the community of modern, civilized nations. As in China, Japanese media in the early twentieth century propagated the idea that their country was "the most leprous country in the world," with an estimated number of 1 million lepers.[46] As a colonizing state, Japan also determined to exterminate leprosy in its colonized Greater East Asia Co-Prosperity Sphere, taking the example of the Culion colony set up by the United States in the Philippines.[47] Leprosy became the disease of national shame for both China and Japan in the same period. The more powerful and centralized Meiji state, however, was more capable than the Chinese Republican government of implementing draconian laws to segregate almost all lepers in prisonlike leprosaria in the early twentieth century.[48] By so doing, Japan seemed to show the rest of the world that it was more civilized and modern than the rest of Asia.

The hysteria in the face of the perceived invasion of the "Chinese" or "Asian" disease in white countries accelerated after Hansen's discovery of the bacillus in 1873–1874, justifying the contagious nature of leprosy. But the real drama came when the famous Belgian missionary working in Hawaii, Father Damien, manifested symptoms of leprosy in 1878, five years after he arrived in the leper colony.[49] His death eleven years later, in 1889, sent off a wave of great panic across the continents. A world pandemic of leprosy seemed imminent. This was also the year of the publication of Wright's *Leprosy: An Imperial Danger,* which warned Europe of the risk of being infected with the disease again. The growing fear of a leprosy pandemic from the 1870s onward soon led to a series of indictments against Chinese immigrants. It was at least one reason behind the Chinese Exclusion Act, passed by the U.S. Congress in 1882.[50] The Chinese were equally indicted by Australia in 1888, and even Colombia contemplated passing a law prohibiting Chinese immigration in 1913, when there was in fact no Chinese immigration into that country.[51] Amid all the brouhaha, the sharpest voice was perhaps that of James Cantlie, a close associate of Patrick Manson's, famous also for his medical education work in Hong Kong, where he established a close friendship with his student, Sun Yat-sen,[52] the future founder of the Republic of China. A leprologist in his own right, Cantlie was a prolific writer on the disease. In the famous prizewinning report "Conditions under Which Leprosy Occurs in China, Indo-China, Malaya, the Archipelago, and Oceania" (1897), he singled out the Chinese coolie as solely responsible for the leprosy pandemic in the Pacific region: "Leprosy is not indigenous in any part of the Pacific, yet there must be some common factor in the three centres which has determined its presence. That fact—indeed, the only common factor—is the Chinaman, and he *is* leprous" (italics Cantlie's). He wrote that Chinese immigrants were totally lacking in "decency and cleanliness" and "one of the evils of this steady migration is the spread of leprosy." For him there was only one way to put the situation under control, "and that is the exclusion or the rigid control of all Chinese coolies."[53] In other words, among the many colored races infested with leprosy, the Chinese were the main world contaminator, as there were more immigrants from China than any other country. As late as 1948, a Chinese employed by the Indian government in Bombay was repatriated for having been found to have the disease,[54] just as patients in British Hong Kong were repatriated to Canton before the Communist takeover in 1949.

The increasing indictment against the Chinese immigrant as a polluter of the world was also a result of the final victory of the contagion theory of leprosy over the hereditary one after Hansen's discovery of the *Mycobacterium leprae* in 1873–1874. The "victory" did not come, however, right after the discovery, but only several decades later.

A Contagious Body? Doubts and Certainties

The important discovery of Hansen did not, as one would have expected, immediately end the discussions on hereditary transmission of the disease. In fact, the idea of leprosy being a hereditary disease was so entrenched in Western medical thought in the nineteenth century that the discovery only served to confuse some and provoke suspicion from others. Medical experts working in China, among others, continued to challenge the contagion theory either by quoting their own observations or by questioning the scientific significance of the discovery.

We have to remind ourselves that medical research in Europe during the second half of the nineteenth century has a complex history, with multiple competing theories. The emerging germ theory, far from being a homogeneous concept,[55] combining new and old premises, was not at all dominant in medical thought and practices before the turn of the twentieth century. The "seed and soil" metaphor continued to contribute to doctors' ideas of the varying receptiveness of the human "soil" to bacteria. The demonstration of the existence of the tuberculosis bacillus by Koch in 1882 did not immediately alter the prevailing understanding of the disease, and many still tried to harmonize the presence of the bacillus with "the fact of heredity." Even when the existence of this bacillus, together with those of leprosy, septicemia, erysipelas, and anthrax had been demonstrated in national tours in the summer of 1882, unconvinced pathologists and surgeons continued to advocate other theories, those they were more accustomed to than the germ theory.[56] And this was almost ten years after Hansen's discovery of the leprosy bacillus. All the debates, doubts, and uncertainties about the nature of many diseases that missionary doctors observed in the colonies were thus inevitable given the complex state of medical research in Europe during the last decades of the nineteenth century.

It is therefore quite natural that many doctors working in China in the 1870s and 1880s were puzzled by Hansen's discovery. The presence of the bacillus did not convince them of the contagiousness of the disease, and the theory of heredity held fast, as in the case of tuberculosis in the early 1880s. Moreover, their observations in China did not seem to support a simple theory of contagion or infection. A Dr. Reid, working in Hankow, reported in 1875 that he was puzzled by the healthy condition of the offspring of lepers, which clearly contradicted the hereditary theory, "although all are alike exposed to contagion."[57] Dr. W. A. Henderson, working in Shandong, also reported, in 1888, that his work on leprosy could not substantiate the contagion theory and urged his colleagues to pull together their findings in order to come to a more convincing conclusion.[58] Patrick Manson, for his part, was rather ruthless in challenging the scientific validity of Hansen's discovery. While working in Amoy, he wrote, in 1881:

> We should be rash to conclude that a bacterium . . . had anything to do with the causation of leprosy. The present is the age of bacteria, and as they are searched for everywhere, and in nearly every disease, they are found everywhere and in every disease. Concomitance and consequence are easily mixed up. Such a degenerate and half-dead piece of flesh as is a leper-tubercle is just the place wherein one would expect to find bacteria. Though one expects to find maggots in a dead body, yet we do not attribute the existence of the body, or its death, to the maggots; neither, when we find bacteria in the tubercles of a leper, should we, without other evidence than mere concomitance, attribute the tubercle and the leprosy to the bacterium. This *bacillus leprae* may, and probably will, turn out a mare's nest, like so many of its predecessors.[59]

The contagiousness of leprosy was further complicated by the confusion with syphilis and the suspicion that the bacillus could be transmitted by means of smallpox vaccination. The alleged similarity between leprosy and syphilis was a subject of controversy in the late nineteenth century, even though mainstream doctors insisted that leprosy was a disease sui generis, unconnected to any other. The answers to a question posed by the London Royal College of Physicians, in a survey conducted in 1867 on the relations between leprosy, yaws, and syphilis, for example, reveal that many doctors working in various parts of the British empire, especially those in India, believed that there was some link between leprosy and syphilis: "I believe leprosy is very often connected with, if not dependent on, syphilis."[60] Some medical doctors continued to believe that leprosy represented the fourth stage of syphilis; Dr. G. L. Fitch, working in Hawaii, was one that spread the idea with great energy in the 1880s. He claimed that if syphilis were still active in its third stage, it then became incurable, passing on to scrofula or leprosy.[61] Such ideas, though refuted by elite doctors,[62] were apparently quite popular in parts of the world, enforcing the belief that the disease was highly contagious. Consul D. B. Robertson reported from Canton in 1867 that "it is a Chinese medical opinion that injudicious mercurial treatment for syphilis may induce leprosy." Similar ideas were put forward by British doctors in Hong Kong.[63]

At the same time, the belief that the smallpox virus and vaccination could transmit leprosy was also a popular idea in China. Transmission of leprosy by inoculation against smallpox (using either human pox or cowpox), according to James Cantlie, was an idea suggested by Europeans.[64] However, one of the first native Jennerian vaccinators in China, Qiu Xi, a disciple of Alexander Pearson, surgeon with the British East India Company, wrote as early as 1817 in his book on vaccination that children to be inoculated should be inspected to make sure they were not carriers of leprosy, lest the lymph they transmitted would help spread the disease.[65] Qiu's recommendation was clearly implemented in the first cowpox dispensary in Canton, as recorded by Benjamin Hobson in 1842: "The government orders two policemen from the lazar house to examine all the children who present themselves for vaccination. If there is any suspicion of leprosy, the child cannot be vaccinated."[66] Cantlie, according to his 1894 report, had asked doctors to discuss this point in their reports on leprosy in places where the disease was believed to be rampant, especially Guangdong and Fujian provinces, where cowpox inoculation was first introduced. Dr. Anna Scott, reporting from Swatow, definitely considered vaccination an important cause: "I have been forced to the conclusion that the vaccination from arm to arm, practised by a class of Chinese (quack) doctors, has caused this very marked increase." A Dr. C. B. Wood, reporting from Honolulu, also believed that arm-to-arm smallpox vaccination "undoubtedly helped to spread leprosy." Many suggested that it was due to the "lymph being obtained indiscriminately and carelessly," a popular belief also observed by Dr. Mouritz in the 1880s in Hawaii.[67] The belief, proven to be totally unfounded, as the leprosy bacillus could not be inoculated by ordinary means on a dermal surface, was nonetheless brought up occasionally in the early Republican medical journals, warning people against inoculation by human pox. Some Chinese doctors seemed to associate the "fetal toxin" causing smallpox, a traditional Chinese medical concept, with leprosy, which was believed to be acquired congenitally. We have already seen this idea played out in the late-Qing popular opera about the leprous virgin.

The many confusing and alarmist ideas related to the contagiousness of leprosy, held by both Western and Chinese doctors in the nineteenth and early twentieth centuries, are understandable in the light of present-day hindsight. Well over a century after Hansen's discovery of the bacillus, modern biomedicine has yet to explain the exact mechanism of the transmission of the bacillus and the varying clinical expressions of infected patients. Leprosy does not transmit easily, and we are still uncertain of the way the bacillus enters the body. This uncertainty bred fear, as various channels of transmission were alarmingly possible. When doctors began to more readily accept the contagion theory in the 1890s, they did not do so on the basis of clear scientific evidence produced by any breakthrough in laboratory research on leprosy, but by submission to the power of changing public opinion, often related to a fear of the unknown. Again, the death of Father Damien in Hawaii seems to have played a decisive role. Dr. Douthwaite's 1892 report clearly illustrates the nature of the change in attitude of some doctors: "I have not been able to obtain evidence in proof of either the heredity or contagiousness of the disease as found here, but the rapid spread of leprosy in the Sandwich Islands, after its introduction from China, shows plainly that under certain conditions it is highly contagious."[68] Obviously it was the power of the Molokai story, especially the death of Father Damien from leprosy in 1889, as reported in the media that converted some to the contagion theory without full scientific proof.

The problem of leprosy in Hawaii was brought to public attention in 1863, twelve years after the first importation of Chinese, with the arrival of 180 coolies, and five years before the first shipment of forty-eight Japanese. In 1865 the Act to Prevent the Spread of Leprosy was passed, legitimizing the strict isolation of lepers in Hawaii. In that year, the Board of Health established a hospital at Kalihikai, about three miles west of Honolulu, which served as a "receiving station," and purchased a portion of land on the windward side of the island of Molokai, known as the Kalaupapa Peninsula, that was soon developed into a 6,000-acre leper colony. Local sheriffs and deputies collected information of cases of leprosy. Anyone suspected of having the disease was transferred to Honolulu, and confirmed cases were shipped to Molokai. From 1866 to 1895, two years after the overthrow of the monarchy and three years before U.S. annexation, the Board of Health reported, in 1896, that the number of admissions each year varied from 43 to 579, with 105 inmates registered in 1866 and 1,087 in 1895. Up to 1885, 97 percent of the inmates were Hawaiian, and 1.8 percent Chinese; from 1901 to 1905, 83.5 percent were Hawaiian 6.8 percent Chinese, and 3.2 percent Portuguese. In fact, afflicted white foreigners were given the choice of leaving the islands to avoid isolation.

Joseph de Veuster, better known as Father Damien, the legendary Catholic priest of Belgian origin, arrived in 1873 at the Molokai colony to begin instructing the outcasts in productive moral behavior. The Board of Health allowed Father Damien to serve as a temporary administrator of the colony, as none of the Hawaiians available were qualified. He contracted leprosy in 1878, was officially diagnosed to have the disease in 1885, and died four years later, on March 28, 1889, on Molokai. For the Catholic Church, he was the hero and martyr who brought civilized life to the colony. More recent scholarship depicts a more complex character with a colonial bias. His having contracted the disease and his death provoked global alarm on an unprecedented scale, and "confirmed" the contagiousness of the disease.[69]

For a level-headed authority such as James L. Maxwell, chairman of the China Medical Missionary Association in the first decade of the twentieth century, however, the contagiousness of leprosy was still, in 1911, an unsettled issue: "We take it for granted that the cause of leprosy is the *bacillus lepra*. It, however, fails to conform to two of Koch's postulates for specific bacteria, i.e., it cannot be cultivated outside the body, or be successfully inoculated into animals. Even inoculation into man has usually failed to transmit the disease. . . .[70] The mode of infection by which the bacillus is carried to man is quite unknown. There is no evidence in favour of any hereditary transmission of the disease or diathesis. It is also extremely difficult to get histories of direct infection."[71] As late as the 1930s, the question of the channel of contagion of the bacillus still haunted most Western doctors. At the fourth International Leprosy Congress in Cairo in 1938, "The tensest moment . . . was the moment Dr. Lagoudasky, of Alexandria, appeared before the Conference. He had experimented on himself by injecting himself with the leprous material from a leper. The result was shown in a frank case of leprosy. This worker has been among lepers for many years. . . . Under great applause for his courageous and self-sacrificial experiment, Dr. Lagoudasky left the auditorium." The report was published in the *Leper Quarterly* in Shanghai.[72] Even though from the report it is not clear if Lagoudasky contracted the disease from inoculation (which is highly unlikely), or from prolonged contact with patients, the drama of the incident simply shows the great tension that still existed between those who claimed leprosy to be highly contagious by contact and those who doubted it. On the question of leprosy in China in this period, therefore, there was no agreement among Western medical experts working in the country on the real cause of the disease, even though the policy of segregation was, by then, generally agreed upon.

If Western medical missionaries were uncertain of the way leprosy was transmitted, the Chinese never doubted the disease's contagiousness, since it had already been described in medical books in the sixteenth century. Moreover, as we have seen, Ming-Qing medical texts were quite specific as to the channels of transmission—by direct and indirect physical contact, by sexual intercourse, and by congenital transmission—of the disease; Shen Zhiwen and Xiao Xiaoting, of the Ming-Qing periods, were as alarmist as any European contagionist on the danger of the ways by which leprosy could transmit from the sick to the healthy. The fear of contagion by physical contact with a sufferer was most obvious, especially in southern China, even well into the twentieth century. Such a conviction was, moreover, noted with great interest by many Western medical missionaries working in China. During the period when the heredity theory was dominant, an astute observer such as Hobson noted, in 1842, "Leprosy is undoubtedly an hereditary disease, but whether it is really contagious I cannot determine. The Chinese affirm that it is, and act accordingly."[73] He also noted, in 1860, that "the true leprosy is considered by the Chinese to be infectious and incurable." He noticed that when a family was infected with it, it shut them off from all direct intercourse with their relations and friends. For him the repulsive appearance of the victim of the disease explained why it was considered infectious, as contact with the victim was feared and avoided.[74] The Chinese fear of contagion only intensified after Hansen's discovery. Dr. J. H. McCartney, in Chongqing, Sichuan province, reported, in 1894, that "the Chinese look upon leprosy as highly contagious and will not allow a leper to mingle with them."[75] Unlike Western medical missionaries, many Chinese elites did not hesitate to make a direct connection between the bacillus and contagion. Xu Ke (1869–1928), the compiler of the famous miscellaneous notes on Qing society *Qing bai lei chao* (1917), described leprosy in Guangdong province as follows: "The climate in Guangdong is hot and leprosy is rampant. The victims bear a microorganism [*wei sheng wu*], making them very contagious."[76] He typically selected from modern biomedicine whatever might help buttress views on the body and diseases that actually came from his own tradition. He was, like many members of the Chinese elite, unaware of Westerners' doubts about the contagiousness of leprosy even after the discovery of the bacillus.

The fear of transmission through sexual intercourse, though considered to be without a scientific basis, also intrigued many Western observers. The idea was firmly held by many Chinese doctors, including Wong Foon, who was again the one who made it well known to Western medical doctors. He wrote in his report in 1873, "The natives here believe that wives of lepers, even when showing no marks of the disease, are capable of infecting healthy people through cohabitation. . . . Hence arises a most common pernicious practice of women, who believe themselves infected, going about in disguise trying to get rid of their poison by clandestine and gratuitous prostitution. This goes by the name of 'selling off leprosy.'" Wong then went on to illustrate his point by giving a series of accounts "showing that there is a great probability of the disease communicable through lepers' wives seemingly unaffected in appearance," from "eyewitnesses," in whom he had "thorough confidence."[77] Wong, knowing that most of his European counterparts would dismiss this belief as absurd, assured them that he had treated a number of male lepers who had confessed that the origin of their illness was from sleeping with women "selling off leprosy," though he himself had not yet seen such a woman.[78]

Mention has been made that this popular belief, emerging not later than the thirteenth century, was the origin of a genre of popular literature with a leprous virgin as its main character, especially in the Qing. Apparently, the introduction of Western medicine did not in the least halt the belief, which continued to have important influence on the behavior of China's southern populations. Manson reported, in 1872, that doctors of Chinese medicine in Amoy recommended to female patients of leprosy a treatment of "selling off" their disease within a period of three to four years.[79] The belief and its associated practices seem to have continued well into the twentieth century. In a Chinese article on leprosy published in a medical journal in 1929, the authors recommended three ways to avoid leprosy: avoid inoculation against smallpox by human pox, likely to be contaminated by leprosy;[80] watch out for men and women attempting to "sell off" their disease; avoid socializing with lepers.[81] James Maxwell also wrote, in 1930, "Perhaps the most serious superstition, and one still found in some regions, is that the patient can be cured and the disease transferred to another person by sexual relations between a leper and a healthy individual. . . . Such ideas die hard and are a real hindrance to any campaign for the conquest of leprosy."[82] Maxwell's reference to "hindrance" to the campaign can be illustrated by incidents of serious social violence prevalent in southern China due to the belief. As late as 1937, there were reports that male and female lepers in parts of Guangdong province were forcing the healthy to have sexual intercourse with them in order to have their disease "transferred." Such incidents provided local military forces an excuse to round up lepers and execute them en masse, with the justification that Western nations also executed people of inferior races.[83] Such extremist acts echoed the concerns of some Cantonese political elites who proposed severe punishment against rapists with the disease, and Western fascist methods such as sterilization of patients in order to exterminate the "racial seeds" (*miezhong*) of leprosy in an "efficient" manner.[84]

The view that leprosy was transmittable by sexual intercourse was rejected by most but not all Western medical missionaries. One rare but important example is that of Wong Foon's managing to convince none other than James Cantlie. In his 1890 report on leprosy in Hong Kong, Cantlie warned that one of the most dangerous channels of transmission of the disease was through the cohabitation of Western males with Chinese women, which, he observed, was more widespread in Hong Kong than anywhere else in the world.[85] In his report on the situation of leprosy in the Pacific region seven years later, his stance on the belief was even firmer. He confirmed that the "selling off [of] leprosy" was "a very common practice in Canton," and concluded that "the present state of our belief may be held to be that 'sexual connection is a means of spreading leprosy.' As a corollary it may be added, that even a single coitus when abrasion occurs may be sufficient to convey infection of leprosy."[86] Cantlie thus appears to have been genuinely concerned about the belief, but his warning could also reflect Maxwell's worries that Chinese lepers with such a belief were tricking innocent people into dangerous sexual relations. It could also simply be an echo of another, more profound Western fear regarding leprosy: the fear of the mixing of races, leading to the degeneration of the white race. Cantlie's concern regarding this point is explicit in his report on Macao, in which he showed his surprise at the relatively small number of Portuguese lepers in the colony, given the fact that "the Portuguese settlers are largely Mongoloid in feature, and yellow-skinned through intermarriage with the Chinese."[87] He definitely would not like to have seen the British in Hong Kong suffer the same fate as the Portuguese in Macao.

Thus, the Chinese fear of the contagiousness of leprosy, uninterrupted since at least the sixteenth century and enhanced by the discovery of Hansen's bacillus, was not checked by the doubts of the medical missionaries on the question, nor challenged by any scientific evidence raised by Western doctors. There was, as we have seen, no agreement among Western doctors working in China as to the way leprosy was transmitted as late as the early twentieth century, thus no dominant theory on the issue. The Chinese, on the other hand, quickly grasped and exploited the semantics of germ theory, which only helped to inflate the danger and fear of leprosy contagion. The dread of the disease only intensified from the late nineteenth century onward. The attitude was apparent in the bilingual journal *Leper Quarterly* (*Mafeng jikan*), published by the Chinese Mission to Lepers (Zhonghua mafeng jiuji hui), which was established in the winter of 1926.[88] In the first issue of the journal published in January 1927, the chairman of the board of a major leprosarium in Canton wrote, in a short commemorative note, that as China was losing ground to the spread of the disease, one had to "vow to eradicate the germ of leprosy in order to cleanse the universe."[89] The emotional language of staging a war against vicious leprosy became typical in the Republican period. The disease was sometimes called the leprosy devil (*mamo*), a formidable and evil enemy.[90] Many Chinese articles published in the 1920s and 1930s on leprosy warned readers of the grave danger of contagion and advised against any mingling or contact with lepers, advocating strict segregation.[91] Basically the attitude was similar to that of Xiao Xiaoting, of the late eighteenth century, except that the regular mention of the bacillus, underscoring the contagiousness of the disease, added a scientific tone to the discussions.

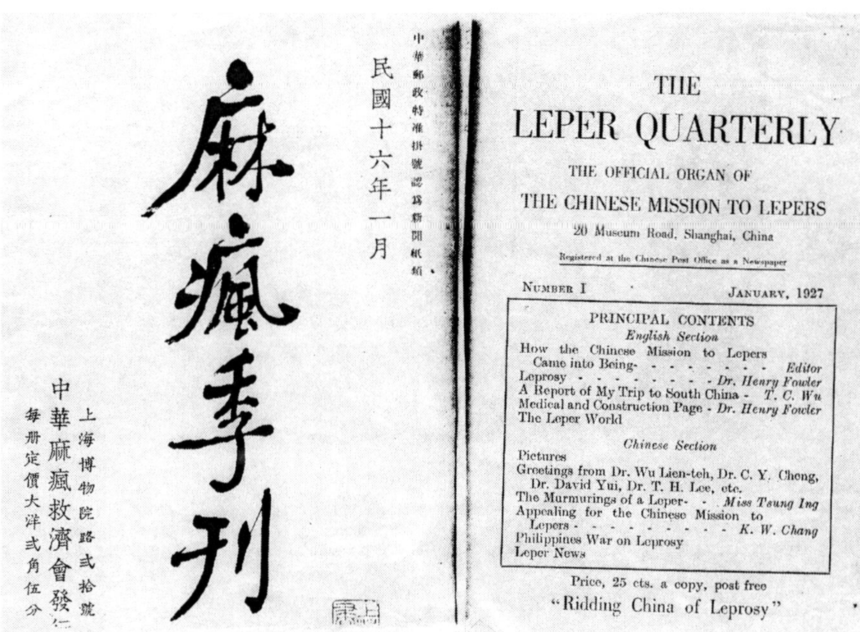

麻瘋季刊

上海博物院路弍拾號
中華麻瘋救濟會發行
每冊定價大洋弍角伍分

民國十六年一月

中華郵政特准掛號認爲新聞紙類

THE
LEPER QUARTERLY
THE OFFICIAL ORGAN OF
THE CHINESE MISSION TO LEPERS
20 Museum Road, Shanghai, China
Registered at the Chinese Post Office as a Newspaper

NUMBER I — JANUARY, 1927

PRINCIPAL CONTENTS

English Section

How the Chinese Mission to Lepers Came into Being - - - - - - - *Editor*
Leprosy - - - - - - - - - *Dr. Henry Fowler*
A Report of My Trip to South China - *T. C. Wu*
Medical and Construction Page - *Dr. Henry Fowler*
The Leper World

Chinese Section

Pictures
Greetings from Dr. Wu Lien-teh, Dr. C. Y. Cheng, Dr. David Yui, Dr. T. H. Lee, etc.
The Murmurings of a Leper - - *Miss Tsung Ing*
Appealing for the Chinese Mission to Lepers - - - - - - - - - *K. W. Chang*
Philippines War on Leprosy
Leper News

Price, 25 cts. a copy, post free
"Ridding China of Leprosy"

Cover of the first issue (1927) of the bilingual journal *Leper Quarterly;* the slogan "Ridding China of Leprosy" appeared on the English cover of almost every issue.

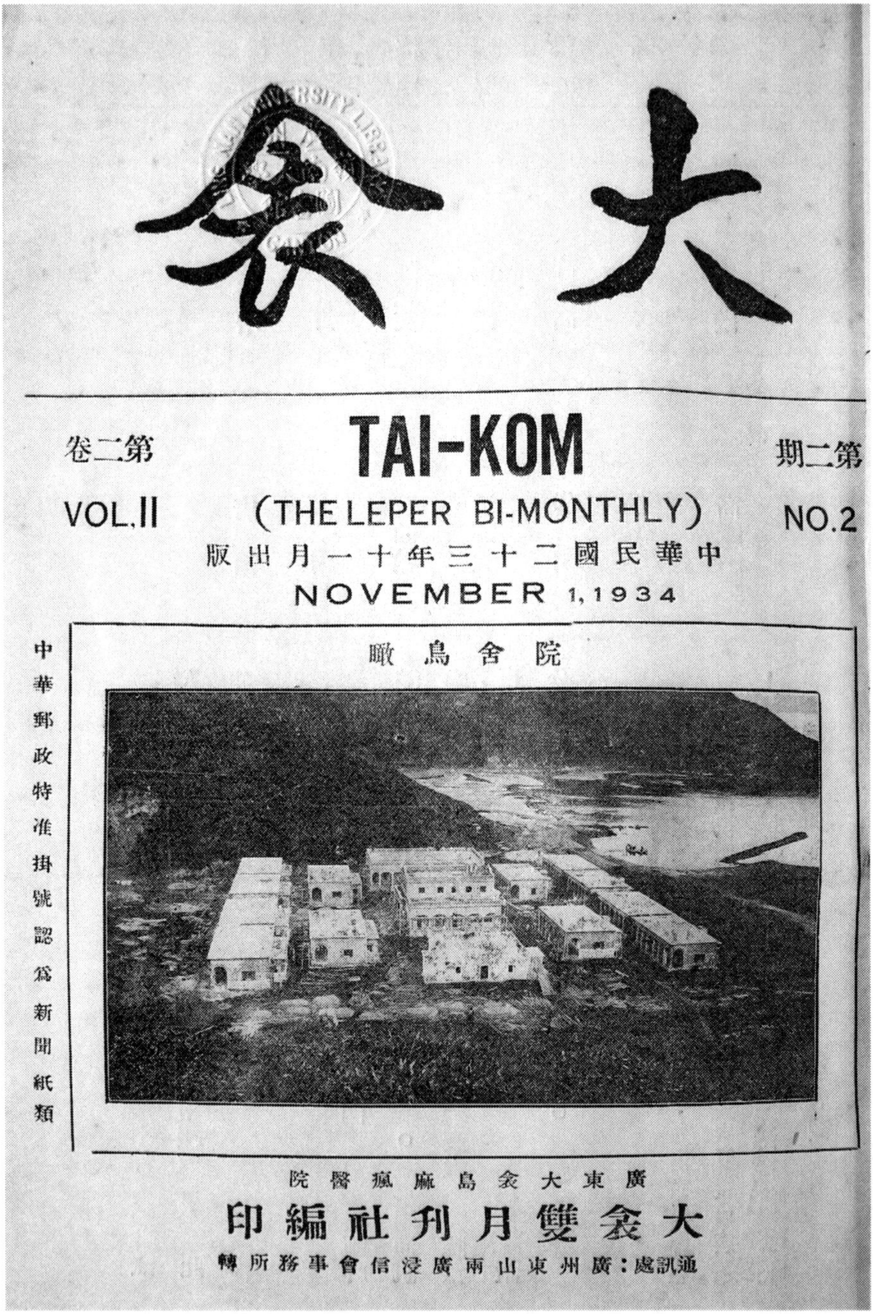
大衾

第二卷 TAI-KOM 第二期

VOL.II (THE LEPER BI-MONTHLY) NO.2

中華民國二十三年十一月出版

NOVEMBER 1,1934

中華郵政特准掛號認為新聞紙類

院舍鳥瞰

廣東大衾島痲瘋醫院

大衾雙月刊社編印

通訊處：廣州東山兩廣浸信會事務所轉

Cover (November 1934) of a journal on leprosy published by the asylum on Taikam (Daqin) island, off the southwestern coast of Macao; it shows a bird's-eye view of the colony on the deserted island. (Courtesy of Sun Yat-sen University, Guangzhou)

On the other hand, Western views on the Chinese role in the perceived growing world pandemic were also made known to the Chinese public in journals. The editorial of one of the early issues of the *Leper Quarterly*, of 1927, claimed that there were 1 million lepers in China, "who are nothing but social parasites and a burden to the nation."[92] The actual number of lepers in China was anybody's guess in the early twentieth century. The high estimates simply reflected the gravity of the situation in the eyes especially of medical missionaries. James Maxwell, for instance, estimated, in 1933, that there were about 3 million lepers in China, about one-third of all lepers in the world. Moreover, "at least half the population of China are included in the areas where leprosy is found."[93] The estimated number of lepers in China in the early twentieth century was often coupled with the problem of Chinese emigration. In the *Leper Quarterly*, for instance, a 1930 article by Maxwell pointed out that China was a country where the disease was endemic, and the increasing number of Chinese emigrants due to international trade was making China a major exporter of the disease. As he put it, "Leprosy in China is not only a problem for China, but one for the entire world."[94] Translated into Chinese, the article was clearly meant to provoke the Chinese reader to exert more pressure on the government to undertake an integrated national policy to deal with the problem, which was Maxwell's consistent position. The way the Chinese reader interpreted such information, however, could be quite different. Such news could increase fear, dread, and a feeling of shame, leading in turn to growing violence and cruelty toward lepers, and policies different from those anticipated by Maxwell.

In general terms, then, despite the limited impact of the discovery of Hansen's bacillus in 1873–1874 on the advancement of the contagion theory of leprosy, events of the last two decades of the nineteenth century gradually culminated in the triumph of the contagion theory. Two especially noteworthy events in this connection were the infection of Father Damien and his death in 1889 and the First International Leprosy Conference in Berlin in 1897, which declared leprosy incurable and that segregation was necessary to halt contagion.[95] The increasingly dominant paradigm of germ theory affected even the most independent thinker. Patrick Manson, a severe critic of germ theory in the 1870s, admitted in his classic *Tropical Diseases*, published in 1898, that "leprosy is a germ disease, and therefore it cannot originate *de novo*. . . . The germ is found in the human tissues and, hitherto, nowhere else. . . . The spread of the disease from individual to individual, and from place to place, can be, and has been, traced."[96] With agreement on contagion, segregation seemed to be a logical way to control the spread of the disease. By the early twentieth century, therefore, despite the persistent uncertainty about the ways leprosy was transmitted, many medical missionaries in

China agreed that more systematic segregation was necessary, although they did not have the same views on how segregation should be implemented. The Chinese medical and political elite, of course, had never doubted the contagiousness of leprosy and had always advocated strict segregation, in the imperial period for the purpose of avoiding contamination and, in the modern period, with the more radical goal of eradicating the bacillus that had brought shame to the nation.

From the mid-nineteenth century onward, for many Western missionaries working in China, leprosy was one of their main interests. They came with their own medical tradition and views on the disease. At the same time, they were intrigued by the way the Chinese themselves interpreted the disease. In fact, many were drawn to the indigenous theory of congenital and sexual transmission, even though it fit awkwardly with their own theories in the mid-nineteenth century. Their tolerance had a reason, however. The prevailing but ambivalent environmentalist paradigm that David Arnold has justly called "a vast metaphor for an ineluctable otherness that European science and medicine found in India and could never entirely gainsay"[97] was also applicable to China. Disease was different in China, too. Tropical disease, the new field of medical knowledge, was in fact constructed on the assumption that bodies and diseases in these "tropical countries" were different. It is interesting to note the similar native environmentalist paradigm of late imperial China, apparent from the sixteenth century onward, according to which the southern Lingnan region was the source region of dangerous, sexually transmitted, chronic, and epidemic diseases exhibiting particularly monstrous symptoms, manifestations of the contamination by the vilest poisons. As explained, late imperial Chinese doctors and literati considered the Lingnan area a miasmatic region inhabited by semicivilized populations, where diseases were different and more horrible than those found to the north. Modern Chinese doctors only used Western germ theory to enforce these traditional views. These views in turn conformed unwittingly to those of Western medical experts, who considered both the climate and environment of China as particularly bad for health, and the Chinese as morally and physically inferior, two reasons that could explain why the country was infested with all sorts of horrible diseases. The similarity of the two views perhaps clarifies why the Chinese social and political elite of the late nineteenth and early twentieth centuries had an intrinsic understanding of Western racist discourse, which they themselves often engaged in to formulate a Nationalist agenda in which the "Chinaman" had to be remade or reformed in order that a new, healthy nation could be built. In a sense, such an agenda was not unlike the old efforts to tame the south, the embodiment of the "other" in late imperial China.

RESHAPING THE BODY POLITIC: SEGREGATION

No one member of the body politic can suffer and other members not suffer with it.
—W. H. P. Anderson, General Secretary, Mission to Lepers, London, 1933[98]

Cantlie's critique of the "Chinaman" being "leprous" and contagious was taken seriously by Chinese Nationalists of the likes of Sun Yat-sen, if not by Sun himself. Cantlie, in a diary entry of December 30, 1890, wrote that he took his student Sun Yat-sen, then twenty-four years old, to serve as his translator when he visited a leper colony in Canton that day.[99] This experience, together with Sun's various other observations of the "undisciplined" body of his countrymen, must have provoked in him reflections on the character of the Chinese race not dissimilar to those of Western racists, reflections he made public in lectures.[100] The Nationalists' determination "to remake the Chinaman and remake the state together," as John Fitzgerald has put it,[101] was indeed the motive behind a series of public health measures, including the establishment of a national network of leprosaria in the Republican era. As T. C. Wu (Wu Zhijian), general secretary of the Chinese Mission to Lepers, wrote in an editorial in a 1927 issue of the *Mafeng jikan,* "To provide relief to lepers [i.e., putting them into asylums] is the most patriotic act."[102] The Nationalist agenda was thus totally different from the "grand rite of purification," as Foucault labeled medieval European leprosaria.[103] Putting lepers away in leprosaria in China was part of a process by which the "leprosy devil" could be completely exterminated. The language was modern and combative. While the infected part of society had to be cut off and left to perish on its own, healthy bodies had to be protected from a dangerous contagion. There was a clear call for stricter social discipline and for an unambiguous expression of authority from the new government, as these were believed to be essential for the improvement of the Chinese race.[104]

China had three different possible models of segregation at the turn of the twentieth century. The traditional leper asylum, which had not totally disappeared; the missionary model; and a lay, "nationalist" model that Republicans associated with what they read and heard about in other parts of the world, such as the Culion colony in the Philippines or Molokai in Hawaii.

The Traditional Model

While many Chinese medical experts and activists held fast to a number of traditional views concerning the disease, few regarded the traditional segregation policy relevant for China's future. In fact, the traditional asylum was forgotten, ignored, or dismissed as useless. Traditional cures, such as the use of chaulmoogra, were also ignored by many elites, who believed it was a new drug brought by Westerners.[105] In addition, many Chinese activists took too willingly the view that China and Chinese society had never done anything for lepers, a bias accepted by many missionaries. A representative opinion was that of A. H. Smith, who, in 1907, declared, "Nothing has ever been done by the Chinese themselves for lepers."[106] Many members of the Chinese elite readily turned a blind eye to the popularity of traditional drugs and the continued existence of a number of old asylums. The famous Cantonese historian Chen Yuan lamented, in 1909, that China had no hospitals for lepers and existing leprosaria were nothing more than places where lepers waited to die; and even these, according to him, were organized not by the Chinese but by Western missionaries.[107]

Such a view continued well into the Republican period. T. C. Wu, a founder and general secretary of the Chinese Mission to Lepers, wrote, in 1927, that "both our government and people have been sadly indifferent about it [leprosy] and no constructive effort has ever been made to cope with the situation."[108] Indeed, Chinese society and the government were often accused of being indifferent and ignorant toward leprosy, not only by missionaries but also by their own elite, who deliberately brushed aside the long tradition of indigenous asylums in order to justify their accusation. Chen Yuan, for instance, admitted in another piece of writing that leper asylums had been established widely during the Qianlong period in Guangdong province.[109] Similarly T. C. Wu, in a 1927 article on the fight against leprosy, mentions in passing that two leprosaria outside the city of Fuzhou, of Fujian, "have existed for a much longer time than we could remember."[110] Neither of them seemed to care to make further comments on the traditional asylum, which they probably dismissed as totally insignificant or irrelevant for the declared war against leprosy.

Such a disdain for traditional institutions was characteristic of the Chinese political elite in the modern period. Unlike Japan, where modernization during the Meiji period provoked a yearning by Japanese society for a disappearing past, the majority of the Chinese elite seemed to reject all that was from the old society, as if it was solely responsible for China's weaknesses and political crises since the mid-nineteenth century. As regards leper asylums in modern Japan, there were petitions in the early twentieth century from leprosy patients for the restoration of organized communities on the model of the traditional *monoyoshi* villages established by Buddhist temples. There was a real nostalgia for the asylums of the past, considered as "something to be proud of before the rest of the world."[111] In contrast, the Chinese elite's rejection of traditional institutions in the early twentieth century seems to have come from their low estimate of China's imperial past, and an excessive enthusiasm for what was considered as Western and scientific. The Chinese attitude explains the scant attention paid to existing institutions for sufferers of leprosy, on which Western missionaries had spilt so much more ink.

Another probable reason for ignoring traditional asylums as a possible model, or even a basis on which modern segregation could be conceptualized, was that the old system was deeply integrated into a social structure that the Nationalists wanted to dismantle and replace with a new social order. The missionary Justus Doolittle provided a detailed account of the organization and functioning of two traditional leprosaria near Fuzhou, probably the same ones observed by T. C. Wu in 1927. Doolittle's account is from 1865, when these institutions were still running in the traditional way. According to him, "A certain number [of inmates] at each asylum has a small stipend allotted them regularly from the government. . . . Each asylum is under the control of a head man . . . [who] has great power over the unfortunates connected with his establishment. . . . These asylums present the appearance of a walled village, having streets, a few small shops, and a school. . . . In case of a poor man becoming leprous, his neighbors are glad to help him in raising the sum demanded by the head man, in order to facilitate his departure [to the asylum]." This sum was thus a kind of "entry fee" ensuring the poor leper of basic room and board. A rich man, on the other hand, would typically bribe the headman so that news of his contracting the disease would be kept from the public and he could then stay at home. The poorest of the lepers were often "obliged to beg in the streets in order to supplement the insufficiency of the Imperial benefaction," which, according to Doolittle, had partly entered the pockets of bureaucrats of all levels. The asylum also employed a doctor, who also charged extra fees for inmates in special need. By and large, the institution seems to have played its designated part. Doolittle interviewed one of the inmates, who claimed that he had stayed in the asylum for fifty-four years.[112] Despite the presence of the most pitiable leprous beggars in the streets, asylums in the Fuzhou region seem largely to have fulfilled their mission of keeping inmates away from public places most of the time, as witnessed by another missionary, S. Johnson, in 1847, who observed, "Leprous individuals are not allowed to roam at large, but I am informed that within the city, four [*sic*] asylums are provided for them, in which they are fed and sustained."[113] When Wong Foon had to write a report on the leprosy situation in Canton in 1873, he interviewed the headmen of existing leprosaria in order to obtain the most up-to-date information, clearly showing that traditional leprosaria were functioning normally then.[114] Missionaries in other parts of China in the mid and late nineteenth century reported similar observations on leper asylums.[115]

In other words, many leper asylums were operating fairly well during the last decades of the Qing dynasty, being self-contained with regular government financial support and money given by individual inmates that maintained some kind of self-management, keeping at least some of the lepers off the street. The traditional asylum depended on several things: a close-knit community that kept track of the health conditions of individual residents, rich and poor; government trust in a headman, always the best informed of the disease situation, serving as middleman between the government and the community; and the acceptance of a certain degree of bribery, seen as a sort of natural evil that kept the system going. The system was also based on the belief that there was no cure for the ailment, and its main objective was to keep the worst contagion out of the community and to provide for poor lepers a minimal living and medical resources.

It is perhaps understandable why the Nationalists would not accept the premises of such a system. First of all, no local middleman could be entrusted, as they would probably be categorized as corrupt feudal local villains or bullies (as characterized by the headman in the late Qing opera described in chap. 3);[116] corruption in whatever form would also have been seen as distinctive of the imperial past. The remaking of China into a new state was to be based on a totally new social fabric and power relations that must not reproduce the old system. The state was expected to intervene in and manage directly whatever new system it created. Moreover, the assumption that leprosy was incurable was unacceptable. The modern body, properly disciplined, should be curable by modern, Western scientific medicine. Medical treatment should be first on the list of priorities, and eradication of the disease from China should be the main objective (see following), even though medical knowledge at that time, Chinese or Western, did not support such optimism. In other words, the idealized vision of modern Chinese society and the unrealistic understanding of medical progress in the curing of leprosy at the turn of the twentieth century excluded the traditional asylum as a feasible model for the Nationalist activists.

The Missionary Model

The missionary asylum, on the other hand, attracted the interest of many Chinese medical and political elites, especially since this model was the most visible at the time, together with Western clinics, hospitals, and other asylums set up by Western missionaries. Protected and promoted by Western colonial powers active in China, they were also considered as bearers of modern Western science and medicine. Missionaries had in fact a long relation with leprosy in China, commencing well before China was forced to permit Western Christian activities on its soil after the 1840s.[117] One of the first leper asylums on Chinese soil was built by Portuguese missionaries in Macao in the sixteenth century. It was part of the Santa Casa da Misericórdia, the major Portuguese Christian charitable organization east of Malacca, established in 1569.[118] According to Spanish sources, lepers in Macao were first accommodated with the poor in the Hospital de San Rafael, set up in 1568 by Spanish and Portuguese missionaries. The following year, a separate establishment, Hospício dos Lázaros, financed by the Misericórdia, was established to take in lepers only.[119] Inmates of the asylum seemed to include both European and Chinese lepers.[120] Besides the Macao institutions, a number of leper asylums established by missionaries, especially by Franciscans in the early Qing, are recorded in Spanish and Portuguese sources.[121] Apparently asylums were established in 1680 in Nangang (probably Nan'an), Jiangxi province, 1681 in Tung Kuan (Dongguan), Guangdong province, 1685 in Sing Ching (possibly Xinxing, Zhaoqing prefecture) and in Xe Lun village (possibly Shilong, in Dongguan district[122]), and 1686 in Chao Cheu (probably Chaozhou). However, these sources show that in most cases, missionaries managed to do evangelical work only among lepers in local leprosaria or outside city walls, or to build simple chapels for lepers. Individual missionary asylums existed only briefly and on a small scale as funding and management were understandably difficult.[123] Moreover, even such limited activities likely diminished after 1732, when Emperor Yongzheng ordered all missionary activities outside of the capital expelled from China and limited to Macao.[124] Other sources indicate that Dominican missionary leper asylums existed in Fujian province during the last years of the Ming and before the 1732 edict.[125]

Most of these asylums were probably small in scale, accommodating from a dozen to a few dozen inmates, like the ones in northeastern Fujian. Moreover, most hospices did not really have proper medical equipment, and inmates were treated mostly by traveling medical missionaries.[126] Only a few were large enough to take in more than a hundred patients, who enjoyed more regular medical care, like the one in Macao, "which contained 115 patients in 1726, though 60 or 70 seems to have been the usual number."[127] In other words, from scarce early Catholic missionary sources, one can conjecture that European lazar houses were established in southeastern China from the mid-sixteenth century onward. Most, however, were set up without leaving written records. We know that many undesirables of metropolitan Portugal, including lepers, traveled overseas in this period to find refuge. The southeastern coast of China was one of their destinations.[128] As the leper house in Macao might indicate, such asylums provided refuge not only to Chinese but sometimes also to European lepers.[129]

After the Yongzheng edict of 1732 and before the massive arrival of modern missionaries in the mid-nineteenth century, individual Catholic missionaries continued their evangelical work among lepers in isolated spots in inland China and went unnoticed by the Manchu court. A French missionary, Father Pottier, for example, established, in a rural area around Chengdu in Sichuan province, a small lazar house, where he cared for some seven or eight lepers between 1773 and 1778.[130] We still know too little about such activities during the long century between 1732 and the opening of China in the mid-eighteenth century. However, the fact that the first Catholic missionaries who arrived in China after the Opium War often picked up work among lepers as one of their first tasks, and that a number of them were known to have died from leprosy[131] may be an indication that there was continuity in that work. However, the early Catholic leper asylums were probably too small, too religious, and their existence too short to rouse the interest of Chinese activists. The major change from the mid-nineteenth century onward was naturally the increasing importance of Protestant missionary work, which soon posed a serious challenge to the Catholics. By the end of the nineteenth century, both Protestant and Catholic leprosaria, like many of their other medical institutions, had taken on a new outlook that the Chinese Nationalists found inspiring.

Early Catholic asylums were small in scale, and they had conspicuous evangelical objectives, as the missionaries' main concern was the number of lepers baptized in the asylums. Late-nineteenth-century leprosaria were bigger, more structured, with subtler and more sophisticated evangelical methods. Major leprosaria, those that could be considered by Chinese elites as possible models, were established only from the late 1880s onward, when the contagion theory was slowly gaining ground and with the growing influence of the international Protestant international organization Mission to Lepers, established by the British missionary W. C. Bailey in 1874 with a special interest in India, where Bailey built his first leper asylum in 1875.[132] By 1893, the Indian mission had set up ten asylums and was supporting eight others; the number of asylums rose to nineteen by 1899, many of which were removed to the outskirts of towns.[133] By the first decade of the twentieth century, not too long after the first international congress on leprosy in Berlin in 1897, activists were quite confident of "a growing world movement for the segregation and care of the approximately three million lepers scattered throughout the world." The mission gave itself the task "to cooperate with governments in order to secure *ultimate world-wide segregation of lepers*" (italics mine). It was active then not only in India but also all over East Asia and was instrumental in the establishment of the National Leprosarium in Carville, Louisiana, U.S.A., in 1917, the only disease-specific institution for the general public ever set up by the American federal government.[134] The series of missionary leprosaria set up in China beginning in the 1880s have to be understood in this international context, as some of the first larger size missionary asylums were established by the international Mission to Lepers. In 1921 the mission opened an East Asian office in Shanghai, which paved the way for the establishment of an indigenous Chinese Mission to Lepers association in the winter of 1926, affiliated with the British and American missions. Even though the Chinese Mission to Lepers claimed it was essentially a lay and patriotic organization, its Protestant association was strong and clear, and many of its board members were fervent Chinese Protestants.[135] The organ of the mission, the bilingual *Leper Quarterly,* began publication in the following year, promoting the setting up of leprosaria and the medical treatment of lepers in China.[136]

According to missionary sources, at least fifty-one leper asylums were set up in China between 1887 and 1940, when the survey was published by the *Leper Quarterly,* eight of which were related to the Mission to Lepers (American or British), eighteen to the Chinese Mission to Lepers, and seventeen others (see appendix).[137] This list is certainly incomplete, with an unknown number of essentially Catholic institutions not recorded.[138] We can see from the organization of some of the early missionary leprosaria their principles of organization. The Pakhoi (Beihai) leper house in Guangdong province was a typical Christian organization. The Pakhoi hospital, established by Dr. E. G. Horder, of the Church Missionary Society, began to take in lepers in 1887 with the assistance of the Roman Catholic Mission, and it had more than 200 patients five years later. It was thus considered by most missionaries and Chinese Christians to be the first leprosarium in China.[139] Male and female patients had separate quarters, and marriage between them was forbidden. They were also not allowed to enter the city, and received compulsory injections as treatment. Religious and economic activities were the main occupations of inmates. For the latter, men produced simple handicrafts such as bamboo baskets, grass sandals, and brooms, whereas women made lace. Their products were first disinfected before the agent delivered them to buyers in England.[140]

In other words, the institution was established for the isolation, medical treatment, and moral and spiritual transformation of inmates through work and religious activities, typical of missionary organizations. The emphasis on practical work for the inmates was probably based on the Christian idea of moral and spiritual discipline. L. Fowler, a prominent China expert, stated, "Indeed, some one has recently described leprosy as 'a disease of laziness.' It is true to state that activity of body and mind under any circumstance is a condition making for the health of anyone; it is specially so in the case of the leper." [141] Moreover, the practice of separating lepers from their kin and traditional community

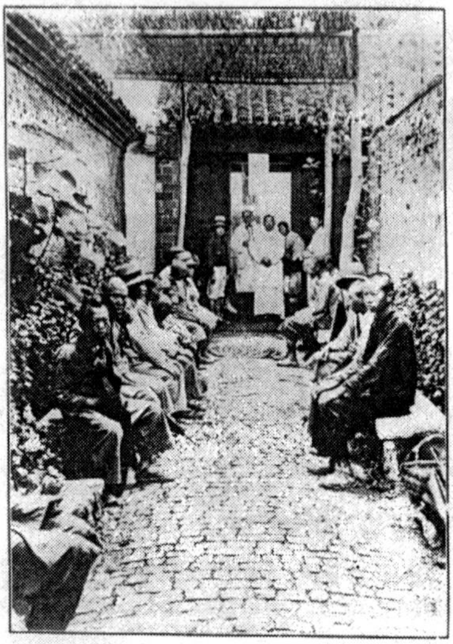

"And the poor have the gospel preached to them." A formal religious service precedes the leper clinic treatments each week.
(Jukao, Kiangsu.)

Leper Quarterly of May 1938 illustrates the importance of missionary religious work in the Rugao asylum in northern Jiangsu province.

provided missionaries with an effective means of evangelization.[142] Similarly, Duncan Main, founder of the leper hospital in Hangzhou, was pessimistic about the prospects for curing incoming lepers but found satisfaction in teaching them to read the Bible and explaining the Gospel to them, which, he thought, brought them hope and comfort. H. Fowler, of the Hiau-kan (Xiaogan) asylum in Hankou, expressed the same sentiment.[143] As in India, missionary leper institutions in the late nineteenth and early twentieth centuries were basically organized for evangelical purposes, as a bodily cure was then, as the medical missionaries well knew, impossible.[144]

Very soon, Chinese Nationalist activists, even Christian ones, decided that the missionary model was in fact also not ideal for segregating lepers. There were several characteristics of the missionary leprosaria that displeased the Chinese: first, the emphasis on religious activities was considered too strong; second, consequently their medical work seemed to be too soft; and third, the isolation of patients was not strict enough. What the Chinese wanted, including those sympathetic to the Christian faith, was an efficient system that would either cure the lepers quickly or eradicate the disease from China in the foreseeable future, or, failing that, strictly separate the sick from the healthy. The Chinese authorities often accused missionary asylums of being too close to urban centers or of letting their inmates go out too easily. Both the Hangzhou asylum of the Church Missionary Society and the Catholic Moximian colony (Kangding) were criticized for their slack discipline of inmates, creating fear and anger among healthy communities nearby.[145]

In fact, the different attitudes of missionaries and local Chinese authorities toward the question of disciplining of patients were obvious at the very beginning of the Republican period. Local authorities often took popular resentment as an excuse to criticize the lax missionary policies. French Catholics working in Nanning, Guangxi, recorded a popular revolt against their relief work for local lepers in 1913 in which the population accused the colony of being too close to the city: "National pride, distrust, and hatred towards foreigners have filled the high officials," who, they believed, were behind the revolt. Violence connected with the revolt finally targeted the lepers of the colony, who were, according to the missionaries' record, rounded up and massacred by the military. A rumor went about saying that anyone reporting a leper to the authorities (so that he/she could be exterminated) would be rewarded with a small amount of money. The missionaries also described a proclamation by a local official that a higher order had been given to kill all lepers in Nanning so that the population would forever be free from contagion.[146] This event was perhaps reported with exaggeration and prejudice on the part of the Catholic missionaries in Nanning, but it serves as an extreme, therefore stereotypical illustration of the deep concerns of the Nationalists regarding the leprosy problem. The disease was a national shame that had to be dealt with radically, as efficiently as possible, and preferably by Chinese hands. Any slackness would lead to contagion, and therefore more cases. The Nationalist model of segregation was ideally one that would eventually put an end to contagion while working toward an effective cure of the disease.

The Nationalist Hybrid Model

The Nationalist model became conspicuous only from the 1920s onward, more than a decade after the Republican Revolution of 1911, led by Sun Yat-sen, that ended the Manchu dynasty but also set in political chaos. The republic was soon usurped by the military strongman Yuan Shikai, who restored the monarchy in 1916 shortly before he died. His death only launched a decade of military anarchy, however, with China torn between warlords. The situation provoked the development of a strong and popular nationalist sentiment, expressed in a series of radical anti-imperialist and anti-Christian movements, and also an unquenchable thirst for Western science and democracy, deemed indispensable for China's much-needed modernization. The Communist movement also grew rapidly during this period. The successful Northern Expedition, led by the Nationalist Jiang Jieshi (Chiang Kai-shek) ended this anarchical state in 1928, and China was finally united under the Nationalist government, until the Sino-Japanese War broke out in 1937 followed by the civil war between the Nationalists and the Communists. It was mainly during the 1920s and 1930s that elites of the Nationalist period experimented on a new model of leprosy asylum.

In general, the Nationalist activists preferred strict isolation of identified patients using military force. One typical example was the taking over of the Swatow (Shantou) asylum from the missionaries by the provincial government in 1922. Replacing an old Christian institution set up in 1867, the asylum was located on a small island about four miles from the city. The colony was by then entirely supported by the municipal government. When T. C. Wu, general secretary of the Chinese Mission to Lepers, visited the place in the spring of 1926, it had forty-one inmates. According to Wu, "A demarcation line, over which no leper was allowed to step, was drawn. A heavy guard was placed to keep order and to prevent the lepers from escaping." Inmates received weekly injections as treatment. On the other hand, the inmates complained that "they have not sufficient food to eat, and some of them have no beds on which to sleep, and no mosquito nets in summer. . . . There was no provision made in the way of recreation, work, or education, so these wretched men and women were kept absolutely idle."[147]

The attitude of the Chinese government toward segregation was even clearer in the case of the nationalization, in early 1927, of the Hangzhou asylum, which had been established by the Church Missionary Society. The new authority made two significant changes to the originally Christian institution. First, "religious meetings and Bible study are now strictly prohibited. Second, a most rigid segregation is being enforced. . . . Inside the asylum, all the gates are locked as though it were a prison. Nominally, lepers are allowed to get out on leave of absence, but when they ask for leave their requests are generally not granted."[148] Despite the fact that these reports on lay institutions, written by Chinese Christians, could have been biased, it is nonetheless obvious that, like the Japanese, strict segregation, considered as the most efficacious way of preventing further spread of the disease, was the preferred model of the Chinese. However, unlike the modern and powerful Meiji government, the Republican state did not have the necessary resources to manage or to sustain such a tough isolation policy. In fact, soon the Nationalists found they had to make compromises by cooperating with the missionaries to come up with a hybrid model, which would only partially meet their goals.

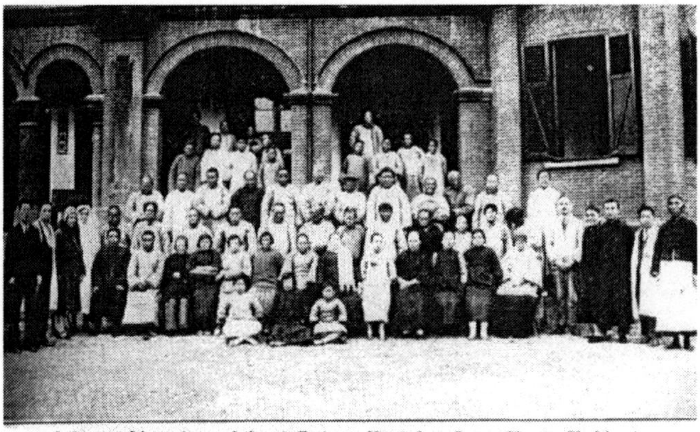
A group of inmates and the staff at our Hangchow Leper Home, Chekiang.
Dr. S. D. Sturton on the right, Mrs. Sturton and Sister S. Morris on the left.

Hangzhou leper asylum, as shown in *Without the Camp: The Magazine of the Mission to Lepers*, no. 160 (October 1936). (Courtesy of The Leprosy Mission International)

The Hangzhou asylum again serves as an example. The takeover by provincial authorities in early 1927 of that institution was temporary, lasting only until June 1928, when the Mission to Lepers regained control. The hospital was restored to its former managers with the intervention of the central government in the early summer of 1928.[149] For the missionaries, those unhappy sixteen months were due to the fanaticism of "certain left wing elements in the provincial government." From mid-1928, the institution was again under missionary management, but obviously with closer cooperation from the provincial government. The mayor of Hangzhou participated in the promulgation of a set of rules related to the discipline of inmates. The agreement seems to have been central to the mission's regaining of control of the institution. A plan for the enlargement of the institution, completed in 1932, was partly due to "the feeling which exists in certain quarters in Hangchow that all lepers should be segregated. This feeling was worked up artificially in the first place by the opponents of our work, but now has the salutary effect of helping us to keep the patients within bounds."[150] Obviously, the requirement of stricter discipline of the inmates and a more severe confinement policy were demanded by the provincial authorities before management was returned to the missionaries. It was also probably not an accident that the weekly injections given to inmates was greatly emphasized after the missionaries regained management. Detailed accounts of the chemical composition of the injections, how they were administered, and the condition of the inmates who had received such treatment were published, probably to show the Chinese authorities that the institution was above all a medical one, while evangelical activities were downplayed.[151]

Another major leper colony run cooperatively between missionaries and the Republican authorities was the Sheklong (Shilong) asylum at Dongguan, near Canton. The institution was the product of the international hysteria over the perceived world pandemic thought to be spread by Chinese emigrant coolies. It was created in 1907 by Father Conrardy (1841–1914), a Belgian member of the French Missions Étrangères de Paris and close associate of Father Damien in Hawaii. He was said to have closed the eyes of Damien on his deathbed.[152] After he left Hawaii in 1896, he went to Portland, Oregon, to study medicine and obtained a degree before going to Canton to start a leper colony,[153] probably on the Molokai model. He chose for a site two small islands (one for men, the other for women) in Dongjiang (East River), about three kilometers down from the Dongguan county seat, or sixty kilometers to the east of Canton. He worked to set up the basic foundation of the colony, including buildings and plantations, until his death from leprosy in 1914.

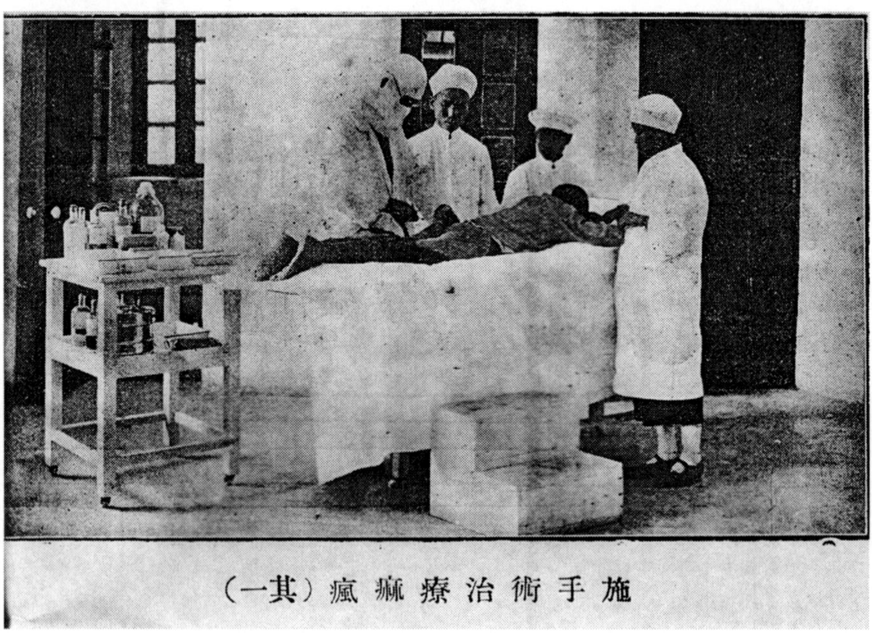

Photo from the July 1933 issue of the journal published by the asylum on Taikam (Daqin) island, emphasizing Western, scientific therapy in asylums. (Courtesy of Sun Yat-sen University, Guangzhou)

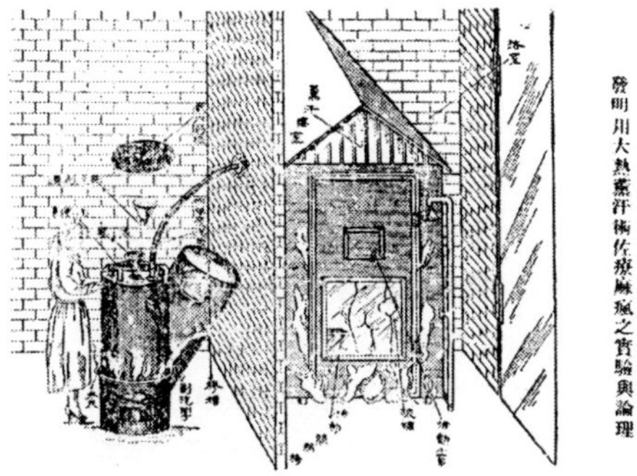

Conceptualization of a modern medicinal steaming machine based on traditional Chinese fumigation therapy, by a Chinese author in the June 1937 issue of *Leper Quarterly.*

In order to realize his Damien dream, Father Conrardy had to make a few political compromises in the early part of the twentieth century, especially since he wanted his colony to serve as a model. During its first years, the asylum was small and not distinguished. In 1910, Father Conrardy managed to keep only twenty-eight inmates, as a bigger institution was beyond his means.[154] The French government did not offer support of the project as Conrardy, although a member of a French mission, was a naturalized American, and, in the eyes of the French Ministry of Foreign Affairs, had always ignored the French Catholic protectorate and turned rather to the Americans for help. His early collaborators, several Canadian Catholic sisters, were, moreover, accused of serving British interests.[155] Competition between French and Anglo-American religious interests in China and the doubts about Conrardy's loyalty to French Catholicism left him with little choice but to ally with the Chinese, with all its consequences. Shortly before his death, in 1914, the provincial government stepped in. An agreement was signed between the Chinese authorities and the Catholic managers. The provincial government was to provide for all building and maintenance costs, besides a stipend of ten cents for each inmate per month, which roughly came to a monthly subsidy of around 1,000 yuan to the colony.[156] In return, the Canton government had the right to send in anyone identified as having the disease by the Bureau of Health. Often the police were responsible for taking patients to the colony. The missionaries were to manage the colony. Due to such active government participation, Sheklong quickly developed into the biggest leper colony in the Republican period in terms of the number of inmates. Rapid expansion actually began in 1913, when the Chinese government sent in some 750 lepers, most of whom had been arrested on the streets of Canton. Later on, lepers repatriated from Hong Kong were also sent there, greatly increasing the population of the asylum.[157] In its prime year of 1922, it had more than 1,000 patients. By 1923, it had treated a total of 3,173 lepers since its establishment.[158] As late as 1940, it accommodated almost 900 lepers.[159]

Its contract with the Canton government, however, left the asylum vulnerable in the 1920s, following the death of Father Conrardy and with the destabilization of the political situation in Canton, eventually leading to the irregularity of Chinese funding.[160] The French government, too, was unwilling to provide diplomatic and financial support to the colony, which had benefited from American Catholic money and Hong Kong government and philanthropic donations.[161] Despite such gifts, financial problems remained a chronic problem for the colony in the 1920s, especially as it attempted to maintain itself as a model colony.

Following his visit to the colony in 1926, T. C. Wu observed, "The colony was perfectly arranged. The place was clean and the roads were flat. Flowers and trees were plenty. All inmates, women and men, children and adults, except those who have lost the extremities of their limbs were required to work, that is, toiling in the surrounding fields. The colony provided seeds, farming instruments and draught animals. Labor was also paid for by the colony, and farm products were sold to cover expenses. . . . There was a school inside the colony. An educated inmate taught some forty students one hour a day. Religious activities were extremely important. . . . The one thing that most disappointed me was that there was no injection of ethyl esters of chaulmoogra. When asked why they did not have the dose, Father Deswazières answered simply that they did not have the money."[162] However, it seems that the priest who succeeded Deswazières in the early 1930s, Marsigny, did manage to contract a doctor in Hong Kong to visit and treat inmates. In fact, financial assistance had occasionally come from France, the United States, and the Vatican during the several decades of its existence. The Hong Kong government later became the other major regular financing party of the asylum, probably beginning in the 1930s, when it began repatriating Chinese lepers found in the British colony to Sheklong. It provided some 80 percent of its regular expenditures, whereas the subsidy from the Guangdong government covered some 20 percent of the entire budget.[163]

The idyllic appearance of the Sheklong colony and the much-publicized cooperation between the Canton government and the French missionaries seem to have made Sheklong one of the best-known "Nationalist" models in Republican China, inspired probably by Molokai or Culion. However, behind this serene facade, there were circumstances indicating harsh political realities faced by the colony. Ill feelings had existed from the very beginning over the subsidy question. The agreement between the Catholic missionaries and the Canton government was a compromise that left no one happy. The missionaries were not satisfied with the amount of money they received from the Chinese at the outset, especially when they compared it with the American subsidy to Molokai, the world-class leprosarium. Even when that modest amount became irregular in the 1920s, they were obliged to take in all the lepers sent in by the Chinese authorities, according to the agreement.[164]

For the Chinese Nationalists, the foreign and religious aspects of the colony had never been to their taste. Providing monthly subsidies to an institution that had acquired a semiofficial status struck them as similar to the imperial government's past arrangements with its leprosaria, only now the headmen were untrustworthy foreign missionaries. The Canton government, however, did not have much choice either. It was under pressure to clear the streets of leprous beggars and receive from neighboring British Hong Kong repatriated emigrants found to be infected with the disease. The agreement with Sheklong, which was only a short distance from the Canton-Kowloon railway, was simply the quickest and easiest solution for Canton. The deep distrust of the missionaries showed itself in the large military force—two squads of armed soldiers—that the government put on the islands, officially to prevent inmates from escaping and patients

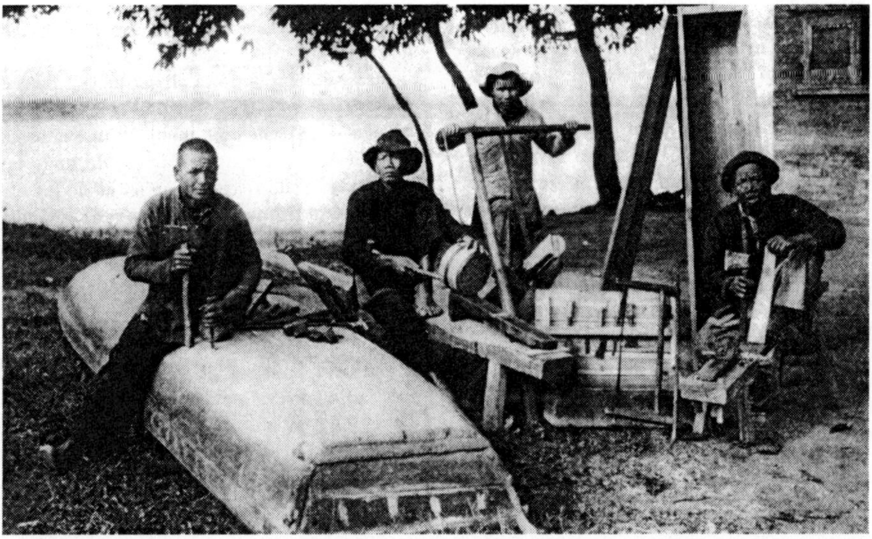

Photo from *Missions catholiques*, no. 58 (1926), showing patients working on their boat in the Sheklong (Shilong) colony, near Canton. (Courtesy of Missions Étrangères de Paris)

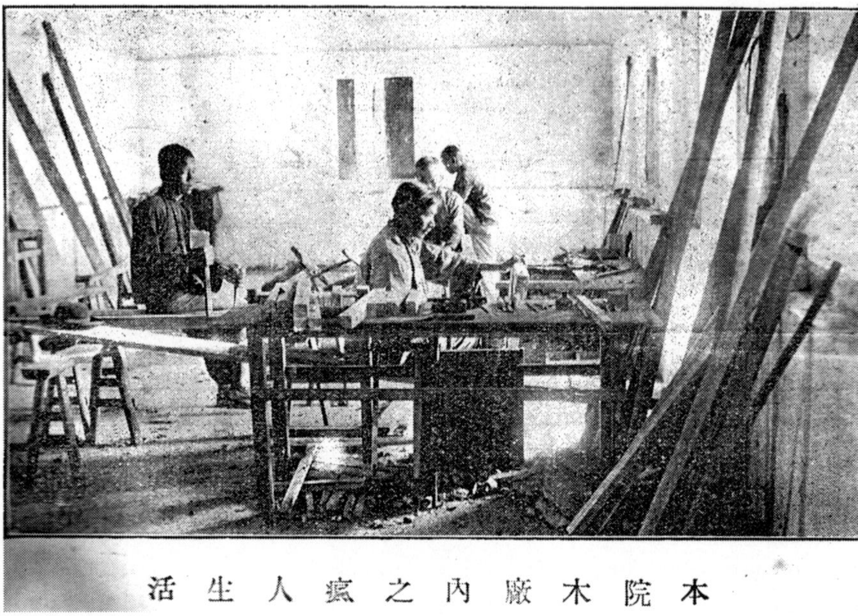

Photo from a 1934 issue of the journal published by the asylum on Taikam (Daqin) island, showing patients doing woodwork. (Courtesy of Sun Yat-sen University, Guangzhou)

of the two sexes from mixing.[165] With that military presence, one also understands why the missionaries continued to honor the agreement even when, as they claimed, the Chinese were not giving the subsidy regularly in the 1920s.[166] In sum, the hybrid model was not exactly what the Chinese had hoped for, as there were too many things that they could not control directly. However, both the Chinese and the missionaries kept up a good face on the enterprise for many years, and it appears to have been one of the more satisfactory asylums in China in the 1920s and 1930s. The model exemplified the sharing of responsibilities between the Chinese government and the missionaries: the duty of the former was to identify and send in patients, whom they kept interned with military force, and the missionaries managed the institution and provided treatment.[167] In this way, the model justified the Chinese state as the sole legitimate source of political power, and the missionaries' evangelical work as a sideline of medical service.

However, as the examples of Hangzhou and Sheklong clearly reveal, cooperation between the two parties was, from the start, shaky, as it was based on convenience and force rather than on true mutual reliance. Distrust and disdain were strong on both sides, each having its own agenda and not always compatible with that of the other. However, the patriotic, Christian Chinese Mission to Lepers did not give up the ideal and set up the National Leprosarium of Shanghai shortly before the outbreak of the Sino-Japanese War, in 1936.[168] It was managed and partly financed by the mission, with contributions from the city government of Shanghai and the Shanghai Municipal Council. The institution was delegated to provide care to lepers of all classes and research facilities for specialists of the disease. It had different norms for charging patients, and fees for the destitute were to be covered by donations. Without official support from the Nationalist government, it was not a state institution like Carville, in the United States, although organizers nonetheless claimed some national status and pressed for financial help from the central government. It was obviously meant to be a showcase for China's civilized effort to combat leprosy in cosmopolitan Shanghai. The institution was, however, constantly under financial pressure until the 1940s.[169] The fact that war broke out almost immediately after its establishment greatly limited its development and reduced its significance as a Nationalist model. Relations between the central government and the missionaries continued to be strained from the 1930s onward, when the relevance of segregation was increasingly questioned by leading medical missionaries in China, while the Chinese state grew more nervous about the apparently unimproved situation of leprosy in the country. Meanwhile, the threat of war approached ominously.

The civil war period between 1945 and 1949 witnessed renewed efforts of the Nationalist government to tackle the problem, often in necessary collaboration with foreign and indigenous Christian organizations. In Yunnan, for example, there were concerted efforts from 1947 to expand the provincial colony in Kunming with the help of the International Mission to Lepers, a Protestant organization that sent in Western medical experts and chemical drugs, notably Promin. The proposed plan was to expand the colony on the site of the former American military hospital. One of the main points the provincial authorities emphasized in these efforts was to "call for the attention of Christian groups to cooperate in the name of Jesus Christ." Similarly in Fujian, the provincial government provided public land to the Christian Xiehe hospital in Fuzhou to establish a bigger leper colony.[170] The local government of Qingdao, Shandong province, also had to ask the Chinese Mission to Lepers for financial and medical help in order to maintain the public asylum after the war.[171] However, these and many other similar efforts were cut short when the Nationalist government lost the civil war to the Communists.

Segregation: Doubted but Desired

James Maxwell, probably the most authoritative and outspoken expert on leprosy in China in the early twentieth century, was always suspicious of the contagiousness of leprosy and never quite believed in the effectiveness of segregation. As early as 1911, he wrote that "the leper asylums at present in China are voluntary institutions and, splendid examples as they are of Christina kindness for the afflicted . . . most of them are of no use whatever as places of isolation."[172] He began to criticize openly the segregation policy pushed by the Chinese government in the late 1920s. In 1930 he coauthored a memorandum with Wu Lienteh to the Ministry of Health in conjunction with the proposal of organizing a Central Leprosy Council, suggesting that "segregation in the strict sense is now undesirable." Using what he thought was the failure of the Culion colony in the Philippines as an example, he emphatically pointed out to the Chinese government that, first, systematic segregation of all lepers was technically impossible, as patients at the early stage of the disease could not be identified and would hide themselves in order to avoid being segregated, thus increasing the danger of undetected contagion; second, the enterprise was economically too burdensome for the Chinese state to support, as the number of lepers, coming mostly from rural areas, was too large; third, the disease was not as contagious as popularly thought, and outpatient treatment, especially at the early stage, and in rural areas, where most leprosy cases originated, should be the focus of the national policy. He recommended the Chinese government reform its present policy after the Indian model, by training schoolteachers or nurses in rural areas to provide simple medical treatment to patients affected with the disease at the early stage. Segregation should be required only for patients at the advanced stage of the illness. He also urged the government to carry out nationwide surveys to find out the exact situation of the disease and to form a council at the national level to deal with the problem.[173] These views were supported by a few missionaries in China, such as F. Reiss, F. Muir, and C. M Galt.[174] C. M Hasselmann, from Manila, spoke to a Chinese audience in 1932 in support of Maxwell's view that compulsory segregation in the Philippines, including the costly Culion enterprise, had "utterly failed" in stamping out leprosy from the Philippines. While the colony had treated an impressive number of patients inside it, it had also scared away more victims of the disease, who went unreported and untreated, and infection continued at large.[175] Reasonable as these views might have been in respect to the nature of the epidemic in China, they were totally insensitive to the nature and limits of the Republican government's political power, the social conditions in the country, and popular opinion.

Abandonment of the policy of segregation and, in its stead, an emphasis on outpatient treatment would have represented for the general Chinese public an unthinkable relapse into the imagined old, anarchical situation responsible for the deplorable spread of the disease. For the state, it implied its incapacity to support a modern, scientific institution and an invitation of a constant public and foreign scrutiny of the omnipresent, ugly, unhealed lesion on the body politic. What Maxwell was suggesting was replacing a highly publicized, costly, and compulsory segregation with an integrated and centralized national policy, one that was in fact much more difficult for China to implement in the 1930s. What Maxwell was thus asking for was nothing short of further exposing the national shame and the state's political and administrative incompetence. On the other hand, Maxwell's stance was controversial in other respects. Missionaries working in the Philippines, colonized by the United States, and on Formosa, a Japanese colony, strongly disagreed with him. Dr. Wade, working in the Culion colony, responded in 1929 that dispensary treatment and voluntary isolation would not ensure a sufficient proportion of the sick population received proper and effective treatment, and that the improvement of living standards and hygiene in the country, necessary conditions for the retreat of the disease, was unlikely to occur under a different system. Instead, he suggested a more elaborate segregation policy, including expanding the "occupational colonies" and an isolation hospital, with the outpatient clinic only a minor part of the system.[176] Dr. George Gushue-Taylor (1882–1953), working on Formosa, similarly doubted the suitability of outpatient treatment in China as suggested by Maxwell and insisted that compulsory segregation was necessary if China wanted to eradicate leprosy.[177] In fact, he indicated that years of outpatient treatment for lepers on Formosa, which had a good and stable government (Japanese colonial) and medical service better than that in most neighboring countries, convinced him that residential treatment was still a better solution for fighting leprosy. His preference for segregation synchronized well with the Japanese colonial government's growing preference for stricter regulation since the late 1920s, that culminated in the drawing up of the national law on segregation of lepers in 1931. In fact, before the colonial government's establishment of its official asylum in 1930 in Taipei, Gushue-Taylor had already begun to gather funds for creating the first missionary leper colony in 1925. The Christian colony was finally set up in the Taipei area in 1932 and was merged with the government asylum after the outbreak of the Pacific War. This asylum continued to function under the Nationalist government after its takeover in 1945.[178] The Japanese policy on leprosy control in the 1930s indeed served as the model for the Nationalist government, which political and cultural elites had criticized for failing to emulate such a model.

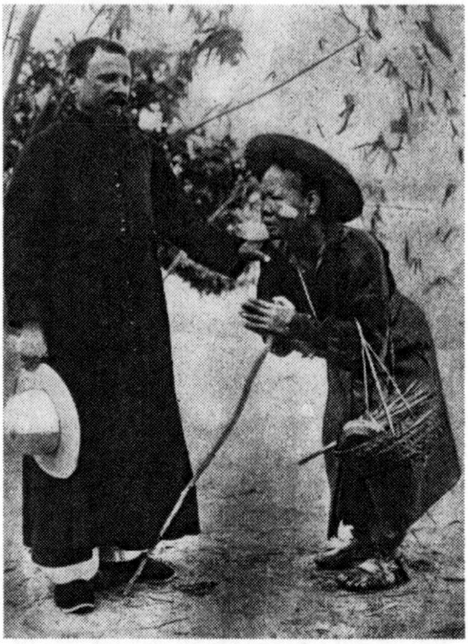

Photo from *Missions catholiques,* no. 61 (1929), showing Father Deswazière, of the Sheklong (Shilong) colony, with a grateful patient. (Courtesy of Missions Étrangères de Paris)

The complexity of the leprosy problem in China left the controversy totally unsettled, with each camp insisting on its own position. Each probably had an idea of what compulsory segregation meant that was often different from that of the others. The Chinese in general understandably disagreed with Maxwell. T. C. Wu, for example, though sensitive to Maxwell's criticisms and suggestions, selectively accepted his suggestions but nonetheless maintained the necessity of segregation. He even recommended the promulgation of further legislative control of leprosy by the Nationalist government to facilitate more systematic segregation, a position clearly inspired by the Japanese policy.[179] The colony in Culion, considered an example of failed segregation by Maxwell and Hasselmann, was publicly cherished as an ideal institution by Chinese activists.[180] Both sides did agree, however, that the Nationalist government was to blame for the disappointing results of leprosy control efforts, whatever the real cause. T. C. Wu criticized the government for not being enterprising enough in tackling the leprosy question,[181] and for providing care to only some 5,000 lepers in institutions out of the alleged 1 million sufferers in the country.[182] He also publicly expressed his dissatisfaction with the government's unresponsiveness to the 1936 establishment of the National Leprosarium in Shanghai.

For Maxwell, the problem was different. In 1938, years after he had proposed, in vain, abandoning compulsory segregation, he uttered in a tone of deep frustration that the government still harbored "the folly of believing that the segregation of the lepers in settlements outside the cities was a public health measure of importance which would eventually rid the country of leprosy," and, despite the impossible economic cost of segregation as shown by the example of the Philippines, "this is the only plan which the public health authorities seem to have in mind."[183] The great disappointment with the central government felt by all parties was clearly expressed at the first National Conference on Leprosy, held in 1933. Delegates to the conference, including a number of foreign missionary experts, thought that the government was shunning its responsibility of dealing with the problem of leprosy, and the minutes of the conference clearly reveal the great anger and frustration of the experts toward its incompetence and indifference and resolved to petition the government to promulgate "modern and human laws for the better supervision and treatment of lepers."[184] Probably what at least some of the delegates had in mind was a lifetime exclusion law, with the goal of confining all lepers, similar to the law passed by the Japanese government

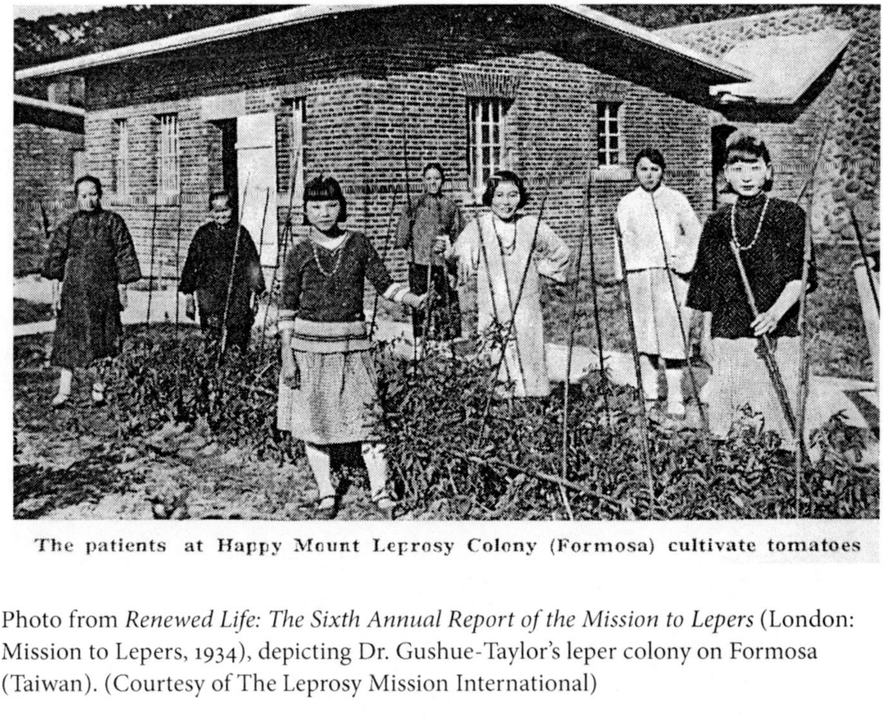

The patients at Happy Mount Leprosy Colony (Formosa) cultivate tomatoes

Photo from *Renewed Life: The Sixth Annual Report of the Mission to Lepers* (London: Mission to Lepers, 1934), depicting Dr. Gushue-Taylor's leper colony on Formosa (Taiwan). (Courtesy of The Leprosy Mission International)

in 1931 that was almost immediately applied to its colony Formosa, and by race-conscious countries like Australia,[185] considered by them as sensible and responsible in its strong policies.

In the end, the relevance of compulsory segregation to the problem of leprosy in China was not really at the center of public debate. All fingers pointed to the incompetence and weakness of the Nanjing government as the main cause of the stagnant or even deteriorating situation of this particular health problem in China. Chinese activists accused it of not giving enough money for the development of the ideal models of segregation. Missionaries in the Maxwell camp criticized it of completely misunderstanding the leprosy problem and of pursuing the wrong policy. All agreed that it had not paid enough attention to passing laws to supervise and manage patients. Meanwhile, the Maxwell's diagnosis seemed to be right, as, despite the establishment of more leprosaria, the number of lepers did not seem to decrease. In fact, no one knew the exact number of lepers in the country, and the government was not ready to carry out a nationwide survey. At the same time, the problems of insufficient funding and management were haunting all the bigger asylums. These problems did not, however, shake the conviction of the Chinese activists of the necessity of segregation. While the traditional model of segregation, which, in the final analysis, produced effects not that different from those of the modern one, was easily dismissed as irrelevant and useless for the situation, the modern hybrid leprosarium somehow seemed to be all the more indispensable. The international movement for segregation was perhaps something the Chinese activists could not resist. But perhaps a more important reason was that, without their being aware of it, the preferred solution for the leprosy problem was also dictated by the weight of tradition. Locking away the contagious leprous body had been, and persisted as, the simplest, most thinkable, and most direct solution for the suffering body politic. The conviction of the necessity of such a system was only reinforced by the new international situation of the modern period, namely, the perceived contamination of the world by the Chinese leper. Compulsory segregation remained at the foundation of the national policy of the much stronger central government after 1949.

FIVE

Leprosy in the PRC

Leprosy can be properly controlled
only through mass movements.
—Jiang Cheng (leprologist, PRC, August 2005)

The epidemiological story of leprosy entered a different stage from the second half of the twentieth century onward. With the growing use of sulfonamides, the disease came under much better control, and the reduced human migrations since the Cold War seem to have calmed the popular fear of global contamination. China could have pursued a significantly different policy on leprosy control from segregation, the favorite option of the Nationalist elites. Nonetheless, the People's Republic of China (PRC) chose to double the efforts to segregate patients in asylums and villages on a national scale, and did so with much greater success than the Nationalist government. Perceived to be a national rural pandemic, and no longer a disease of the south, leprosy became, probably for the first time in Chinese history, officially targeted by the central government as a major contagious disease. Firmly established in the political agenda, leprosy control, centering on the construction of a national network of segregative villages, became, above all, a persuasive illustration of a successful and efficient government. The PRC revealed itself through this health policy as a regime of a notably distinctive character, one with unprecedented central political power aimed at full national integration possessed of every modern means. In a sense, this policy had been the dream of many Nationalist activists. Perhaps the PRC, in the early 1950s, had little choice but to pursue this nationalistic dream based on political rather than purely medical considerations.

This chapter does not pretend to provide a complete picture of the leprosy situation in post-1949 China. A huge amount of information kept in local archives, most not easily accessible when this project began, even now has not yet been examined. Most of the available sources, and the authorities, emphasize the "success" of leprosy control, and materials on this aspect are abundant. On the other hand, a number of delicate issues remain difficult to clarify, especially those related to the early period. One wonders, for instance, how some of the repressive and extremist attitudes and measures supported by local political leaders toward patients in parts of the country so well publicized in the 1930s and 1940s persisted or changed in the 1950s and 1960s. We have good reasons to believe that traditional beliefs concerning the disease persisted well after 1949.[1] A survey in Hong Kong, south China, and Taiwan in the 1960s also revealed this trend.[2] This might have had an important influence on the conceptualization of the nationwide leper village system and on local control practices, revealing meaningful regional differences, observable even today, that are regrettably underdocumented in this study. With such shortcomings in available sources, I can only attempt to provide a general picture of the leprosy control story and explain its political and social implications during the past five decades, from the flamboyantly optimistic state-building period before 1958 to one of radical revolutionary fanaticism, from the Great Leap Forward to the Cultural Revolution, followed by the gradual opening of the country in the 1980s to a market economy and to the outside world.

GENERAL DEVELOPMENTS, 1950S–1990S

One of the first tasks that the PRC undertook in regard to leprosy control that had been neglected during the Republican period was the organization of systematic regional surveys, which formed the basis of the first national statistics on the problem. In 1956, the "preliminary figure" of sufferers in the entire country was said to be between 380,000 and 390,000. There were, moreover, some 160 institutions treating or accommodating about 20,000 of the sufferers, plus more than one hundred outpatient clinics.[3] The figure of between 380,000 and 390,000, in fact, remained more than preliminary and became the official national figure of the 1950s, even though surveys carried out in individual provinces (see following) suggest that this official figure was a low estimate. Indeed, important experts working in China, such as the American leprologist George

Hatem (1910–1988), celebrated as a heroic fighter of leprosy in the PRC, stated publicly that he believed the national number in the early 1950s was as high as 500,000, an opinion shared by many missionaries of the Republican period and by the World Health Organization (WHO).[4] At any rate, by the latter half of the 1950s, leprosy had been clearly defined and dealt with as a rural pandemic, and the program to prevent and treat the disease was included in the "essentials of national agricultural development," published by the central government in 1956. In 1957, the Ministry of Health announced a national plan for leprosy control, with three main emphases: surveys, segregation, and treatment.[5]

Provincial surveys carried out in the 1950s revealed regional differences of the leprosy problem. Figures available to us show that the problem was especially serious in a number of provinces: Guangdong counted more than 140,000 sufferers in the early 1950s;[6] Jiangsu province between 50,000 and 60,000 in the same period; Shandong more than 50,000; Fujian more than 15,000, which is likely an underestimate;[7] and Guangxi more than 10,000, again, a figure lower than expected.[8] Other available statistics, being cumulative and not specific in time, also indicate fairly high prevalence rates in provinces such as Hunan, Hubei, and Jiangxi.[9] Xikang was estimated to have had more than 10,000 sufferers in the early 1950s. We do not have provincial figures for such regions as Zhejiang, Yunnan, Guizhou, Sichuan, Tibet, and Liaoning, where leprosy was considered to be widespread.[10] Provinces with high prevalence rates occurred all over China, with pockets of seriously infected areas in mostly poor, rural regions. Even though we do not have all the provincial figures, from what is available, we can tentatively conclude that a reasonable national figure in the 1950s would be somewhere between the official figure of 380,000 and 500,000, the number suggested by Hatem.

According to WHO's definition of the elimination of leprosy (a prevalence below 1 per 10,000 population), the PRC reached that target on the national level in 1982. Subnational elimination was accomplished at provincial, municipal, and autonomous regional levels by 1992.[11] In 1988, experts believed that leprosy could be eliminated in China by 1997, with the country's own, stricter criterion for leprosy elimination of a prevalence below 1 per 100,000 population.[12] By the year 2000, there was about 10 percent of counties or cities where this higher target had not yet been reached.[13] The confidence of the PRC in putting the disease under effective control was manifested in a series of national congresses on the question in 1990 and 1995, culminating in Beijing's hosting the Fifteenth International Congress on Leprosy in 1998, where the PRC's success in controlling the disease was enthusiastically applauded.[14] By and large, the fight against leprosy begun in 1949 had become a success story.

As for drugs, during the first thirty years, China relied heavily on dapsone (DDS), administered essentially by domestic doctors. You Jiajun, a famous leprologist of Shandong Qilu University and leader of the national leprosy program from the 1950s, along with cadres of the Ministry of Health concentrated their efforts on developing sulfone drugs, until at least 1956. The national Xinhua drug company began to produce sulfones on a large scale beginning in 1951. Apparently a few new drugs were tested and proved to be effective in Shandong, where You worked, although some were found to be too strong.[15] The plan for more production of sulfones to treat leprosy was confirmed by an article published in the *People's Daily* in January 1956 and in major medical journals.[16] DDS remained the most important Western drug used to treat leprosy until the application of MDT (multidrug therapy) in the 1980s, marking the beginning of the final stage of the leprosy control program. MDT was introduced by WHO and was first tested in Yangzhou prefecture and Sichuan and Yunnan provinces in 1982. Three years later, a specific WHO MDT treatment plan was introduced, and nationwide implementation began in 1987.[17] Thereafter, various provinces received aid and MDT drugs from WHO and other foreign countries and foundations.

The story of leprosy control in the PRC was a complex one involving a top-down policy-making model promoted by a strong state, which was at times interrupted, at other times enhanced by the series of tumultuous political movements during the first decades of the regime. It also involved technical questions, such as the administration of different chemical drugs, sometimes combined with traditional Chinese herbal ones, or innovations within traditional therapeutics. Given the size and complexities of the country, the program was never a truly uniform one. Regional or even local variations, in terms of economic power, social structure, and cultural heritage, were important elements affecting the implementation of the policies.

National Policy

Leprosy, like schistosomiasis and venereal diseases, as a rural, chronic and infectious disease affecting mostly poor peasants, was an ideal candidate as a targeted disease in the national health campaigns of the PRC. It was widespread enough to be dealt with on a national scale, and its chronic nature and associated stigma provided fertile ground for prolonged mass propaganda and mobilization. In every aspect, it was a worthy enemy for the PRC state, inspiring strategies on every administrative level to integrate rural health programs with production policies and political campaigns. Establishing an integral national health policy was a main task of the PRC after 1949. It is clear that the regime consciously conceived the policy as a key element in its state-building strategy. The purpose of the policy was not only the improvement of the population's general health but also the fulfillment of socialist ideals and national pride. For the latter reason, health policy was often designed to coordinate with major political campaigns.

One important aspect of the national health policy was to target particular groups of infectious and endemic diseases thought to be the most common and damaging to the Chinese population, especially in rural areas, and then to mobilize all political and social resources to combat them. There were naturally local variations of targeted diseases, but leprosy, like venereal diseases, remained at the top of the national list for a long time.[18] As early as 1950, the Ministry of Health had publicly called for special attention to be paid to leprosy control. A research group on leprosy was set up in Beijing in the early 1950s, headed by You Jiajun, who, in 1951, organized the first national training course for doctors specializing in leprosy. This course was attended by medical trainees from the provinces from the 1950s until the early 1980s, some of whom were in turn able to organize training courses back in their provinces.[19] Similar courses were later organized not only in the capital but also in the provinces.[20] Beijing was determined to maintain a reasonable number of leprosy specialists on all administrative levels.[21]

Besides the training courses, the Ministry of Health also provided, as early as 1952, special incentives to encourage workers to participate in leprosy control programs. Medical personnel dealing with leprosy, together with those who worked in national minority areas (i.e., in economically backward regions), in hospitals for acute contagious diseases, and in TB hospitals and clinics, received a special state subsidy on top of their pay, equivalent to 10 to 20 percent of their regular salary. There was obviously a lack of such personnel in the early 1950s, and the subsidy was a way to attract more medical expertise into these areas.[22] Consideration of strategies in leprosy control continued in the early 1950s, and, in 1953, a first national meeting on the prevention and treatment of leprosy was held, emphasizing the importance of both prevention and cure.[23] The announcement of a National Plan for Leprosy Control came in 1957, and, in the following year, segregation, in the form of leper villages, was integrated into the Great Leap Forward movement.[24]

The pace of development varied from province to province. As early as 1951, Fujian province had begun to set up clinics and hospitals in Fuzhou. Beijing urged the provinces to establish their own Leprosy Preventive Plans, and by 1956, fourteen provinces were said to have complied.[25] Basically, the implementation of leprosy control policies in the provinces followed, from the 1950s to the 1980s, the main lines defined by the central government. Most provinces, especially those where leprosy was considered rampant, dutifully observed the 1957 national guidelines demanding local authorities carry out surveys and implement segregation and treatment at the same time.

The 1957 plan, centering on a national network of rural leper villages and urban clinics and hospitals, called for the mobilization and coordination of several governmental departments: (1) the Ministry of Civil Affairs, responsible for the relief program; (2) Security, for the supervision of crimes involving lepers; (3) Agriculture, for organizing production in leper villages; (4) Health, for implementing surveys and prevention and cure of the disease; (5) the Women's Federation and Youth Corps, for promoting propaganda and mass mobilization; and finally (6) local party and government units for the actual organization of leper villages.[26] Again, one can see here the tremendous political value of the program of leprosy control, especially that of leper villages, in piecing together the various parts of the state machine on all administrative levels.

By the end of 1980, there were, according to official figures, 1,199 leper hospitals and villages, involving more than 9,000 specialized workers.[27] Though official figures did not distinguish between hospitals and villages, it is clear that the majority of the institutions were likely leper villages. In other words, from the 1950s to the early 1980s, the PRC's leprosy prevention policy centered on the establishment of rural leper villages, basically cheap, segregative, conveniently "self-sufficient" units with basic medical services provided by mobile or regular teams.

In order to consolidate leper villages, official policy encouraged patients to enter voluntarily. There were various forms of enticement to persuade sufferers of the disease to enter these villages. One was the conferring of the status of urban residents (*shangkou liang*), even though the villages were situated in rural areas. In theory, therefore, village residents enjoyed the same privileges as urbanites in terms of household registration and job allocation.[28] An even more attractive enticement was the monthly stipend village residents received. It is unclear if this was a regular practice in all leper villages, as no instructions were given in the 1957 national directive. However, individual examples indicate that at least some villages provided inmates with monthly stipends as early as the 1950s. When the provincial authorities of Guangxi took over the village in Suilu from the missionaries in 1951, each patient received a monthly stipend of four yuan from the provincial government. The same amount was given to patients of the Beihai (Pakhoi) asylum, originally set up by French missionaries.[29]

The national average for such stipends between 1957 and the early 1980s ranged from six to nine yuan a month.[30] In some cases the degree of physical incapacity of patients was used to determine the amount of stipend. In Kaiping, Guangdong province, for instance, from 1957 to 1981, totally crippled patients received nine yuan; the partially crippled received six yuan.[31] There was a marked increase in the amount of stipends for patients of leprosy from the 1980s. In Kaiping, in 1982, the monthly stipend for a totally crippled patient increased from nine to twelve yuan a month, and that for a partially crippled resident rose from six to nine yuan. The amounts rose further, to twenty-two and nineteen, respectively, in 1985.[32] For Sanshui district, of the same province, it is recorded that before 1982, each patient in a leper village received a stipend of seven to nine yuan a month, provided by the production team. From 1983–1984 onward, the amount rose to nine to twelve yuan, reaching nineteen to twenty-two yuan from 1985 to 1986.[33] Patients in other provinces also received an increase in their stipends.[34] The reasons behind the sudden increase of stipends in the 1980s were never specified. It was probably a strategy to lure otherwise unwilling patients to come forward for MDT treatment. The increase could also have been a result of the decreasing number of patients in such villages as a result of the success of MDT, and possibly a consequence of international subsidies from organizations such as WHO. Soon after the increase of stipends in the late 1980s, the number of leper villages, owing to their subsiding importance, fell steadily.

Other enticements for patients to enter leper villages at the initial stage included free medical care and basic necessities for their livelihood in the village, although they were supposed to work for their own living thereafter. In Kaiping district, Guangdong, for instance, from 1959 onward, each commune was to have a specialist who would distribute care and medicines to segregated patients.[35] These specialists were normally trained in the special courses organized by the central and provincial governments in the early 1950s, mentioned earlier.[36] They were to provide help to leper villages during their regular tours. Medication was also distributed by mobile medical teams organized by local governments. In Anhui province, the provincial leprosy hospital organized five mobile teams to provide care and medicine for neighboring villages from 1967 to 1971.[37]

However, exaggerated publicity on the advantages of entering a leper village seem to have created disillusionment in the late 1950s, so that cadres were later cautioned not to overdo the propaganda.[38] Such exaggeration was in fact necessary, as it was a difficult task to persuade reluctant patients to enter the segregated villages. A 1958 report relates that those who were not seriously sick were afraid of aggravating their situation by living with more seriously ill patients, who, they thought, would be economically dependent on better-off patients. Some worried that entering a leper village would deprive their own families of their labor. Others were concerned that their spouse would divorce them if they left home. Even though organizers reported that, after showing the families the remarkable facilities of the leper villages and explaining to them the principles of segregation, many willingly entered villages,[39] it is still difficult to understand fully why they would finally consent. The available sources fail to provide convincing answers to such an attitude change.

In a 1966 report, it is said that leper villages were far from being the place many patients desired to spend the rest of their lives. An internal document of the Health Bureau of Jiangsu province reported that most city dwellers refused to live in leper villages. One sufferer complained, "These villages are not like hospitals. Why should we come here? Living conditions are not as good as in towns." Many came with great expectations, thinking that they would receive full medical care, as advertised by the government, but they were disillusioned after a few days and left. Peasants were also reluctant to enter leper villages, as they preferred to receive medication at home, where they could still perform their domestic duties. Reports of the lack of funding of leper villages in the 1950s and 1960s throw light on their poor living conditions and the reluctance of peasants to remain in them.[40] In many parts of China, therefore, in the late 1950s and 1960s, the number of patients isolated was less than expected. In Jiangsu province, for instance, less than 50 percent of known cases was segregated in leper villages in the mid-1960s.[41]

There were cutbacks in the services provided by commune clinics during the Great Leap Forward, lasting until the early 1960s. This setback, however, only prompted Mao Zedon to make his famous June 26 directive in 1965 ordering the massive relocation of medical resources to rural areas, which triggered a series of drastic policies, such as sending large teams of medical personnel to the countryside and the implementation of the Barefoot Doctor program during the Cultural Revolution.[42] This feature of the PRC public health policy remained in force until the era of liberalization beginning in the 1980s.

Despite the early setback, leper villages, together with other institutions devoted to leprosy control, did contribute to the final dramatic retreat of the disease after the 1980s by providing a basic national network of treatment centers, down to the village level, that permitted a relatively thorough and systematic application of dapsone in the early decades and MDT from the 1980s onward. After having partially fulfilled their mission of segregating the "contagious," they became an indispensable infrastructural component of the implementation of drug treatment. Without the initial network of leper villages, clinics, and hospitals at various administrative levels set up beginning the 1950s, the "vertical program of leprosy control," allowing a relatively efficient administration of antibiotics and chemotherapy, would not have functioned so smoothly in the 1980s.[43]

Synchronizing with Major Political Movements

The development of leprosy control in the PRC underwent adaptation in almost every key stage of the turbulent political history of the country during its first four decades, and it became an inextricable part of its initial state-building process. The control policy closely synchronized with the outbreak and aftermath of the Korean War in the early 1950s, the Great Leap Forward in 1958, the Cultural Revolution in the mid-1960s, and, last but not least, the economic reforms beginning in the 1980s.

The Korean War

Leprosy control was intimately related to the Korean War in two stages: at its outbreak in 1951, and in its immediate aftermath. By 1951, in retaliation for the American intervention in Korea, the PRC began to confiscate churches, hospitals, schools, and philanthropic institutions originally sponsored by American and European missionaries. Beijing ordered all such institutions to become "self-sufficient" and "independent," cut off from all foreign financial subsidies, and the religious personnel working for such institutions were told, in early April 1951, to "study politics."[44] Since a great number of the leprosaria in China were missionary institutions set up in the late nineteenth century and thereafter, this political act became an important landmark for the nationalization of leprosy asylums and hospitals, big and small, in rural and urban areas.[45] In Guangdong province, for instance, beginning in September 1951, eight missionary leprosaria were taken over by the government, two of which were transformed into provincial hospitals specializing in the disease.[46] This wave of confiscation of foreign property allowed the Chinese government to take complete control of the nationwide network of leprosy institutions, facilitating the implementation of central policies right down to the grassroots level via provincial and county hospitals and clinics. On the other hand, the exodus of foreign specialists, nurses, and other medical personnel aggravated the problem of the lack of such resources, which was already being felt at the beginning of Communist rule.

The lack of resources was, however, partly compensated by the state after the outbreak of the Korean War. Many rehabilitation hospitals were built at the time to accommodate sick and wounded soldiers. Some were later turned into leprosy asylums to care for soldiers, cadres, and urban professionals and students with the disease.[47] The Korean War was also an element behind the first Patriotic Hygiene Campaign, in 1952. The campaign, focused on the extermination of pests, was launched to counter the first "germ war" said to have been launched by the imperialistic United States against China and Korea.[48] Shortly afterward, in the years of intensive collectivization between 1955 and 1965, the emphasis of the Patriotic Hygiene Campaign shifted to the national development of agriculture,[49] by improving hygiene conditions in rural areas.[50] It was in this context that the organization of leper villages was first integrated into the national program. As an institution to accommodate "contagious patients among the masses,"[51] leper villages became an important part of the public health program in the countryside.

The Great Leap Forward and Cultural Revolution

A great number of leper villages were organized during the years of collectivization, especially the two or three years after 1958. There are, however, indications that some leper villages were set up before the announcement of the 1957 national plan in provinces where the disease was rampant. Of course the English term "leper village" in the Chinese context was not new. It was used, in its English form, in an article by the French doctor Durand-Fardel in 1877, referring to a number of "villages where lepers were confined" on the outskirts of Canton city he learned of in the winter of 1875–1876 during his first visit in China.[52] James Cantlie called the indigenous leper asylum that he visited in 1894 with Sun Yatsen a "leper village."[53] *Mafeng cun,* as the Chinese term for "leper village," was almost nonexistent, however, before the 1950s. Indigenous institutions for leprosy sufferers were called *mafeng yuan* (leper asylums) by Chinese writers. Activists in the Republican period sometimes translated the term "leper colony" literally as *mafeng zhimindi* to more closely evoke the idea of a leper village. Chinese Christians were especially attracted to the idea of a colony of sufferers of leprosy who participated in production, considered a healthy physical activity and an important strategy for making an institution economically self-sufficient.[54] Christian activists were convinced that physical labor and economic self-reliance were two necessary conditions for the physical and spiritual health of inmates, and this Christian ideal was finally realized in the form of the leper village by the Communists. However, for PRC experts, the idea of the leper village was borrowed, above all, from Latin American experts. The contribution of Dr. S. Schujman, a leprologist from Carasco Hospital in Rosario, Argentina, who first visited China in 1956 and trained Chinese experts in 1958, was said to be decisive. Many experts consider leper villages set up in China in the 1950s and 1960s a version of the Argentine model.[55]

Leper villages in the PRC were in fact at the bottom of a hierarchical structure of segregative institutions for leprosy defined by the 1957 national plan for leprosy control. Following the plan, leprosy hospitals on the provincial level accommodated sick soldiers, cadres, employees of urban enterprises, and students. On the county level, there were clinics or "stations for leprosy control" or smaller hospitals.[56] Villages were directed to isolate sick peasants in the countryside. The Bureau of Health of Zhejiang province, for example, directed in 1957 that the two provincial leprosy hospitals, limited in the number of beds but obviously with better medical resources, only accommodate active military officials (*xianyi junguan*), government cadres, employees of enterprises, and students of institutions of higher education, whereas peasants were to be taken in by local leper villages set up on the edges of the patients' natural communities, in old temples, or in abandoned houses in remote areas. An important requirement was that these villages had to be "economically self-supporting," according to the principle of the collectivization movement.[57]

The acceleration in the building of leper villages really began in 1957–1958, at the height of the Great Leap Forward. In Guangdong at this time, the major counties began to set up leper villages, such as Kaiping, Jieyang, and Sanshui.[58] By 1959, seventy-four leper villages were said to have been established in Guangdong province. By 1962, there were 130 hospitals and villages.[59] Fujian held two meetings in 1958/1959 on leprosy control and ordered all counties and municipalities with more than thirty contagious cases establish a village. Many such villages were called rehabilitation villages (*kangfu cun*), later changed to leprosy control stations (*mafeng bing fangyi zhan*). The aim was to attain the total segregation of patients by 1962.[60]

In a 1959 article full of political propaganda promoting the Great Leap Forward, He Biao, Vice Minister of Health, reported that in less than one year in Shandong province, more than seventy leper villages had been established, "solving the age-old problem of isolating contagious patients of leprosy and achieving the goal of basically controlling contagion." Fujian, Guizhou, Shaanxi, Henan, Jiangxi, Hunan, and Jiangsu were all said to have made similar plans to set up networks of leper villages within one or two years.[61] By 1963, Fujian province had established a hierarchy of institutions for leprosy control: one hospital at the provincial level, ten at the county or municipal level, with twenty-four leprosy control stations and three specialized outpatient clinics at Xiamen, Quanzhou, and Zhangzhou that provided medical services to leper villages in their surrounding regions.[62]

The central government dictated three main requirements for the setting up of leper villages. Their location should be in naturally isolated spots with mountains or lakes separating patients from healthy communities. Organizers were encouraged to occupy old Buddhist or Daoist temples, lineage halls, or abandoned houses for that purpose.[63] Second, they should be organized as administrative villages combining medical treatment with agricultural production. Last, they were to be directly supervised by local party authorities.[64] The last point was stressed in official documents of the late 1950s and 1960s, demonstrating the political importance of this rural institution. According to the official policy, the size of leper villages should be flexible, accommodating from several dozen to several hundred patients, on land provided by county governments. Medical treatment was to be given free, while inmates were expected to participate in agricultural production.[65] The emphasis on flexibility in terms of size was in fact a way to enforce segregation under any circumstances. In some cases, leper villages could be created for as few as two to three patients. Out of the twenty-six leper villages still functioning in 1985 in Anhui province, twenty-two had fewer than ten patients, with the smallest having only two patients (in Dangtu), and many others housed only three to five patients. The biggest had thirty-one patients.[66]

Self-sufficiency was one "merit" of the villages that was most frequently mentioned in propaganda materials. The provincial authorities of Zhejiang, for instance, wrote in a 1957 report that, according to experiences in Shandong, Hunan, and Gansu, leper villages were the best form of prevention of contagion because the expenses of these "administrative villages" could be covered by the production of the villagers.[67] To achieve self-sufficiency, organizers of leper villages during the Great Leap Forward relied on cadres from communes to manage their work and production.[68] In Bailu village, Huiyang county, Guangdong province, for example, at its establishment in 1954 and under the management of fifty-eight cadres, its 431 patients were mobilized to form an agricultural cooperative (*nongye she*), subdivided into two production teams, each with three to four subgroups.[69]

This merit of leper villages as an integral part of the national agricultural production movement was again stressed in a talk by the leprologist You Jiajun in the People's Congress in the spring of 1960. You described leper villages as an "easy to establish, simple, and manageable" institution that coordinated perfectly with the "general line" of collectivism. Based on his experience in Shandong province, he considered leper villages with medical services provided by mobile teams as the "only and most appropriate" measure for the prevention and cure of leprosy in China, whereas hospitals were "too expensive, time-consuming, and unable to catch up with the present situation."

This period was also marked by a national emphasis on the return to traditional drugs and therapies. In the summer of 1956, the Minister of Health made the self-criticism in the First People's Congress that Chinese medicine had been neglected by experts. Highlighting the efficacy of traditional drugs became a politically correct discourse. Even You Jiajun, a Westernized doctor, stressed the importance of using both Western chemical drugs and traditional Chinese recipes.[70] He wrote in early 1960 in the *People's Daily* that, as four years were required for a complete therapeutic cycle for chemical drugs, which was long, Chinese drugs were recommended to be used in tandem with Western chemical drugs, since they seemed to be able to work according to a shorter cycle. You added, however, that there were not yet any "conclusive results" of experimentation on Chinese remedies, as "neither the dose nor the duration of the treatment could be specified."[71]

The use of Chinese drugs not only partly complemented the more expensive Western chemical drugs but also nourished the PRC's nationalistic discourse by elevating the status of traditional medicine, once denigrated by Republican intellectuals in a different nationalist discourse, to the same level as Western medicine. The necessity of applying traditional recipes to treat leprosy was explicitly stated in the 1957 national plan. There was a stated preference for the use of herbal drugs, with less discussion of other traditional methods, such as acupuncture, fumigation, and baths, which had been important in the traditional treatment of *li*/*lai*.[72] At the same time, a number of so-called effective recipes were being distributed to the Health Bureaus of various provinces. Jiangsu province, for instance, kept a report of fourteen traditional recipes compiled from old medical texts and said to be proven effective in Liaoning, Zhejiang, and Guangdong. These recipes almost exclusively had the function of "dissolving toxins, activating Blood, dissipating Wind, and expelling Dampness." Less-serious cases were to be treated with drugs that expel Wind and Dampness, two external pathogens believed to be the main causes of *li*/*lai*/*mafeng*; the seriously sick were to be given drugs that dissolve toxins or activate stagnant Blood, accumulated inside the body after years of illness. Indeed, the drugs commonly used in traditional recipes for the treatment of *li*/*lai*, such as chaulmoogra seed, flavescent sophora root (*kushen*), *Ledebouriella* root (*fangfeng*), fleeceflower root (*heshouwu*), ephedra (*mahuang*), dried silkworm larvae, scorpions, ginseng, pubescent angelica root (*duhuo*), Pallas's pit viper, earthworms, and so on, were commonly called for in the recipes. One of the recipes even included realgar, a toxic mineral that had fallen out of fashion in late imperial recipes, except for extremely serious cases.

Ingredients were mostly ground into powder and made into pills for swallowing. It is likely that some of these pills were distributed by leprosy control stations or clinics to various leper villages as curatives. Most of the recipes could be traced back to important traditional medical texts, and many were compiled in the Qing imperial compendium *Golden Mirror of Medical Orthodoxy* (see chap. 1), which remained a major medical reference book for most doctors of Chinese medicine in this period.[73] It is interesting to note that the belief in the efficacy of viper for the disease was still strong and viper wine was mentioned in some recipes.

New recipes based on traditional therapeutic principles were also developed in the 1950s and 1960s. One of the most quoted and appreciated drugs was *saofeng wan* (pill that sweeps Wind away), a recipe developed by the No. 6 Hospital, Zhejiang province, and based on old recipes in medical texts; it called for twenty to thirty ingredients, including chaulmoogra seed, flavescent sophora root, *Ledebouriella* root, fleeceflower root, angelica root, viper, and others.[74] Another indigenous herb, *leigong teng* (*Tripterygium wilfordii* Hook), said to be effective,

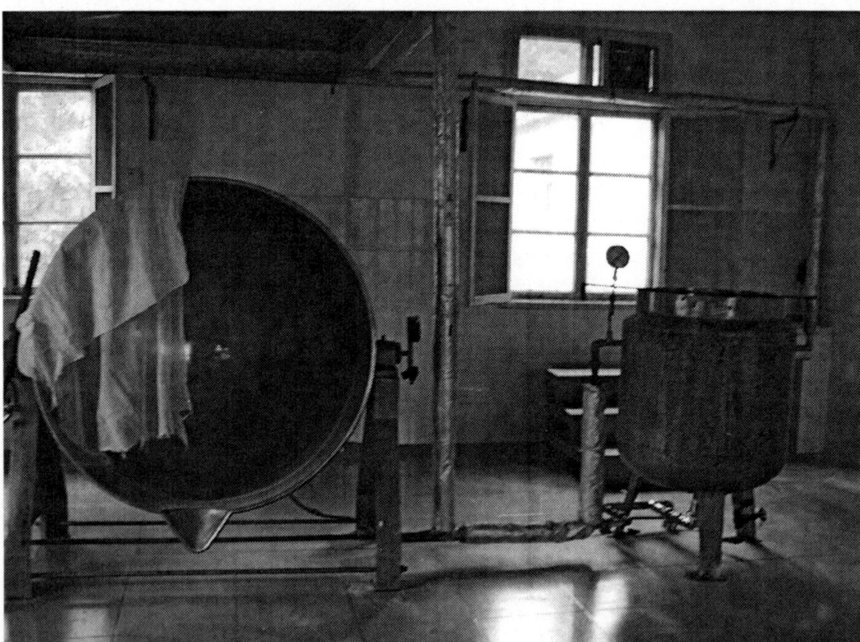

Equipment for processing the Chinese herb *leigong teng* (*Tripterygium wilfordii* Hook), at Wukang asylum. (Photo by author, August 30, 2005)

was first used by Chinese doctors in Gutian district, Fujian province, in 1962. An official report on the uses of the herb was finally presented in 1984, at the Twelfth International Leprosy Congress. The Wukang asylum (Zhejiang province) still operates the machines used in the fabrication of this drug for its patients (see following).[75] Guangdong experts claimed to have discovered the efficacy of *daxue teng* (Caulis Sargentodoxae) in the 1950s and 1960s.[76]The application of Chinese remedies was also accompanied by a draconian regime of food taboos, including fish, chicken, pork, goose, beef, lamb, bamboo shoots, mustard leaves, rape, taro, and ginger, which obviously left patients with an extremely limited choice of permissible foods.[77] Handbooks for barefoot doctors in the 1970s also recommended Chinese remedies, alongside chemical drugs (when available) for patients of leprosy, including the traditional viper wine.[78]

It is hard to evaluate the actual contribution of Chinese therapeutics in the leprosy control program of this period, as they were used together with chemical drugs. They were probably effective in treating some of the external symptoms of certain cases, and they were perhaps often the only drugs available in remote rural areas. According to Jiang Cheng, an expert active in leprosy control, despite the official appreciation of Chinese therapeutics, "they have not played a central role in the control program during the past decades."[79]

The Cultural Revolution seemingly had a disruptive effect on the leper village network, although mentions of such events in written records are usually brief. From these occasional descriptions, however, one can well imagine the deterioration of the situation. The most common fate of leper villages during the Cultural Revolution was abandonment. In Hubei province, it was reported that, during the peak years of the movement, patients simply left their villages.[80] Most of the time abandonment was the result of the total disorganization of the villages and the suspension of medical provisions. Sometimes the chaos nurtured serious conflicts between patients and the healthy villagers of neighboring communities.[81]

Worse still, there was allegedly serious abuse of village assets in some cases. In 1967, the 200 patients in the Sishan leper village in Anhui province became "revolutionaries" and expelled all the medical personnel, whom they labeled "capitalists." They consumed all the stored grain, killed all the pigs, and divided up all the cash among themselves. When the food and money ran out, they set up a casino inside the village and invited residents of nearby villages to gamble. This situation lasted for at least two years, and the village came under complete control again only after the fall of the Gang of Four in the winter of 1978.[82] This may be a case of villagers seizing the revolution as an opportunity to vent long-standing discontent. Similar events occurred in urban hospitals in the same province. In the Anhui provincial leprosy hospital in 1965, for example, patients "escaped, obtained an audience with the higher authorities, and filed complaints [against the hospital]," thus creating long-lasting political struggles inside the hospital. The "chaos" was temporarily settled only by the military taking over in August 1967.[83]

Despite such disruptions during the Cultural Revolution, the network of leper villages survived. As mentioned, with Mao Zedong's June 26 directive in 1965, the state policy to divert medical resources to rural areas, with the implementation of the Barefoot Doctor program, was maintained. Thus, from then until the aftermath of the fall of the Gang of Four, beginning in the 1980s, rural leper villages continued to receive regular state support and subsidies.

Liberalization and the MDT Program

Even though in the early post-Mao liberalization era WHO considered China as having eradicated leprosy, with the average national prevalence rate just below 1 per 10,000, China's struggle with the disease did not end. China considered the norm too low and set for itself the new target of a prevalence below 1 per 100,000. Moreover, an average *national* prevalence of 1 per 10,000 meant that, in the pockets where the disease was endemic, the prevalence rates were much higher.

The optimism revealed in the setting up of such a goal was understandable in this new era of political and economic reforms and the opening up of China to the international community. This new political era was particularly marked by key economic reforms, in particular the "household contract responsibility system" (*chengbao zeren zhi*), which allowed peasants to keep surplus produce after they had paid their taxes and reserves to the government. This was the beginning of the PRC's "free market," which reversed the revolutionary ideal of the Great Leap Forward. These reforms also implied the beginning of a "free market" for medical care, where the "spirit" of Mao's June 26 directive would be abandoned. In other words, the original rationale of the leper villages would soon disappear, in terms of their ideological role (as self-sustaining health-care and economic units) and medical character (as rural beneficiaries of state-managed, free medical resources). Their function as instruments to eradicate leprosy in rural China, however, persisted. The system had to, once again, accommodate the new political trend. The contract responsibility system was said to run on a local three-tier hierarchy (county-district-village), and was applicable to leprosy control in the summer of 1985. Medical bureaucrats of the lower administrative units were to "contract" with their superiors and be responsible for the control program under their jurisdiction. They were to be awarded with bonuses if their performance was satisfactory.[84]

Shortly after WHO declared China had eradicated leprosy in 1982, the PRC began to stop diverting medical assets to rural areas and put more weight on an urban-based public health policy, emphasizing cure over prevention as part of the liberalization process,[85] marking the end of an era of revolutionary idealism. The focus of leprosy control shifted, in the 1980s and 1990s, to the implementation of the international program of MDT, consisting of treating patients with a combination of several chemical drugs according to the type of leprosy for a period of six to twelve months, coinciding with the economic reforms and open-door policy led by Deng Xiaoping. In 1985, a national meeting in Nanjing on leprosy control announced the coming of the new era.[86] In the same year, the China Leprosy Association and the China Leprosy Control and Research Center (in Canton) were also established. From that year onward, Chinese experts began participating in international academic conferences and congresses and the PRC became more actively involved in WHO programs.[87] Starting in 1988, China began to celebrate, like many Western countries, World Leprosy Day, in January.[88] The PRC had become a major actor in the international community on the question of leprosy control.

MDT required close monitoring of drug administration, and the contract responsibility system appeared to be particularly effective for overseeing its implementation. The new leprosy control policy of "prevention and cure within society," beginning in 1986 and emphasizing in-home treatment of patients,[89] was in accordance with the loosening of the leper village as a productive *and* segregative unit. The new policy was part of a new five-year plan, conceived in 1985, the year a national Research Center for the Prevention and Cure of Leprosy was established.[90] At the same time, China began to accept foreign aid. The resources of regional hospitals and clinics were soon reorganized and pooled together under the supervision of local medical officials, who were now eligible for further financial rewards for "good performance." An increasing number of patients underwent a strict regime of treatment in specialized urban hospitals, leper villages, or at home under the supervision of medical professionals.

There were, in the 1980s, many accounts of the successful implementation of the contract responsibility system with MDT treatment. In Cixi, Zhejiang province, for example: "Beginning in December 1986 , a provincial hierarchical network of leprosy control was set up on the county [*xian*], district [*qu*], and village [*xiang*] levels. There were twenty-seven villages, which had their own doctors [specialized in leprosy]. From 1987 onward, these doctors were responsible for delivering the drugs to every known patient once a month and overseeing the taking of those drugs." After six months to a year of treatment, most patients were cured. They were then monitored for another ten years.[91] Reports of success were many. In Zhangzhou, Fujian province, medical doctors at the county and village levels were rewarded with handsome bonuses because the administration of MDT treatment was proven effective: 96.5 percent of patients were receiving the new treatment in 1986.[92] Reports from Guangdong province also showed that the implementation of MDT, starting in 1987, was a success, as the work of experts on all administrative levels was closely supervised under the new system.[93] The program was implemented even in peripheral regions like Tibet and Yunnan. In Tibet, it was said that, in 1988, 99 percent of patients received MDT, thanks to the contract responsibility system. In Kunming city, Yunnan, the reporter stressed the efficacy of treating patients in their own homes.[94]

Implementation of MDT was further facilitated by the availability of foreign financial and material aid. After having rejected foreign aid, especially from the industrialized world, for more than thirty years, PRC policy makers began, in the late 1980s, to work closely with international organizations such as WHO, and with foreign philanthropic societies.[95] Jiangxi, for instance, received free drugs from Japan in late 1987, and Guizhou was one of WHO's expensive targets of its LEC (leprosy elimination campaigns) in the 1990s. Private foundations like the Damien Foundation donated 2 million RMB (renminbi) worth of medicines and equipment to Fujian province in 1988.[96] These are only a few of the many cases of foreign aid flowing into China for the implementation of MDT to control leprosy from the 1980s onward, so much so that, by 1989, MDT coverage in China increased a staggering 95 percent.[97] The trend continued into the 1990s. In Guangdong province, a Sino-British cooperation program was launched in 1990, to operate until 1998, for promoting control of the disease. In the early 1990s in Yunnan, provincial authorities worked with Belgium on a patient rehabilitation program.[98]

LOCAL IMPLEMENTATION OF NATIONAL GUIDELINES

Despite the top-down nature of the control policy and the highly centralized government of the early decades of the PRC, there was significant local variation in the implementation of the national policy. This depended not only on the differences in prevalence rates but also particularly on the economic power of local governments, and often also on the bureaucratic and ecological characteristics of each locality.

Surveys

As mentioned, surveys were a key part of the PRC's leprosy control program, but there seems to have been no fixed methodology of conducting the surveys, and each province, district, or town, had its own preferences in terms of method. For provinces believed to have a higher concentration of sufferers of leprosy, large-scale systematic surveys on the provincial level were done early on. Fujian province, for instance, claimed to have carried out surveys on the provincial level from 1956 onward, and from 1958 until the 1980s, the province carried out five such surveys. Some of these were said to be general surveys, involving the entire provincial population, others were screening surveys in schools, or "track surveys" (*zhongdian di xiansuo diaocha*), meaning studies carried out by tracing known sufferers' family members, neighbors, colleagues, and friends. On the county level, surveys were said to have been carried out annually or biannually, and apparently several dozens of such surveys were carried out.[99] In Jiangxi province, an unknown number of general surveys were undertaken between the 1950s and 1980s. It is said that, in one of these surveys, during the 1950s, 6,629 new cases were identified, and in the 1960s, a single survey revealed 8,364 new cases, showing the thoroughness of such enterprises. By the end of 1992, a cumulative total of 17,232 cases had been uncovered by surveys in the province.[100] Gansu, as a province with traditional low prevalence rates, carried out four surveys on the provincial level, from 1957 to 1983, involving close to 98 percent of the entire provincial population. A 1965 survey revealed 2,955 new cases, and morbidity was found to be 0.23 per 1,000, which was high. From 1949 to 1965, the total number of cases uncovered by surveys reached 4,137.[101]

The more important surveys seem to have been carried out on the county level, especially in provinces where the problem appeared to be serious. In Guangdong province, for example, many counties kept records of frequent surveys carried out from the 1950s onward. It is said that provincial authorities constantly pressed county governments to identify new cases and family members of patients in the Canton area as high-risk groups were examined regularly after 1950. Kaiping district was said to have implemented annual track surveys between 1956 and 1958.[102] In Shaoguan district, the first of seven general surveys was conducted in the spring of 1958, covering 95.8 percent of the population older than two and identifying more than 600 new sufferers.[103] Several counties of Jiangsu province also carried out thorough general surveys from the 1950s onward. Nantong, for instance, began surveying in 1956, and, by the early 1970s, the surveys had become large scale. Track surveys began in 1977, mobilizing barefoot doctors and health officials of production teams. These later surveys were said to have identified 736 patients in sixty-two communes and 308 production teams.[104] In Jiangdu district of the same province, a total of fourteen surveys were undertaken between 1963 and 1983, five of which were general surveys carried out between 1971 and 1980. In the 1971 general survey, 122 new cases were identified, and prevalence was as high as 1.83 per 1,000. These surveys revealed that Jiangdu county had high prevalence rates in the early 1960s. In 1963, the rate was 1.78 per 1,000, with some areas as high as 25 per 1,000. General prevalence peaked in 1969 (1.87 per 1,000), and the worse period was 1963–1976,[105] that is, at the height of the Cultural Revolution. In the small county of Cenxi, Guangxi province, one large-scale general survey was taken in 1972, followed by smaller family visits conducted in the 1980s. In sum, surveys done in the entire province between 1956 and 1959 in fifty-three cities and counties revealed 5,136 new cases, and, as of 1990, the total number of cases discovered amounted to 26,297, with a high concentration among national minorities, especially the Yao (with a prevalence of 1.10 per 1,000).[106]

Some of the early surveys were carried out partly to justify the segregation policy. One such survey, done in Zhejiang province shortly before 1955, for instance, showed that contagion within the family accounted for 15.66 percent of all cases, whereas contagion within the same or neighboring villages accounted for, it was claimed, 53.82 percent. The same surveys revealed that, from 1948 to 1952, the average morbidity was 0.1 per 1,000, meaning if nothing was done, there would be 22,000 new cases in the province every year.[107] These figures supported the policy of strict segregation as a necessary preventive measure and reflected the persistent fear of contagion. Right after the publication of the national plan for leprosy control in 1957, a national congress on leprosy was held in 1958, with the resolution of "obliging patients to be segregated in hospitals, outdated errors having to be abolished."[108]

The belief that public surveys could not reveal all the cases, the perceived need for a more thorough knowledge of the epidemic situation of the disease, and the taste for greater mass mobilization soon inspired a bonus system or report system, adopted by a number of local governments, that effectively exploited popular dread of the disease. The principle of the system was encouraging members of the public to reveal suspected or known unreported cases. For each reported case proven to be correct, the reporter was awarded a bonus. The system, used apparently to compensate for the inadequacies of the surveys, was implemented in some but not all counties and provinces from the late 1950s onward. Hubei province, for example, adopted the system in 1960 and operated it until the 1980s, awarding ten to thirty yuan for each confirmed report of a leprosy case. In some counties, such as Tianmen, the price per head could be as high as

200 yuan.[109] In Fujian province, the Fuzhou municipality began, in spring 1963, a system of leprosy reporting (*mafeng bao bing zhidu*) that encouraged citizens to reveal unreported cases. Bonuses for correct reports began being awarded in the 1970s.[110]

The majority of counties and provinces, however, seem to have begun the practice only from the 1980s onward. The Kaiping municipality in Guangdong province, for instance, began giving a bonus of ten yuan for a valid report in 1980. Twenty such new cases were said to have been revealed under the bonus system between 1980 and 1985.[111] Jiangsu province began awarding a bonus varying from ten to thirty yuan for each correct report in 1981.[112] One year later, Anhua district, Hunan province, began handing out a bonus of ten to fifteen yuan for each verified case.[113] Although the bonus system was not adopted in all counties and provinces and, where it was, not at all times, it was apparently a fairly widespread method employed to supplement the survey system. In the earlier periods, it obviously had the "merit" of rousing popular sentiment for "combating" the disease, a possibility that had never been considered by former political regimes. Its increased importance from the 1980s onward was certainly related to the integrated effort to uncover otherwise hidden cases for an exhaustive implementation of MDT, believed to be essential for the ultimate elimination of leprosy from China.

Leper Villages

The fear of contagion was the main social and political force behind the initial establishment of leper villages as an essentially segregative institution. In Fujian province, where incidents of sufferers being buried or burned alive, or starved to death, sometimes even by close relatives, were abundant until at least the 1960s,[114] the total segregation of contagious patients of leprosy was one main public health objective from 1958 to 1962. The provincial authority later claimed that it had segregated 80 percent, or close to 10,000 of its patients between 1950 and 1970.[115] In Guizhou, two years after the establishment of the first eight leper villages, in 1957, it was claimed that, by 1959, 54.35 percent of the almost 900 contagious cases in the autonomous region had been segregated.[116] In Jiangxi, a first leprosy segregation station was set up in the winter of 1957 in an old temple in an isolated mountainous spot in Nanchang county, "with no natural villages in the neighborhood, which is convenient for segregation." It started as a village for thirty-nine patients, and in two years, by 1959, ninety-one had been segregated.[117] These are just a few examples to demonstrate the great enthusiasm of local authorities to follow the central directive to set up segregative villages to prevent contagion.

Given the size and complexities of China, however, there is no standard format of leper village, despite the central control plan of 1957 and the many directives distributed by provincial cadres on the principles of the organization of such villages. There was, first of all, a significant time lag among the various villages. Some, especially those in provinces considered most affected, were set up before the launching of the central plan. In Guangxi province, for instance, leper villages had been established as early as 1952. In the twenty years between1952 and the 1970s, a total of sixty villages had been established in the province.[118] In Gansu, a leprosy prevention team was established in 1953 by the provincial Bureau of Health, and a first village was set up in Wudu district, which was said to have treated eighty-six patients.[119] On the other hand, in southwestern provinces such as Yunnan and Guizhou, the segregation of patients seems to have lagged behind that of most other provinces. In Dali county, Yunnan, it was not until 1980 that the authorities accommodated the greatest number of patients (1,195). In Guizhou, some villages were set up as late as the mid-1970s.[120]

This time lag had much to do with the different economic situations of the provinces. For rich provinces, the expansion and consolidation of the control program was often directly financed by the provincial government. In Jiangsu province, for example, a 1964 proposal on the establishment of leper villages immediately resulted in a provincial investment of 1 million RMB to jump-start the program. Consequently four hospitals at the municipal and county levels and thirty-six villages were set up. By 1971 another twenty-five villages had been established, and the original forty institutions were expanded, which continued through 1974.[121] Each patient in Jiangdu county, Jiangsu province, during the thirty years since 1950 was said to have cost the government and the collectivity an average of more than 1,200 yuan.[122] Similarly, Zhejiang province was reported to have spent, in 1951, roughly 100,000 RMB to set up the first control institutions. The expansion of hospitals and villages in the years between 1978 and 1980, costing 4.65 million RMB, was also financed by the provincial government.[123] Anhui province spent more than 1.9 million RMB between 1956 and 1986 on one of its bigger leper villages, Sishan village.[124] Comparatively, the slow development of the control programs in the southwestern parts of the country was due partly to their more backward economic situations, especially before the 1980s.[125]

Another important factor affecting the timing of the establishment of leper villages was the intensity of local resistance. In regions where the disease had a long history of stigmatization, social violence against sufferers was particularly strong and could be a serious obstacle to the setting up of leper villages. In Shaoguan and Qujiang counties (Guangdong province), for instance, attempts to establish leper villages encountered serious resistance from the local populations.

It was reported that all projects for such villages conceived in 1956 and 1957 fell through due to serious opposition from local residents. When a spot was finally decided upon for a village accommodating patients of eight nearby districts, several hundred local peasants, wielding bricks and sticks, protested angrily in front of the cadres' office. This put an end to the project. A leper village was finally set up in the winter of 1957 near the government office of a village in Qujiang county, which began to take in patients the following summer. The report does not explain how this project survived local protests,[126] but a good guess might be that the site was small and remote and protected by the nearby seat of village government.

The fear of contagion could, however, be both an obstacle and a help in organizing leper villages. Reports in 1957–1958 for Guangdong province often mention peasants' superstitious beliefs that vicious *chong* will fly out from the bodies of patients and infect the healthy, that healthy women in the neighborhood risk being raped by patients trying to rid themselves of the disease, and that all patients of the disease are necessarily bad people. These were the reasons for which peasants were said to have resisted the organization of a leper village in Sihui county, Guangdong. The peasants finally relented, however, when they were told by the cadres that "the purpose of the village was to segregate patients in order to avoid contagion."[127] We might never know how exactly public opinion was turned around, but apparently such superstitions and the dread of contagion were often the reasons for which some early villages were located in extremely remote areas, their remoteness leading in some cases, however, to their premature closing.[128]

More significant was that even the cadres themselves sometimes resisted government policy due to the same bias toward sufferers of the disease. It was well known that many cadres refused to work in cooperatives or villages that had leprosy patients. In an internal document of Jiangsu province, of 1965, for example, it is reported that some patients were violently expelled from their villages by cadres. Many of the patients, who had become petty criminals as a means of survival, were eventually arrested by the local police, who turned a blind eye to their torture by other, healthy criminals detained in the same place. Many of these rejected sufferers found their last stop in leper villages, giving the institutions a bad name. Some luckier patients, after being kicked out of their communities, started their own agricultural enterprises in remote places, without any party supervision, and became rich. This phenomenon was highly criticized as serious sabotage of socialist collectivism.[129] Dreaded, and ostracized by the population, including cadres, sufferers of leprosy, whether persecuted or economically successful, constituted a serious predicament for the regime, which could not tolerate any marginal behavior.

The fear of contagion on the part of cadres and local governments is fully revealed by a document of the Bureau of Health of Jiangsu province, dated May 8, 1967, in which the bureau quotes the reply from the Ministry of Health to a question posed by the governments and cooperatives of several districts in Jiangsu as to whether cotton produced by inhabitants of leper villages was contagious. The ministry answered that leprosy bacteria could not survive on cotton, and even if the cotton was contaminated, the germs would be killed after being exposed to the sun. The ministry added, "We should disseminate [knowledge that would] eliminate the social fear of leprosy," revealing the strong persistence of the fear, which was hindering the execution of official policy.[130] Similarly, in the 1960s and early 1970s in a rural area of Baokang county, Hubei province, the responsible cadres forced not only sufferers of the disease to be interned in a leper village but also their healthy children and spouses, for a period of ten years.[131]

However, persuading patients to enter leper villages remained a central challenge in the establishment of leper villages. The official tactic, as we have seen, was to encourage them to enter voluntarily by propaganda or persuasion, or by material enticements such as stipends. Some organizers, however, found coercion a more efficient method. Rongchang county, Sichuan province, for example, from the 1960s until 1985, routinely dispatched envoys from the county leprosy control station in special vehicles to round up anyone identified to have contracted the disease for internment.[132] Not only urban patients were closely monitored but rural ones were also not spared. In Shaoguan, Guangdong province, for instance, after the establishment of a leper village in 1958 in a remote rural area, organizers began searching for patients who had taken refuge in the mountains before 1949 and forcing them to enter the village. "After unyielding education of these 'stubborn patients' [organizers managed to] intern them in the village one after the other."[133] Persuasion and coercion were probably also used in Gansu in 1953. During that year, doctors went into the surrounding villages in an attempt to "discover" new cases to be brought to the hospital to be treated in isolation. By the end of 1953, a second hospital had been set up. The first one took patients from sixteen different provinces and cities, including Beijing, in 1955. By 1958 there were 933 resident patients. The second one accommodated a maximum of 700 patients in 1966.[134]

Once established, each village was supposed to run on its own according to rules of management fixed by a committee of residents after consultations with experts and cadres. On the question of the separation of the sexes, for instance, You Jiajun, in his review of leprosy control in 1956, emphasized the importance of separating male and female patients in leprosy hospitals.[135] But this was not systematically followed by all local authorities. Some villages insisted

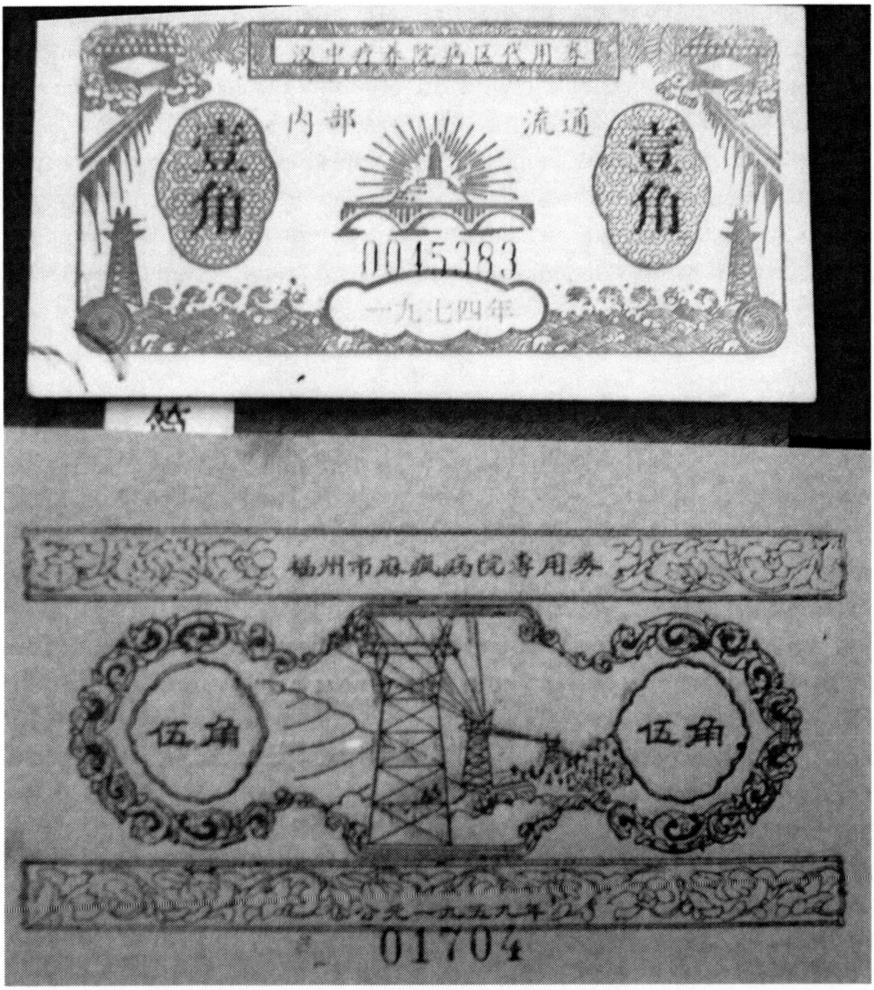

Examples of currency used exclusively inside Chinese leper asylums in the 1970s. (Collection of Dr. Jiang Cheng)

on separation of the sexes,[136] while others simply stipulated in their regulations that patients should not "fall in love, get married, or have sexual relations."[137] Some allowed married couples to live together, and others required patients to be sterilized.[138] Moreover, each province decided on its own medical and social criteria for the release of patients.[139] The differences in disease status among the provinces also determined how patients were treated. In Shanxi province, where the prevalence rate has always been low, the only leper village was set up in 1958 in a rural community in the southeastern part of the province, accommodating about thirty patients, most of whom were said to be migrants from Shandong province. The relative rarity of the disease provoked great fear among the local population when a new case was found in the late 1990s. The patient was immediately abandoned by his family and was treated by a doctor equally fearful of the contagiousness of the disease. The pressure on the patient was so great that he soon committed suicide. His body remained unattended for days, as no one dared to bury it for fear of contamination.[140] Such attitudes were rare after the 1980s in regions where the disease has been more common.

Treatment

As mentioned, the central government imposed a combination of Western and Chinese drugs at the early stage of leprosy control. There were nonetheless local variations of this official policy. During this period of political tension and experimentation in treatment, some doctors attempted to invent new methods to treat the disease by combining Chinese materia medica and Western technology. This was marked in regions where the disease situation was serious and where traditional medicine was strong. A Cantonese doctor by the name of Chen Zhiping, for instance, claimed, in 1960, that, using new instruments, he had extracted and purified ingredients contained in "secret recipes left by my grandfather" that he used experimentally on patients by injecting the drug under their skin, into their muscles, and into their veins. He baptized his new invention Di li ping, and it earned considerable attention from Guangdong province, which financed a research group in 1959 to experiment on the invention. Chen criticized the use of DDS as being too toxic and the therapeutic cycle too long. He claimed that the first results of his experiments showed that his new drug was effective and less time-consuming, even though, he admitted at the end of his report, there was insufficient control in his experimentation. Nonetheless, he considered his invention a worthy gift to be presented to the country on National Day, 1958, the high tide of the Great Leap Forward.[141] There were probably other, similar attempts during this period of fanatic idealism and nationalism characterized by extreme confidence in traditional and indigenous technologies.[142] Few of them, however, seemed to be really successful in treating leprosy in any sustained and radical way. The introduction of MDT in the early 1980s finally ended all experimentation.

Reports from individual provinces show the same evolution of strategies for treatment from the 1950s to the 1980s. Yunnan province claimed to have gone through three stages of development: From 1921 to 1951, chaulmoogra oil was the major drug, considered "one brought by the missionaries." Its use stopped in 1954 and was replaced by derivatives of sulphones and dapsone, such as Tb1 (thiosemicarbazone). During the third stage, chemotherapy, including the use of MDT, became the major treatment from 1987 onward, after partial application in 1984. It is interesting to note that this provincial report makes no mention of the use of traditional Chinese drugs during the four decades.[143] Such mention is usually not left out, as, for example, in the 1989 report on Fujian, which describes a four-stage development of drug use for leprosy since 1949: first dapsone and its derivatives were used; then such derivatives were used together with traditional Chinese medicines; the third stage was characterized by the use of dapsones with Chinese drugs and other (unspecified) Western treatments; and the fourth and final stage was dominated by the general application of MDT.[144] Clearly, by the late 1980s China had openly embraced MDT treatment and had more or less abandoned research into and the application of Chinese drugs.

Example of the Wukang Asylum

Although there was no "standard" development of leper villages in the PRC, it is nonetheless interesting to look at one village, whose long story covers the late Qing to Republican and PRC periods. Wukang leper village grew out of the Hangzhou hospital founded by Duncan Main, of the Church Missionary Society, in 1887, in Hangzhou city, Zhejiang province, mentioned in chapter 4.[145] Leprosy patients of this hospital were moved from the hospital, in 1903, to a location outside the city on the edge of West Lake. The asylum moved again in 1915, when the area had become a tourist site, to a remote hill called Songmu chang (Pine Grove), where two separate buildings, for male and female patients, were built and where able-bodied patients were required to labor in the open air.[146] Except for the brief interruption of the unhappy nationalization of the asylum by the provincial authorities in 1927 (see chap. 4), the hospital remained in the hands of missionaries until 1952, and Stephen Sturton (1896–1970) and James Maxwell were the two main missionary doctors responsible for the asylum when the Communist took over China in 1949. At that time, other than the two doctors, there were one manager and three helpers, with ninety-eight patients; and the institution was receiving a regular monthly subsidy of £130 from England, plus daily rice rations from the provincial government.[147]

An elderly patient who had been interned at the age of eighteen in 1950, and who was interviewed on August 31, 2005, told us that he had stayed in the Songmu chang asylum for four months before it was moved to an isolated farm in Shangbo (Cypress) village, in Wukang, about ten kilometers west of Deqing county. The patients were then divided into two groups. Those who could work, like himself, stayed on the farm to labor. The more handicapped ones were hospitalized in a nearby Buddhist temple. The elderly patient still remembered James Maxwell coming from Hangzhou city to treat patients at both sites, with the help of two Chinese doctors who translated for him, until his death in 1951. Patients of leprosy in the army, on the other hand, were treated in an older Buddhist temple, less than a kilometer from Shangbo, which was, when the whole institution was taken over from the missionaries in 1952, named Rehabilitation Hospital No. 6 and reserved for the military of the east China region. There were more than 200 soldiers suffering from the disease, and, by 1955, a total of 550 beds were available for military and nonmilitary patients,[148] clearly showing the seriousness of the disease situation in this part of Zhejiang province. It was only in the early 1970s that patients interned in the various parts of the asylum were grouped together in the No. 6 hospital in the old Buddhist temple, where today's Wukang asylum is.

The same patient recalled that at Shangbo village there was a church with "foreign preachers," until the takeover in 1952, when the foreigners left and the Chinese doctors who had worked for Maxwell took over the medical service. Maxwell's doctor-translator, Gao Lu, was a twenty-four-year-old graduate from Shandong Medical in 1949 and is now a retired doctor in his mid-eighties. Gao told us that he signed a contract to work in the Hangzhou leprosarium after he had finished his internship in March 1950 because "the salary of doctors treating leprosy was higher [than that of the average doctor]." Dr Gao took over the medical service, with a Dr. Xu (who died in 1957) after Maxwell's death. According to Dr. Gao, during the 1950s and 1960s, the asylum maintained a good stock of drugs sent from England, "which were of better quality [than the Chinese drugs]." He admitted at the same time that, in the 1950s, some Chinese drugs, such as "Wind-repelling pills," were used together with English chemical drugs and DDS (B663) made in Shandong. They stopped using chaulmoogra in 1954, and, beginning in 1957, the asylum started to make the famous Chinese herbal remedy *leigong teng* (*Tripterygium wilfordii* Hook).

With the rapid economic growth and urbanization of the province beginning in the 1980s and the systematic implementation of MDT, the number of patients fell rapidly. In the summer of 2005, 120 patients, mostly cured, remained in the asylum. The average age was around sixty-eight, with the oldest eighty-five and the youngest twenty-eight, a young woman from Guizhou who had recently married a resident of Hangzhou, shortly before she was diagnosed with the disease. There were twelve nurses and other workers serving these patients, and about four doctors taking shifts to take care of their various medical problems.

Each patient received a monthly stipend from 260 to 360 RMB, depending on the financial capacity of the government of their native place.

The Wukang asylum is certainly not a typical leper village, with its apparent affluence, revealing the exceptional economic power of Zhejiang province, which finances most of the expenses. The asylum is composed of rows of bungalows built in 2001 or so, adjacent to the old Buddhist temple where the military hospital once was. Two patients share a room with a toilet. There is also a canteen where patients can order their lunches, though most do their own cooking on common stoves, or in the common kitchen. There is also a small convenience store run by one of the patients, and neighboring peasants daily carry vegetables and other farm products for sale to the patients. According to workers in the asylum, local peasants are no longer fearful of the contagiousness of the disease, proven by the growing community in the neighborhood in recent years. There was even a widow of sixty-five who chose to marry a patient of sixty and live with him inside the asylum. Nonetheless, the leprosy control experts are still on the alert. The bonus system used to uncover hidden cases is still maintained: for each valid report, 200 yuan is given.

After some 120 years since its establishment, the Wukang asylum is still functioning as an institution for patients of leprosy, although now in a completely different political and social context. The faint memory of the early missionaries can be heard now only from old patients and retired doctors. The influence of Protestantism can hardly be detected, except on the walls of the room of a quiet patient where calligraphy of Bible quotations is displayed, though he is not old enough to have known the missionaries of Maxwell's time. The relaxed atmosphere of the asylum clearly shows that the disease is no longer considered a major threat to the health of the local population, and the national pride at the success of the disease's control has replaced the shame the malady induced in former times. Nonetheless, the institution's administrators seem not to have any plans to close the institution anytime soon. On the contrary, the ongoing investment of energy and resources seem to suggest that such asylums will continue to function in the foreseeable future.

SHOWCASE OF A HALF-CONQUERED DISEASE

Both WHO and the PRC government, as well as most experts involved in the control policy during the past decades, consider the fight against leprosy a successful one, especially when China's case is compared with the situations of India and Brazil, where the disease is still prevalent. The discourse on the contagiousness

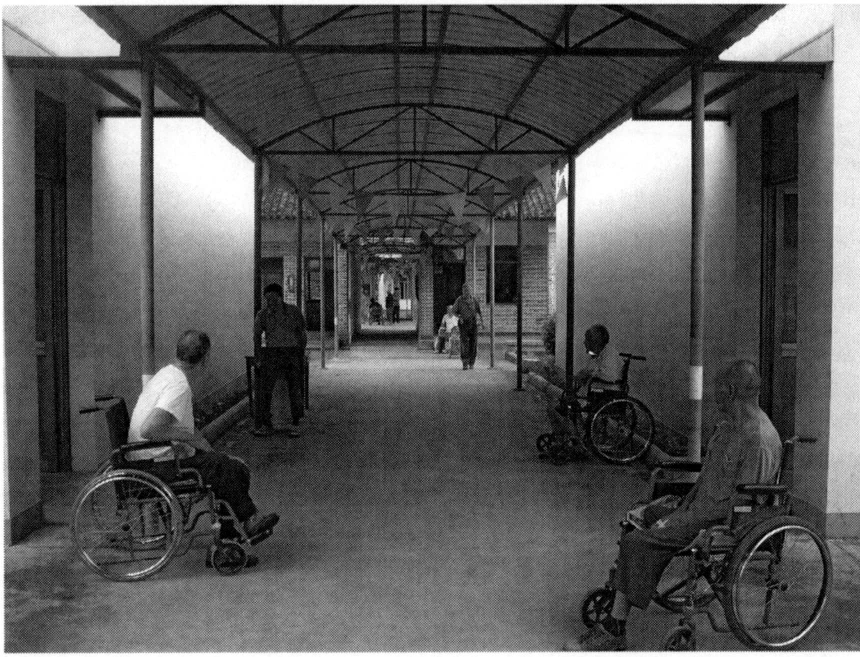

Glimpse inside the Wukang asylum; most inmates are elderly cured patients who consider the place their retirement home. (Photo by author, August 2005)

of the Chinese leprous body, so loud in the early half of the twentieth century, has finally faded to the point that it has almost been forgotten in many places. However, the lesson of leprosy still haunts a good number of medical doctors and social workers in China, who do not quite agree with the point of view that the leprosy problem has been entirely overcome.

Persistent Stigma

One major problem has its source in the central government itself. Despite the seemingly rational attitude of the Ministry of Health in connection with the issue of leprosy, tolerance for sufferers of the disease was definitely not displayed in governmental rules and regulations. Patients were legally discriminated against in important professions, and in civil law. In the regulations drawn up in 1952 regarding the licensing of medical doctors of Western and Chinese medicine, dentists, and pharmacists, there are four categories of people forbidden to take the national licensing examinations: criminals deprived of their political rights, those under the age of twenty, the mentally sick or physically crippled, and, finally, patients of leprosy.[149] It is extraordinary that sufferers of a chronic disease were singled out and barred from participating in certain trades. Moreover, as late as 1980, patients of leprosy were deprived of marriage rights by the civil law passed in the Fifth People's Congress. This rule was emphasized time and again, in 1992 and in 1994, in another set of regulations concerning the "health of mothers and children," despite opposition from specialists published as early as 1986.[150] This legal ban against leprosy sufferers marrying was officially lifted from the new civil law concerning marriage only in April 2001.[151] In other words, even during the last phase of the eradication of leprosy in China, the central government, like its imperial predecessor, still deprived sufferers of leprosy of their basic civil rights.

These legal restrictions partly revealed the persistence of the fear and suspicion surrounding leprosy despite the dramatic effects of, first, DDS and then MDT and the rapid decline of the prevalence rate during the past thirty years. One illustration of this lingering fear can be seen in a piece in the *People's Daily* of 1984. A series of crimes in Sichuan, Hebei, and Hunan were committed by people with false documents from leprosy hospitals indicating that they were patients. Using the documents, the criminals extorted money from local government bureaus, claiming that they were entitled to subsidies for travel and accommodation on their way to seek treatment from other clinics. Often they grouped into several dozens and made terrible scenes or resorted to violence if their requests were not met. Because people feared being infected, they usually got their way.[152] This was exactly the same strategy patients of leprosy had used during the late imperial period to make a living: exploitation of society's irrational fear and disgust of the disease. The old negative social attitudes toward patients of leprosy had thus hardly changed. They might even have spread as a result of the establishment of the nationwide network of leper villages and clinics.

The persistence of the stigma was particularly visible on the local level. In many regions, patients, including even those who have been cured, and their descendants are still discriminated against as carriers of a horrible disease. The stigma persists usually in regions where the control policy began relatively late, such as the southwestern provinces, or where the disease is rare, such as Shanxi province. An anthropological study in 2003 of a leper village in the southwestern region of the Yi national minority, in Sichuan province, revealed that more than a hundred cured patients and ninety of their healthy offspring had been rejected by their families and original communities and so preferred to remain in the leper village, which is still shunned by nearby communities. The healthy children of patients can marry only among themselves, as the disease is still believed to be hereditary.[153] In Tibet today, there are cases where villagers refuse the return of cured patients, who are sometimes violently treated. Schools also refuse to accept their healthy children.[154] In parts of Shandong province, another region where leprosy has a long history but is well under control today, the disease remains much dreaded by local populations. It is said that in Guangrao county, residents keep away from the place where a leper asylum once stood, and rumors of black magic carried out with things once used by lepers are still current. Local residents remember that, during the days of the existence of the asylum, people were wary of cheap eggs for sale, for fear that they had been laid by chickens raised by asylum patients and were thus contagious. By and large, although the asylum no longer exists, the disease still haunts residents of the neighborhood as something mysterious, loathsome, and highly contagious.[155]

Although such fears have faded in many regions, negative impressions linger. Many still harbor a feeling of disgust toward those who once had the disease, and the majority are still reluctant to socialize with them.[156] A 1986 survey revealed that only 45.5 percent of patients of the disease got married, with a divorce rate of 18.3 percent, significantly high relative to the Chinese standard of the period (5.7 times more than the average).[157] Another survey, done in the Yangzhou area of Jiangsu province in the mid-1980s, showed that only 24.5 percent of the healthy population would accept unconditionally cured patients returning to their families and workplace, whereas 46.2 percent admitted that they would avoid associating with families and children of patients. The authors of the survey concluded pessimistically that social bias and discrimination was extremely strong: "It is stronger among cadres than among the masses, stronger in the cities than in the rural areas, stronger among the younger and the more educated."[158] Another survey, conducted in 1989, revealed that 57.8 percent of people found leprosy "repulsive," and only 10.5 percent would be willing to continue seeing close friends and relatives with the disease.[159] These attitudes apparently continued until at least the early 1990s.[160] The situation might perhaps have improved thereafter, especially with the elimination, in 2001, of the article in the PRC marriage law forbidding patients of the disease to marry and campaigns, throughout the past decade, to destigmatize the disease.[161]

Persisting Leper Villages

Even though the goal of the elimination of leprosy has been largely attained during the last two decades, in 2005 there were still 662 leper asylums and villages in China, with the largest number in poor, mountainous regions, where the disease, traditionally serious, is still prevalent, such as places in Yunnan (120), Sichuan (80), and Guangdong (90).[162]

Table 5.1 The Distribution of Leper Villages (as of June 15, 2005)

Province/Municipality/Region	Number of Leper Villages
Beijing	0
Tianjin	0
Hebei	1
Shanxi	0
Inner Mongolia	0
Liaoning	1
Jilin	1
Heilongjiang	0
Shanghai	2
Jiangsu	39
Zhejiang	14
Anhui	17
Fujian	17
Jiangxi	59
Shandong	50
Henan	1
Hubei	43
Hunan	32
Guangdong	90
Guangxi	36
Hainan	15
Chongqing	11
Sichuan	80
Guizhou	21
Yunnan	120
Tibet	3
Gansu	3
Shaanxi	3
Qinghai	2
Ningxia	0
Xinjiang	1
Total	662

Chinese authorities admitted in the 1990s that "treatment of the disease lagged behind world development in the 1960s and 1970s. The aim now [in the 1990s] is to eradicate the disease by the year 2000. Leper villages, however, will not disappear for least thirty years after 2000, because many patients still live in them."[163] The continued functioning of these villages in parts of China can be explained by several facts: first, they are still considered necessary as a segregative institution in areas with high prevalence rates; second, in regions where the disease is basically under control, they are now welfare institutions for the cured elderly, often crippled patients who no longer have their families; third, they are considered necessary by a number of experts who are alert to the possible comeback of the disease.

In 1999, 15 percent of all counties still had a prevalence rate of more than 1 per 100,000, with 2,000 new cases discovered annually on top of the 6,000 existing patients.[164] The situation is worst in western regions such as Tibet, Yunnan, and Guizhou, where leper villages remain an indispensable tool of control, even though the conditions of the villages in these regions are actually poor and deteriorating. Not only the number of uncured patients remains high, but also the social fear of the disease, which is still so great that patients are often rejected by their communities. In Tibet, for instance, where prevalence rates vary between 1 and 10 per 10,000 (east and south of the region) and medical resources invested in leprosy control have drastically declined since the announcement of the eradication of the disease in China, the number of patients is actually increasing. They have, moreover, nowhere to go except leper villages, often constructed about twenty or thirty years ago. Experts who surveyed the problem in Tibet in 2003 suggested that leper villages should be renovated and resources for leprosy control be restored.[165]

The problem of accommodating elderly and crippled ex-patients has been a general one for almost all leprosaria, even in countries where the disease has been declared eliminated. In Japan, for example, the legal liberation of patients in 1996 did not lead to the closing of the remaining fifteen state-run leper colonies, as most of the patients, elderly and without families, decided to remain in the colonies.[166] The existing leper villages in China serve the same purpose of accommodating elderly patients.[167] As of 1999, over 20,000 cured patients, representing one-tenth of the total number, still lived in leper villages all over the country.[168] We have seen how the Wukang asylum, in Zhejiang province, now serves essentially as a "retirement" home for the cured elderly, with a couple of new cases of immigrants from poorer provinces. In more remote areas, like Shaanxi province, in 1994, there were still 326 cured elderly patients forced to stay in the villages since they had been completely cut off from their own families.[169] It will indeed take another two or three decades for this generation of patients to disappear.

In contrast, the demand in Taiwan for the continued presence of leprosaria comes less from a material and more from a cultural need. The Taipei Lesheng (Happy Life) leprosarium, established by the Japanese colonial government in 1930, housing more than 300 cured, elderly patients, recently made headlines as a symbol of social injustice and a landmark in Taiwan's cultural history. Social activists were resisting the government's plan to tear down the building and remove the patients to a new nursing home for the construction of a mass transit line. The resistance is an ongoing social movement that highlights the society's growing consciousness of its colonial past and collective guilt over the victimization of patients.[170]

The Return of Leprosy?

More important, for certain Chinese specialists, the continued existence of leper villages is a medical necessity for making sure all early cases are treated in time and completely before these patients are allowed to move on in their lives. Otherwise, the return of the disease is, to them, a real threat. The problem was felt in parts of the country as early as the 1980s, when the optimism of eradication was reigning and the policy was shifting toward the gradual closing down of villages. In Baoying, northern Jiangsu, more than 6 percent of patients at the early stage of the disease and under treatment left the region and could not be followed.[171] This inevitably rendered control more difficult. Those working in Shandong in the early years of the twenty-first century have warned that "the eradication of leprosy is only a momentary achievement, and not definitive. At present, new cases continue to appear. In some villages, there are new cases every year. The return of the disease is serious."[172] This opinion is shared by experts working in Shaanxi, Fujian, Guangdong, and Guizhou provinces. A doctor in Shaanxi asked, in 1994 the question, "Where will leprosaria go in a market economy?" expressing the concern that, with the financial difficulties in sustaining the old public health network, the danger will be that, once the disease makes a comeback, most likely in the poorest areas, there will be no system to cope with the situation. Similarly, in Fujian, once a badly affected province, experts claimed, in 2003, that "there is the possibility that the disease could recur at any moment."[173] Expressing a similar concern, an expert in Canton stated, in 1999, that, after the "initial eradication" of the disease, institutions, specialists, and funding should remain unchanged so that new patients could be identified and treated as early as possible in order to achieve the goal of "total elimination" of the disease.[174] In Guizhou, as recent as 2003, local experts strongly recommended an increase in funding of leprosy elimination campaigns (LEC), designed by WHO, as there was still a significant number of hidden cases in rural areas of the province.[175] Jiang Cheng, an active leprologist, has also warned that a premature declaration of the eradication of leprosy in China would drain resources from existing clinics and villages, having the undesirable results of neglecting current cases.[176] All these factors might result in an increase of new cases. Are these alarms legitimate, or are they voiced simply to remind the state of the importance of maintaining a centralized and just public health policy at a time when state health care in rural areas is disintegrating?[177] It is difficult to tell at this stage, but leprosy control certainly remains one important indicator of the PRC's health-care system in the twenty-first century.

Leprosy control and leper villages in rural China today no longer occupy a central position in the PRC's public health concern, as new problems such as AIDS, SARS, avian flu, and the recurrence of old problems such as schistosomiasis and VD have become much more pressing. However, the evolution of the policy on this once frightening disease clearly reveals the character of China's public health problems. The eradication of leprosy as a rural scourge, announced in 1982, was shown to be not simply the result of effective therapeutics but also of the successful maintenance of a nationwide rural public health infrastructure constructed during the series of mass political movements between the 1950s and the 1980s. The present fear of the disease's return or of the spread of new diseases is due not so much to the lack of modern drugs or international aid but to the rapid disintegration of such an infrastructure since the late 1980s. Once again, the ups and downs of the leprosy problem will indisputably follow closely the PRC's political and economic evolution.

Under the PRC, leprosy has become a truly national concern and no longer a miasmatic disease of the semicivilized south as in late imperial and Republican China. In interesting ways, the history of leprosy control in the PRC closely reflects the changes in the political foci of the regime. It spotlighted the rural interest of the early PRC regime defined by Mao and corresponded perfectly to the series of political movements launched since the 1950s. The methods of control also satisfied the official nationalist discourse for the strengthening of China after a century of national humiliation. It was in the 1980s that the political agenda mapped out in the late Qing play *Bing yu yuan* (see chap. 3) was finally and effectively implemented. From the 1980s onward, the general acceptance of MDT, introduced by WHO, and of financial aid from foreign organizations and governments to eradicate leprosy also fit in perfectly with the PRC's liberalization and open-door policy promoted by Deng Xiaoping. The successful control of the disease in the 1990s marked China as being finally a modern nation-state, triumphantly entering the international community of nations and realizing the long-awaited end of an era of humiliating experiences. There is no disease that could better define China's body politic in the modern and contemporary era than leprosy.

But is leprosy already a thing of the past? That is again not only a question of medical progress but also a critical problem of political choice for the PRC. As the rural public health infrastructure, an essential factor in the eradication of leprosy, began quickly disintegrating from the early 1990s onward, the PRC seemed to consider such successful policies as leprosy control as indicators of the emergence of a prospering rural world that no longer needed special state subsidies, a position radically different from the one in force up to the late 1970s. However, with the gradual realization that old and new, chronic and acute epidemics are seriously damaging the health, thus also the economy of rural populations, the policy of leaving the problem of rural health to the market economy seems to have come under serious revision since 2005. The threat of the return of leprosy, a disease that cannot be eradicated by means of a vaccine, is as real as the rapid spread of AIDS, the return of VD and schistosomiasis in rural regions, and other health problems linked to a quickly deteriorating environment. The new direction of the PRC's rural public health policy in the twenty-first century will determine if leprosy is really going to become a thing of the past.

Epilogue

Leprosy, China, and the World

Much of this volume has traced the long history of leprosy as it evolved inside China over many centuries. As in the medieval history of leprosy in Christian Europe, early Chinese understandings of the disease were mediated by religion, allowing sufferers the possibility of redemption through Buddhist or Daoist salvation or Confucian good works. When, after the twelfth century, elite Chinese doctors stopped talking about *li/lai* as an environmental, Wind pathogen, popular healers, identified with "external medicine," gradually filled the vacuum with an account of *mafeng* as a contagious disorder manifested in skin symptoms. In their accounts of *mafeng,* an incurable disease of the far south, transmitted by bodily contact or inheritance, Chinese sources after the sixteenth century offered a picture that has recognizable convergences with European models of leprosy in the early modern period. State authorities even resorted to the unusual strategy of segregative measures, producing leper asylums that seemed quite familiar to early Western missionaries. Nonetheless, much in my narrative highlights what is distinctive in the medical, social, and religious history of leprosy, whether it is the perspective of Asian religious traditions, the late imperial split between elite and popular healers, the sexualization of *mafeng* in popular folklore, or the Ming-Qing construct of the disease as the plague of an ethnically different and inferior southern "other."

In the nineteenth century the Chinese and Western histories of leprosy converged. This is when China faced Western imperialism, and the disease became a national issue in part because it was also at the same time a global one.

The trauma brought by Western medical men, especially leprologists, was not related to any new medical understanding of the disease. The trauma was the realization that leprosy was now considered by the West as a Chinese disease. The Chinese elite had now to face the common Western view that "leprosy is smeared over the face of China as butter on bread—not in spots, but found just about everywhere."[1] That the disease was dubbed the Chinese disease in Hawaii or that a popular term in Capek's prewar novel *The White Plague* (1937) for a horrible epidemic was Peking leprosy[2] clearly shows the common association of leprosy with China that had developed by the early half of the twentieth century. The West changed the traditional Chinese self-image by imposing the interpretation that, if leprosy was indeed a disease of darker-skinned, semicivilized races—a view easily understood given the late imperial Chinese conception of the disease—China, with its amazing number of patients, was thus at the margin of the Western civilized world. The Chinese had to face the fact that they were now the inferior, Oriental, "other."

China was not, however, the only Asian nation traumatized by such a view. Even the successfully modernizing Japanese state, which defeated China in 1894, with an estimated 30,000 sufferers at the end of the nineteenth century, considered its leprosy problem "nothing but a national disgrace." Japanese authorities consequently opted for such drastic measures as absolute segregation, mandatory sterilization, and abortion to eradicate the blight.[3] These policies were also tried or adopted in parts of Japanese colonized East Asia, such as Taiwan, Manchuria, and Korea. "Cleaning up the continent" was one of the objectives of such policies.[4] In sum, it is clear that the meaning of the leprosy problem in China and Japan from the late nineteenth century on was largely dictated by Western views on race and degeneration, rather than by new, confirmed medical knowledge. China's problem with leprosy was nonetheless different from that in Japan. Unlike Meiji Japan, the Chinese were too overwhelmed by military defeat and protracted internal civil war and revolution to carry out any state programs for control of the disease in the late nineteenth and early twentieth centuries. Whereas Japan sent only small numbers of overseas emigrants to specific locations in the Americas, Chinese migrant labor moved around the world, which put China at the center of attention of forces mobilized against leprosy as an international public health crisis seen in a global context.

Developments and events building up to the intense internationalization of the leprosy problem began with the discovery of the bacillus in 1873–1874 by

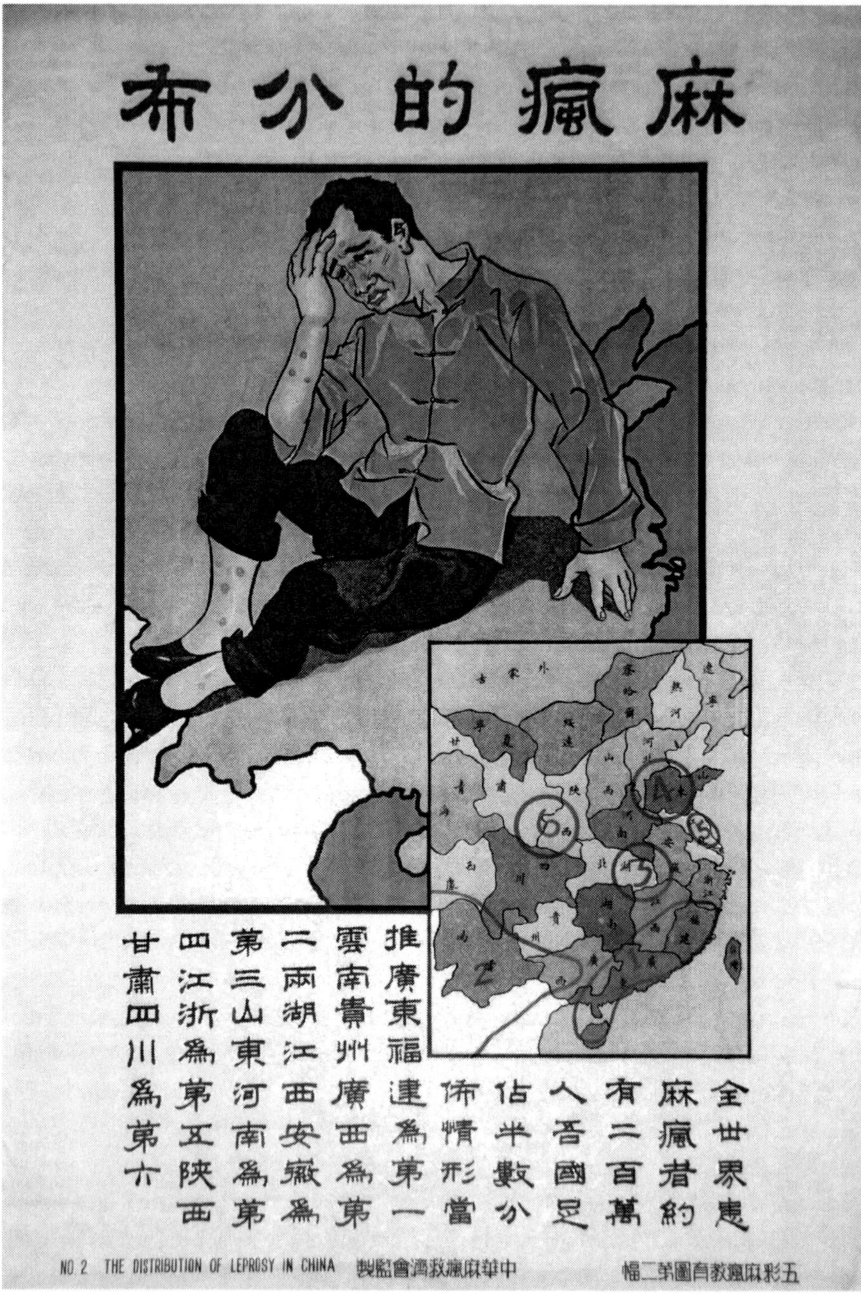

Poster printed in Shanghai in the 1930s showing the distribution of the disease in China; the sick man sitting on the map of China illustrates the seriousness of the epidemic in the nation. (Courtesy of Yale University)

G. H. Hansen, which strengthened the emerging biomedical contagion theory of the disease. But the turning point was probably the widely publicized news that the Belgian priest Father Damien, working on Molokai, was infected by the disease, in 1878, five years after he arrived in the Hawaiian leper colony, leading to his death eleven years later, in 1889.[5] The alarm provoked by Father Damien's illness was evident in Henry Wright's influential book *Leprosy and the Imperial Danger,* published in 1889, which argued that a global pandemic was imminent. Fear and concern finally pushed European contagionists to organize the First International Leprosy Conference in 1897, at which leprosy was declared incurable and segregation was recommended to all countries as the best measure to stop its spread. By this time, germ theory had gained ground in Europe, and the contagion theory of leprosy quickly came to dominate popular discourse.

Recent studies have made clear that a key activist of this first conference on leprosy, Jules Goldschmidt, of France, was especially concerned with the danger of the Chinese emigrant worker, who, in his view, "will never accept modern civilization." Another founder of the first conference, the American Albert Ashmead, insisted that the disease must be prevented "from being brought by emigration."[6] Such alarmist views of the danger of emigration from "leprous countries" continued to be propagated by certain Western leprologists and finally received official recognition in the Third International Conference on Leprosy, at Strasbourg, in 1923, where a proposal to prevent and deny entry of "alien" lepers was approved unanimously as the first resolution.[7] Clearly globalization and labor migration under colonialism, the spread of the germ theory of disease, and the emergence of influential worldwide public health organizations all fostered the internationalization of the leprosy problem during the first decades of the twentieth century.

Moreover, China's leprosy was considered particularly dangerous to global health. The actions by the Japanese state to eliminate the disease were obvious, but nothing seemed to be occurring or even planned in China. The estimated number of patients in the country was alarming, from half a million to 3 million in the late nineteenth and early twentieth centuries, and these numbers were coupled with the idea of endless tides of emigrating coolies, "uncivilized" carriers of the disease to all parts of the world. Such a view of the global spread of leprosy was promoted not only by the likes of Goldschimdt and Ashmead but also by James Cantlie, the reformer and ally of Sun Yat-sen, father of the Chinese Republic established in 1911. Cantlie was himself a leprologist, as noted in chapter 4.

Was this alarm justified? Was the perceived pandemic of leprosy at the turn of the twentieth century real? The disease was indeed widespread in many countries. In China of the early twentieth century, leprosy was doubtless a real public health problem, with at least half a million patients throughout the country, concentrated especially in poor, rural regions. Many sufferers, in order to survive, begged or committed petty crimes in urban centers, something that had been going on since at least the late imperial period but which was now visible to the outside world. The political and social dislocations of the late Qing and early Republican periods certainly aggravated the situation. Similar problems were observed in almost all Asian, Latin American, and African countries at the time, only to different degrees; no estimate of the total number of worldwide sufferers of the disease existed, however.[8] As recently as the mid-1980s, there were reported to be about 11.5 million cases, a low estimate, in the world, with a heavy concentration in South and Southeast Asia, parts of Africa, Latin America, and the western Pacific. It was not until the 1990s and the worldwide application of multidrug therapy, promoted by WHO, that these global numbers began to fall significantly.[9] The situation half a century earlier, when there was no effective drug to control the disease, could only have been much worse. Despite the early discovery of the bacillus, no vaccine could be developed to prevent its spread, and the exact mode of its transmission remained mysterious.

In hindsight, the overview and explanation given by WHO on the situation in 1980s shows that the idea of an early twentieth century world pandemic was basically fictive. WHO described the disease as one that had been endemic in most parts of the world for more than 1,000 years; the only exceptions were the Pacific Islands and Australia, where the disease had been introduced more recently. Historical reports of epidemics in specific locations described short-lived phenomena, with the conventional pattern of endemic leprosy quickly reemerging. The reason frequently given to explain such epidemics, "the arrival of a single lepromatous immigrant," was "often traceable by hearsay." Using comparative genomics, scientists today conclude that, whereas the disease was introduced to Asia and Europe from East Africa thousands of years ago, in the New World it was most probably brought by Europeans and North Africans during the past 500 years, whereas in places such as the French West Indies and New Caledonia, the disease was introduced through the settlement of different human populations and in more recent years.[10] In other words, the global pattern of the occurrence of leprosy at the turn of the twentieth century was the result of successive human migrations over thousands of years. There was nothing to suggest the possibility of a sudden large-scale outbreak of leprosy across national borders causing a global pandemic in the early twentieth century. Leprosy declined gradually in Europe, Hawaii, Japan, and the United States by natural means.[11] The patterns of natural decline began long before chemotherapy was available. "In England, France, Hawaii, the Netherlands, and northern continental USA, it is clear that the secondary attack rate of leprosy in people closely exposed to the many immigrant or few native lepromatous cases is far lower (approaching zero) than the rate observed in endemic populations." WHO suggests that this "implies that the risk factors associated with such contacts have changed over time."[12]

However, at the height of the global leprosy panic, the "hearsay" of "the arrival of a single lepromatous immigrant," often a Chinese worker, was typically quoted as the origin of leprosy epidemics in many places, such as Hawaii, California, and Australia, as we saw in chapter 4. Such rumors, together with the increasing conviction that the disease was highly contagious, especially after the infection and death of Father Damien, helped to construct the crisis atmosphere. The conveners of the First International Leprosy Conference, the French doctor Jules Goldschmidt and the American Albert Ashmead, were explicitly concerned about the danger of Chinese and Indian emigrants. Goldschimdt warned, in 1896, of "the danger of a new pandemic of leprosy . . . on the European continent," just prior to the international event,[13] echoing Wright's alarm over the "imperial danger" in 1889 and James Cantlie's pinpointing the Chinese coolie as the main contaminator of the Pacific region. Such worries were not scientifically grounded. The unprecedented concern over a world pandemic was essentially based on irrational fear fed by a combination of the current ideology on race and degeneration and an exaggeration of the disease's contagiousness, an effect of its mysterious nature, in a modern context of intensive global trade and human migrations. In this sense, the interest of the history of leprosy is again shown to lie not only in its unique medical characteristics but also especially in its political, social, and cultural implications.

A century after the global public health campaign against an "imminent" leprosy pandemic, leprosy has turned into a museum piece. It is one of the few diseases that human societies memorialize with exhibitions. Besides the major leprosy museum at Bergen, Norway, whose Leprosy Archives were included in UNESCO's Memory of the World, in June 2001, there are leprosy museums in Carville (U.S.A.), Acworth (Mumbai, India), Kumamoto (Kyushu, Japan), Münster (Germany), Molokai (Hawaii) , Culion (the Philippines), and probably a few others. The National Center for Leprosy Control in Nanjing, China, is also preparing an exhibition space with archival materials.[14] In Taiwan, activists are fighting to prevent the government from tearing down the colonial leprosarium, now seen as a historical monument.[15] In trying to comprehend its colonial past, the postcolonial world seems to be making every effort to retrieve the leper from "bare life," a life devoid of value or sovereignty,[16] by evoking human rights and identity, especially when publicly commemorating their past plight, not the least in museums.

Leprosy's long history and unique place in many religious systems, and its remarkably persistent "suitability for the purpose of stigmatization" make it a most "natural" museum item.[17] In modern history, its role in medical development and in colonial politics, and its intricate metaphorical association with the body politic of modernizing nations magnified its universal historical significance. In this postcolonial era, as a powerful reminder of questions related to human suffering and dignity, and to social injustice, it reemerges as the subject of heated public discussions. One can imagine each of the mentioned museums laboriously excavating "facts," reconstructing, and amplifying a distinct kind of historical memory to justify or to explain the present.[18] The history of leprosy clearly has both universal and local interests that impel the worldwide movement of public commemoration of the victims' tragic past.

At this stage, one could try to imagine how a Chinese museum of Hansen's disease would present its archive to the public. A major theme would certainly be the success story of the eradication of the disease in the late twentieth century, in contrast to the misery of patients in the late imperial and Republican periods, concerning which pictures, texts, and various materials are quite abundant. This would probably be shown as a glorious chapter in the state-building history of the PRC. Unlike Japan's painful soul-searching process in reviewing past policies toward patients that so clearly infringed upon human rights,[19] China's narrative would likely be much more positive and forward looking. On the other hand, China's constructed memory of leprosy in the past would also be significantly different from that in India, the British colony par excellence in the nineteenth century, where the disease was also a serious public health problem but seemed to have little association with national pride. In India, colonial policies were conceived along class rather than racial lines, conscientiously protecting the liberty of the upper and middle classes, resulting in a very loose confinement of patients, which was interestingly different from the policy in Hong Kong, another British colony but a Chinese society, where lepers were first systematically repatriated to Canton and then, from the 1950s onward, confined in an asylum on an island when the border with China was closed.[20] While the sacrifice of human rights for the benefit of nation building is irrelevant to India's historical narrative on leprosy, would China begin to question its past preference of strict segregation as the best policy for the successful eradication of the disease and, above all, as a valid indicator of responsible government, now that the leprosy problem is no longer a central issue of national pride?

Another aspect that would deserve mention in the museum would be the role attributed to Western missionaries in late nineteenth and early twentieth centuries, prior to the Communist takeover. It would be most interesting to see how the stories of these missionary institutions would be judged in the museum. Were they simply tools of Western imperialists, oppressors of Chinese patients? Were they Christian humanists or disseminators of modern Western medicine and public health? Or all of these? The Chinese museum story of leprosy would be revealingly different from the version told in a Christian mission museum.

Even harder to imagine is the way the history of the disease in the long imperial period might be presented. A simple strategy would be to treat this entire history as "feudal," meaning backward and irrational. The southern custom of "passing on" the *lai* ailment through erotic sex would probably fall into the category of feudal and superstitious practices, as shown in the modern opera described in chapter 3. There might, however, be more sophistication in the treatment of the place occupied by the ailment in the Buddhist, Daoist, and Confucian traditions, as this could be closely linked to medical thought and practice in premodern China, a tradition that the PRC has always extolled as a precious cultural heritage, essential to China's national identity. The PRC's complex relationship with China's imperial past would be revealed in the presentation of the disease's earlier history.

A delicate point at the end of the exhibition on the history of leprosy in China would be the historical "lesson" for present and future public health issues. It is unclear if the lesson would be used to define strategies for the contemporary epidemics of HIV or even SARS, where the issues of stigma, segregation, and quarantine, and investment in rural public health infrastructure in a new era of a market economy and globalization would be central. How the historical lesson would be learned depends not only on its relevance to contemporary problems but also on the political and economic complexities of a more prosperous but not more democratic China.

With the official global number of reported cases of leprosy drastically reduced to around 290,000 at the beginning of 2005,[21] leprosy is now well known to be a curable disease and does not provoke fear in most parts of the world. There is some truth in what Susan Sontag wrote about leprosy in 1989, that the disease, once "most fraught with meaning" like AIDS of the late 1980s, had become "just an illness."[22] The recent organization of leprosy museums and archives also implies that the ailment is now of the past. Now everyone can talk freely about it, without feelings of horror, guilt, or shame.

However, very few diseases have a history that is rich enough to sustain so many museums, which seems to indicate a collective and universal psychological need to understand the atrocity humanity has inflicted upon innumerable patients in the past. These museums belong with those commemorating the Holocaust, or other modern genocides. Local variations of the history of leprosy, on the other hand, add to the complexity of the message such museums attempt to convey, often linked to present-day problems of health in specific sociopolitical contexts. In this sense, leprosy will never be exactly "just an illness" like the others, and its history will remain open-ended.

Appendix 1

List of Leprosaria and Clinics in China (March 1940)

Location	Name of Institution	Superintendent	Year Established	Responsible Organ	No. of Inmates	No. of Outpatients
Hangchow (Hangzhou), Chekiang (Zhejiang)	Kwang-Chi (Guangji) Leper Home	Dr. S. D. Sturton	1887	Church Missionary Society, Mission to Lepers, London	108	
Amoy (Xiamen), Fukien (Fujian)	South Fukien Leprosy Clinic	Dr. E. S. Cheong	1931	Amoy Leprosy Committee		100
Diong-Loh (Changle), Fukien	Diong-Loh Leprosarium			Joint Committee of Government, Gentry and Missions	31	
Foochow (Fuzhou), Fukien	Chacang Christ's Hospital Leprosy Clinic	Dr. S. L. Chiu	1939	Missions		50
Hankong (Hanjiang), Fukien	Lilian Gamble Leper Home for Women	Miss Pauline E. Westcott	1901	Woman's Foreign Missionary Society of Methodist Episcopal Church	46	
Hankong, Fukien	Hankong Leper Church	Mrs. E. F. Brewster		Woman's Foreign Missionary Society of Methodist Episcopal Church		
Hinghwa (Xinghua), Fukien	Hinghwa Leper Church	Mrs. F. S. Carson		Methodist Episcopal Mission, North		100

Kutien (Gutian), Fukien	Kutien Leper Asylum	Dr. H. N. Brewster		Mission to Lepers, London	60	
Shima, Fukien	Shima Leprosy Clinic	Mr. Lim Ping- Siang		Private		100
Yenping (Yanping), Fukien	Westminster Leprosarium, Alden Speare Memorial Hospital	Dr. G. L. Downie	1919	Methodist Episcopal Mission	20	
Hengchow (Hengzhou), Hunan	Leprosy Clinic, Presbyterian Mission Hospital	Dr. Frank W. Newman		American Presbyterian Mission, North		150
Paoking Mission (Baoqing), Hunan	Paoking Leprosy Clinic	Rev. J. H. Stanfield		English Methodist Missionary Society		150
Sinhwa (Xinghua), Hunan	Sinhwa Leprosarium	Dr. Margit Mortensen	1934	Chinese Mission to Lepers, Norwegian Missionary Society, local government	17	7
Hankow (Hankou), Hupeh (Hubei)	Hankow Leprosy Clinic, Union Hospital	Dr. H. W. H. McClelland	1939	Hankow Rotary Club and Union Hospital		43
Siaokan (Xiaogan), Hupeh	Siaokan Leper Hospital	Rev. H. F. Wickings	1890	Mission to Lepers, London	90	
Lanchow (Lanzhou), Kansu (Gansu)	Leper Home, Borden Memorial Hospital	Dr. R. A. H Pearce	1920	China Inland Mission; Mission to Lepers, London; Chinese Mission to Lepers	64	
Nanchang, Kiangsi (Jiangxi)	Nanchang Leprosarium	Rev. L. W. Holland	1931	Chinese Mission to Lepers, American Methodist Mission, local government	166	

List of Leprosaria and Clinics in China (March 1940)

Location	Name of Institution	Superintendent	Year Established	Responsible Organ	No. of Inmates	No. of Outpatients
Jukao (Rugao), Kiangsu (Jiangsu)	Jukao Leprosy Clinic	Dr. Lee S. Huizenga	1933	American Mission to Lepers, Chinese Mission to Lepers, Christian Reformed Church		200
Nantungchow (Nantongzhou), Kiangsu	Nantungchow Leprosy Clinic	Dr. G. L. Hagman		United Christian Missionary Society		40
Shanghai, Kiangsu	Shanghai Leprosy Clinic	Dr. Lee S. Huizenga	1938	Chinese Medical Association, Chinese Mission to Lepers		53
Shanghai, Kiangsu	National Leprosarium of Shanghai	Dr. Lee S. Huizenga	1935	Chinese Mission to Lepers, National Medical College of Shanghai	110	
Taichow (Taizhou), Kiangsu	Taichow Leprosy Clinic	Dr. R. B. Price		American Presbyterian Mission, South		
Tsingkiangpu (Qingjiangpu), Kiangsu	Leprosy Clinic, Tsingkiangpu General Hospital	Dr. L. Nelson Bell		Southern Presbyterian Mission		
Lungchow (Longzhou), Kwangsi	Lungchow Leprosarium	Dr. Lo Tsong		Provincial government		

Chaoyang, Kwangtung (Guangdong)	Leprosy Clinic, Chaoyang General Hospital	Dr. B.C. Chang		Chinese Mission to Lepers, American Baptist Foreign Mission Society		40
Hoihow (Haikou), Hainan, Kwangtung	Hainan Leprosarium	Dr. N. Bercovitz	1931	Chinese Mission to Lepers, government and public	152	
Kityang (Jieyang), Kwangtung	Leprosy Clinic, Bixby Memorial Hospital	Dr. Marguerite Everham	1935	Chinese Mission to Lepers, American Baptist Foreign Mission Society		170
Kongmoon (Jiangmen), Kwangtung	Leprosy Clinic, United Church of Canada Mission Hospital	Miss R. M. Isaac	1939	United Church of Canada Mission		12
Lo Ting (Luoding), Kwangtung	Lo Ting Leprosarium	Dr. M. Edna Wallace		Pok Oi Hospital, Chinese Mission to Lepers	20	
Pakhoi (Beihai), Kwangtung	Pakhoi Leper Settlement	Maj. H. L. Wright	1886	Church Missionary Society, Chinese Mission to Lepers, government	210	63
Sheklong (Shilong), Kwangtung	St. Joseph's Homes for Lepers	Rev. Bishop A. Fourquet	1907	Mission Catholique, Canton; Chinese Mission to Lepers; Kwangtung provincial government	800	
Swatow (Shantou), Kwangtung	Eastern District Leper Asylum	Mr. Lim Ching-khi	1922	Kwangtung provincial government	174	

List of Leprosaria and Clinics in China (March 1940)

Location	Name of Institution	Superintendent	Year Established	Responsible Organ	No. of Inmates	No. of Outpatients
Swatow, Kwangtung	Leprosy Clinic, E. P. Mission Hospital	Dr. H. R. Worth		English Presbyterian Mission		27
Taikam (Daqin), Kwangtung	Taikam Leper Colony	Rev. John Lake	1919	Southern Baptist Convention	124	
Tsingyuen (Qingyuan), Kwangtung	Wai Wah Leper Home	Rev. W. L. Winter	1932	Boat Mission, Chinese Mission to Lepers	74	
Tungkun (Dongguan), Kwangtung	Tungkun Leper Asylum	Rev. W. Grundmann	1905	American Mission to Lepers, Rhenish Missionary Society, Chinese Mission to Lepers	330	20
Yeongkong (Yangjiang), Kwangtung	King's Mother's Leper Village	Dr. W. H. Dobson	1917	American Presbyterian Mission, North	56	
Pichieh (Bijie), Kweichow (Guizhou)	Salachi Leper Home	Miss M. C. Welzel	1933	China Inland Mission, American Mission to Lepers, Yunnan provincial government, Chinese Mission to Lepers	59	

Tenghsien (Tengxian), Shantung (Shandong)	Leper Home, Mrs. Sarah Watters Memorial Hospital	Miss A. D. Dodds	1919	Mission to Lepers, London	142	
Tsinan (Jinan), Shantung	Tsinan Leprosarium	Dr. H. J. Smyly	1926	Mission to Lepers, London; School of Medicine, Cheeloo University	50	25
Tsingchow (Qingzhou), Shantung	Tsingchow Leprosarium	Mr. Chung Hsiao Wu	1936	English Baptist Mission; Mission to Lepers, London; Chinese Mission to Lepers	21	51
Tsingtao (Qingdao), Shantung	Tsingtao Leprosy Clinic	Rev. R. G. Coonradt	1939	Church of Christ in China, Chinese Mission to Lepers		25
Weihsien (Weixian), Shantung	Leprosy Clinic, Shadyside Presbyterian Hospital	Miss Ruth A. Brack		American Presbyterian Mission, North		40
Yenchowfu (Yanzhoufu) Shantung	Yenchowfu Leper Asylum, St. Joseph's Hospital	Rev. Father Procurator Kubischok	1928	Catholic Mission, Chinese Mission to Lepers	49	
Shensi (Shaanxi)	The Sixth District Leprosariuam, Shensi					
Chengtu (Chengdu), Szechwan (Sichuan)	West China Leprosarium	Dr. Chao	1939	West China Union University	1	

List of Leprosaria and Clinics in China (March 1940)

Location	Name of Institution	Superintendent	Year Established	Responsible Organ	No. of Inmates	No. of Outpatients
Chaotung (Zhaotong), Yunnan	Chaotung Leper Home	Dr. Oliver Lyth	1933	Local government, Missionaries Memorial Hospital, Chinese Mission to Lepers	32	2
Kiulungkiang (Jiulongjiang), Yunnan	Kiulungkiang Leper Asylum	Dr. D. C. Nelson		American Presbyterian Mission, North; Chinese Mission to Lepers	140	
Kunming (Kunming), Yunnan	Kunming District Leprosarium	Dr. Hsu Piao-nan		District government of Kunming	40	
Kunming, Yunnan	Kunming Municipal Leprosarium	Dr. Hsu Piao-nan		Yunnan provincial government	60	
Kunming, Yunnan	Leprosy Relief Corps	Dr. H. Y. Yao	1939	Yunnan Provincial Health Administration, Chinese Mission to Lepers		

Leper Quarterly, March 1940; repr., *Chinese Recorder* 71 (July) 1940: 465–471.

Appendix 2

Indigenous Leper Asylums in Late Imperial China Recorded in Gazetteers

County	Year Established	Name of Asylum	Source
Fujian Province			
Minxian	1518	Yangji yuan	1868 Fujian tongzhi
Jinjiang	Ming	Cunxu yuan	Same as above
Tong'an	Ming	Cunxu yuan	Same as above
Longxi	Early sixteenth century	Laizi ying	Same as above
Huian	Early sixteenth century	Cunxu yuan	Same as above
Changle	1567–1572, 1638 extension	Yangji yuan	1737 Fujian tongzhi
Zhangzhou	1737	Laizi ying	Same as above
Nanjing	?	Puji tang	Same as above
Nanping	Qing	Yangji yuan (quota: 42 inmates, 12 outpatients)	1737 Fujian tongzhi, 1868 Fujian tongzhi

Indigenous Leper Asylums in Late Imperial China Recorded in Gazetteers

County	Year Established	Name of Asylum	Source
Shaxian	Qing, reconstructed after fire of 1724	Yangji yuan	Same as above
Jianning	Qing	Yangji yuan	Same as above
Zhenghe	1735	Mafeng yuan	1868 Fujian tongzhi
Jiangle	1735, reconstructed on old site dated to the Ming	Yangji yuan	Same as above
Shaowu	1758	Yangji yuan	1900 Chongzhuan Shaowu fuzhi
Liancheng	1743	Mafeng yuan	1938 Liancheng xianzhi
Guangdong Province			
Guangzhou (Canton)	Ming	(Quota: 174 inmates, 134 out-of-province patients, 33 additional)	1806 Yangcheng guchao
Haiyang	Before 1744	Laimin suo (quota: 128 inmates, 519 outpatients)	1762 Chaozhou fuzhi
Chaoyang		Laimin suo (quota: 170)	Same as above
Boluo	Before 1764	(Quota: 140 after 1764, 67 before 1864)	Same as above
Jieyang	Before 1731	Laimin suo (quota: 85, another 65 at a newer site)	1731 Jieyang xianzhi, 1762 Chaozhou fuzhi
Huilai	Before 1762	Laimin suo (five different sites, quota: 171)	1762 Chaozhou fuzhi
Chenghai	Before 1762	Laimin suo (two sites, quota: 66)	Same as above
Puning	Before 1762	Laimin suo (quota: 113)	Same as above
Haifeng	1756	(Three sites)	1864 Guangdong tongzhi
Shunde	1731	Mafeng yuan	1853 Shunde xianzhi, 1864 Guangdong tongzhi
Xinhui	Mid-sixteenth century	Pinzi yuan	1690 Xinhui xianzhi
Nanhai	Before 1609	Yangji yuan	1609 Nanhai xianzhi, 1691 Nanhai xianzhi

County	Year Established	Name of Asylum	Source
Panyu	1797		1864 Guangdong tongzhi
Zengcheng	1736	Mafeng yuan	1801 Zhengcheng xianzhi
Dongguan	1639		1639 Dongguan xianzhi
Enping	1738	Feng yuan	1934 Enping xianzhi
Gaoyao	?	Feng yuan (quota: more than 400)	1826 Gaoyao xianzhi
Xinxing	1685?		1834 Zhaoqing fuzhi
Leizhou	Before 1614	Yangyi yuan	1614 Leizhou fuzhi
Jiangxi Province			
Fengxin	1774	Yiji tang	1824 Fengxin xianzhi
Wuning	1743	Mafeng yuan	1873 Nanchang fuzhi
Nanchang	?	(Quota: 40)	1920 Nanchang jishi
Dayu	1736	Puji tang	1875 Nan'an fuzhi buzheng
Zhejiang Province			
Jingning	After 1483	Yangji yuan	1872 Jingning xianzhi
Hubei Province			
Hanyang	1731	Mafeng yuan	1868 Xuji Hanyang xianzhi

Notes

INTRODUCTION

1. F.-O. Touati, *Maladie et société au Moyen Age: La lèpre, les lépreux et les léproseries dans la province écclesiastique de Sens jusqu'au milieu du XIVe siècle* (Paris: DeBoeck University, 1998); F.-O. Touati, "Historiciser la notion de contagion: L'exemple de la lèpre dans les sociétés médiévales," in *Air, miasmes et contagion: Les épidémies dans l'Antiquité et au Moyen Age*, ed. Sylvie Bazin-Tacchella, Danielle Quéruel, and Évelyne Samama, 157–187 (Langres, Fr.: Dominique Guéniot, 2001); F. Bériac, *Des lépreux aux cagots: Recherches sur les sociétés marginales en Aquitaine médiévale* (Bordeaux: Fédération historique du sud-ouest, 1990); Carole Rawcliffe, *Leprosy in Medieval England* (Suffolk, U.K.: Boydell Press, 2006).

2. R. Edmond, *Leprosy and Empire: A Medical and Cultural History* (Cambridge: Cambridge University Press, 2006), 8.

3. V. Møller-Christensen,"Evidence of Leprosy in Earlier Peoples," in *Diseases in Antiquity*, ed. D. Brothwell and A. T. Sandison, 295–306 (Springfield, Ill.: Thomas, 1967); G. D. Lu and J. Needham, "Records of Disease in Ancient China," in ibid., 222–237; J. K. Kinnier Wilson, "Leprosy in Ancient Mesopotamia," *Revue d'assyriologie* 60, no. 1 (1966): 47–58.

4. A. Nakayama and N. Sivin, *Chinese Science: Explorations in an Ancient Tradition* (Cambridge, Mass.: MIT Press, 1973), 306.

5. K. McLeod and R. Yates, "Forms of Ch'in Law: An Annotated Translation of the *Feng-chen shih*," *Harvard Journal of Asiatic Studies* 41, no. 1 (1981): 152–153. There is also a tentative and unannotated translation by D. Harper in *Early China* (3 [1977]: 104), quoted by Derk Bodde, "Forensic Medicine in Pre-imperial China," *Journal of the American Oriental Society* 102, no. 1 (1982): 9–14. For a discussion of the descriptions in this document, see chap. 1.

6. M. Stol, "Leprosy: New Light from Greek and Babylonian Sources," *Jaarbericht Ex Oriente Lux* 30 (1987–1988): 22–31; E. Lieber, "Old Testament 'Leprosy,' Contagion and Sin," in *Contagion: Perspectives from Pre-modern Societies*, ed. L. Conrad and D. Wujastyk, 99–136 (Burlington, Vt.: Ashgate, 2000); D. Wright and R. Jones, "Leprosy," in *Anchor Bible Dictionary*, ed. D. N. Freedman (New York: Doubleday, 1992), 278. Robert Biggs has claimed that "evidence now suggests the occurrence of true leprosy in Palestine in the Byzantine period, but we would not at present be justified in suggesting its occurrence in ancient Mesopotamia at an ealier time" ("Medicine, Surgery, and Public Health in Ancient Mesopotamia," in *Civilizations of the Ancient Near East*, ed. J. M. Sasson [New York: Scribner, 1995], 1917).

7. The term seems to have appeared once or twice in earlier poetry and medical texts, but most likely it was not commonly used before the sixteenth century.

8. Shen Zhiwen, *Jiewei yuansou* (*Sources of Relief*) (1550; repr. facs., Shanghai: Shanghai guji chubanshe, 1997), see chap. 1, 1816 Wuxi Sundetang ed.

9. M. Vaughan, *Curing Their Ills: Colonial Power and African Illness* (Stanford, Calif.: Stanford University Press, 1991); W. Anderson, "Leprosy and Citizenship," *Positions* 6, no. 3 (1998): 707–729; W. Anderson, *Colonial Pathologies: American Tropical Medicine, Race, and Hygiene in the Philippines* (Durham, N.C.: Duke University Press, 2006), especially chap. 6; S. Kakar, "Leprosy in British India, 1860–1940: Colonial Politics and Missionary Medicine," *Medical History* 40 (1996): 215–230; M. Worboys, "The Colonial World as Mission and Mandate: Leprosy and Empire, 1900–1940," *Osiris* 15 (2001): 207–218; J. Buckingham, *Leprosy in Colonial South India: Medicine and Confinement* (New York: Palgrave, 2002); A. Bashford, *Imperial Hygiene: A Critical History of Colonialism, Nationalism and Public Health* (New York: Palgrave, 2004).

10. Z. Gussow, *Leprosy, Racism, and Public Health: Social Policy in Chronic Disease Control* (Boulder, Colo.: Westview, 1989); P. Moblo, "Institutionalizing the Leper: Partisan Politics and the Evolution of Stigma in Post-Monarchy Hawai'i," *Journal of the Polynesian Society* 107, no. 3 (1998): 229–262; S. Burns, "From 'Leper Villages' to 'Leprosaria': Public Health, Nationalism and the Culture of Exclusion in Japan," in *Isolation: Places and Practices of Exclusion*, ed. C. Strange and A. Bashford, 104–118 (London: Routledge, 2003).

11. D. Obregon, "Building National Medicine: Leprosy and Power in Colombia,

1870–1910," *Social History of Medicine* 15, no. 1 (2002): 89–108; K. Jung, "'Colonial Modernity' and the Hegemony of the Body Politic in Leprosy Relief Work" (unpublished document, 37 pp.).

12. S. Parry, "Of Vital Importance to the Community: The Control of Leprosy in the Northern Territory," *Health and History* 5, no. 1(2003): 2.

13. Bashford, *Imperial Hygiene,* 88.

14. P. Moblo, "Blessed Damien of Moloka'i: The Critical Analysis of Contemporary Myth," *Ethnohistory* 44, no. 4 (1997): 696–697; N. Shah, *Contagious Divides: Epidemics and Race in San Francisco's Chinatown* (Berkeley: University of California Press, 2001): 99. See details in chap. 4.

15. The Australian health officer John Ashburton Thompson (1846–1915), for instance, believed that leprosy could have been introduced into Hawaii by immigrants of different ethnic groups during a long period before the end of the eighteenth century. Arthur Mouritz, a physician with the leper settlement of Molokai, showed that leprosy had existed in Hawaii before the arrival of the Chinese coolies. J. A. Thompson, "Leprosy in Hawaii: A Critical Enquiry," in *Mittheilungen und Verhandlungen der internationalen wissenshaftlichen Lepra Conferenz zu Berlin im October 1897* (Berlin: Hirschwald, 1897–1898), especially 2:274, 280–281; A. A. St. M. Mouritz, *The Path of the Destroyer: A History of Leprosy in the Hawaiian Islands* (Honolulu: Honolulu Star-Bulletin, 1916).

16. Bashford cites the Canadian Immigration Act of 1885, which imposed a restrictive head tax on Chinese people, the 1881 Chinese Immigration Restriction Act passed in New Zealand, and also a series of similar acts, beginning in 1881 and continuing until 1888, in other parts of Australia, and the statutory exclusion of Chinese by the U.S. government beginning in 1882 (*Imperial Hygiene,* 142).

17. See chap. 3.

18. J. Fitzgerald, *Awakening China: Politics, Culture, and Class in the Nationalist Revolution* (Stanford, Calif.: Stanford University Press, 1996), 11.

19. R. Rogaski, *Hygienic Modernity: Meanings of Health and Disease in Treaty-Port China* (Berkeley: University of California Press, 2004), 238.

20. See Rogaski's description of the discourse of the "father of Chinese eugenics," Pan Guangdan, in the mid-1930s (ibid., 240–244).

21. For a recent discussion of the epithet, see Yang Ruisong, "Xiangxiang minzu chiru: Jindai Zhongguo sixiang wenhua shi shang di 'Dongya bingfu'" (Imaging National Humiliation: "Sick Man of East Asia" in Modern Chinese Intellectual and Cultural History), *Guoli Zhengzhi daxue lishi xuebao* 23 (2005): 1–44. Yang argues that the anxiety about the decline of physical prowess of the Chinese people grew during the early twentieth century and that this epithet, used to describe the weakness of the Qing state in the late nineteenth century, was later used to imply the physical weakness of the Chinese people.

22. See David Arnold's fine analyses of the interaction between Indian society and

Western medicine in the colonial period: *Colonizing the Body: State Medicine and Epidemic Disease in Nineteenth-Century India* (Berkeley: University of California Press, 1993); *Science, Technology and Medicine in Colonial India* (Cambridge: Cambridge University Press, 2000).

23. My account here is a summary of the following texts: R. McGrew, "Leprosy," in *Encyclopedia of Medical History* (New York: McGraw-Hill, 1985): 161–165; A. Carmichael, "Leprosy," in *The Cambridge World History of Human Disease,* ed. K Kiple (New York: Cambridge University Press, 1993): 834–839; "Microbiology of Leprosy," WHO, http://www.who.int/lep/disease/microbiology/frconten.htm (accessed February 10, 2004); WHO Study Group, *Epidemiology of Leprosy in Relation to Control,* WHO Technical Report Series 716 (Geneva: WHO, 1985): especially 19–29; WHO Regional Office for the Western Pacific, *Overview and Epidemiological Review of Leprosy in the WHO Western Pacific Region, 1991–2001* (Manila: WHO, 2003): especially 69.

24. The treatment consists of combinations of a number of chemicals, including rifampicin, dapsone, and clofazimine, and also ofloxacin and minocycline. The dosage, combination, and duration of treatment (from six to twelve months) vary according to the type of leprosy. See http://www.who.int/lep/disease/disease.htm, 1.

25. WHO Regional Office for the Western Pacific, *Overview,* 28.

26. There is notably a Franco-British team working on such a project, financed by the American Heiser Foundation and the French Fondation Raoul Follereau. See N. Brunel, "Lèpre: Découverte franco-britannique," *Label France* 44 (2001): 48.

27. WHO, *World Health Organization Leprosy Elimination Project Status Report 2003 Draft* (Geneva: WHO, 2004): 10, 14.

28. Although the relation of leprosy to HIV has not been well studied, it is now recognized that HIV infection is a cause of an increase in pulmonary tuberculosis. The close relation between leprosy and tuberculosis (BCG vaccination is effective for the prevention of the leprosy bacillus) makes many experts nervous about the possible link between HIV infection and lepromatous leprosy. See "Microbiology of Leprosy," WHO, http://www.who.int/lep/disease/microbiology/factors.htm (accessed February 10, 2004), 2.

29. For a discussion of the liberal position of British colonialists who were against enforced segregation, see Bashford's quote of a prominent British expert, Leonard Rogers (*Imperial Hygiene,* 89–90). Such a position was also taken by James Maxwell, the expert in China.

30. Buckingham, *Leprosy in Colonial South India,* 178–186, 191; Kakar, "Leprosy in British India," 220–221.

31. G. Woods, "The Demographic Effects of Introduced Diseases, and Especially Leprosy, upon the Hawaiian People" (paper read at the Ninth International Medical Congress, Washington, D.C., September 9, 1887), quoted by R. D. K. Herman in "Out of Sight, out

of Mind, out of Power: Leprosy, Race and Colonization in Hawai'i," *Journal of Historical Geography* 27, no. 3 (2001): 328.

32. Bashford, *Imperial Hygiene,* 89, 93–94; Parry, "Of Vital Importance," 5.

33. Burns, "From 'Leper Villages' to 'Leprosaria,'" 108; the quotation is from Saitō Yoshio, a Diet member who, in 1902, proposed a leprosy prevention law.

34. Ibid., 111, 113–114, 117. On enforced abortion, see *Lianhe bao* (United Daily [Taiwan]), January 28, 2005, A14, a translation of a report from Agence France Presse (Tokyo, January 27, 2005) to the effect that, between 1924 and 1956, many female sufferers were forced to abort, and the fetuses were kept as laboratory samples.

35. I. Kikuchi, "Hansen's Disease Patients: Responses to Stigma and Segregation in Kumamoto, Japan," *International Journal of Dermatology* 33, no. 2 (1994): 142–143.

36. "The Lepers of Japan," *Economist,* February 24, 1996, 64; P. Pons, "Les lépreux japonais vont retrouver la liberté," *Le Monde,* February 6, 1996. More recent research on Japanese leprosy control policies attempts to modify this Foucauldian version of Japanese history by looking at other, "softer" versions of leprosaria set up by British missionaries. See Hirokawa Waka, "Hansen byōsha no ryōyō keitai ni kansuru kōsatsu: Gunma Ken Agatsuma Kusatsu chō Yunosawa Buraku no jirei kara" (A Study on the Care of Patients of Hansen's Disease Based on the Yunosawa Leper Village in Kusatsu, Agatsuma District, Gunma Prefecture), *Buraku mondai kenkyū* 173 (2005): 22–42.

37. Moblo, "Blessed Damien of Moloka'i"; Moblo, "Institutionalizing the Leper"; Herman, "Out of Sight"; Anderson, "Leprosy and Citizenship"; Anderson, *Colonial Pathologies.*

38. Quoted in Worboys, "Colonial World as Mission and Mandate," 217.

39. Li Wenzhong, ed., *Xiandai mafeng bing xue* (*Modern Leprology*) (Shanghai: Shanghai kexue chubanshe, 2006), 14; e-mail message to author from Dr. Jiang Cheng, leprologist in Nanjing, February 22, 2005.

40. Vaughan, *Curing Their Ills,* 86, 92, 97.

41. Burns, "From 'Leper Villages' to 'Leprosaria,'" 116.

42. The journal published by the Chinese Mission to Lepers, *Leper Quaterly,* began, in 1927, publishing occasional short letters, novels, and essays by patients. In April 1940, a bilingual quarterly called *Chenguang jikan* (*Morning Light Quarterly*) was created by a patient, Zhuang Jianxiong (1914–1941), with two other patients in the Shanghai asylum. This journal, also supported by the Chinese Mission to Lepers, combined articles on medical knowledge of leprosy, literary creations by patients, and pieces on the "virtue of self-support." See Jiang Cheng, "Mafeng bingren chuangban di zazhi: 'Chenguang jikan'" (A Journal Created by Patients of Leprosy: *Morning Light Quarterly*), *Zhongguo mafeng zazhi* 8, no. 1 (1992): 44. More recently a long novel by a cured patient who claimed to have survived leprosaria of the pre- and post-1949 periods in Guangdong province reveals the harsh realities inside these institutions. Lin Zhiming [1929–], *Feiyue mafengyuan* (*Fly*

Over the Leprosarium) (Hong Kong: Legend Publishing, 2000) (This is a reprint of an earlier book, *Kunan buzai renjian* [*Hardship Is Not Found in the Human World*], published by Huacheng chubanshe, Canton).

On the other hand, a considerable amount of archival materials at the Lesheng asylum in Taipei, established by the Japanese colonizers in 1930, may contain writings by its patients. Such documents have not yet been systematically classified and analyzed.

Very few of the mentioned sources, which could shed light on the formulation of the modern identity or subjectivity of patients, have been available to scholars.

43. Chin Hsien-yu, "Colonial Medical Police and Postcolonial Medical Surveillance Systems in Taiwan, 1895–1950s," *Osiris* 13 (1998): 326–338; Liu Shiyong, "Qingjie, weisheng yu baojian: Ri zhi shiqi Taiwan shehui gonggong weisheng guannian zhi zhuanbian" (Sanitation, Hygiene, and Health Protection: The Changes in the Conceptualization of Public Health in Taiwan During the Japanese Occupation Period), *Taiwan shi yanjiu* 8, no. 1 (2001): 41–88; T. Henry, "Sanitizing Empire: Japanese Articulations of Korean Otherness and the Construction of Early Colonial Seoul, 1905–1919," *Journal of Asian Studies* 64, no. 3 (2005): 639–676.

See also the research of Wataru Iijima on the development of Japanese colonial medicine in the colonies: "Infectious and Parasitic Disease Studies in Taiwan, Manchuria, and Korea under the Japanese Empire: Brief History on Japanese Colonial Medicine" (paper presented at the conference "Ideas and Practices of Hygiene in Han Societies from the Traditional to the Modern Periods," Academia Sinica, Taipei, November 22–24, 2004).

44. D. Chakrabarty, *Provincializing Europe: Postcolonial Thought and Historical Difference* (Princeton, N.J.: Princeton University Press 2000).

45. W. Anderson, "Postcolonial Histories of Medicine," in *Locating Medical History: The Stories and Their Meanings*, ed. F. Huisman and J. Warner, 285–306 (Baltimore: Johns Hopkins University Press, 2004).

1. *LI/LAI/DAFENG/MAFENG*

1. A few such works are Huang Shengbai, "Shuo li" (On *Li*), *Yiyao xue* 12 (1929); Wang Jimin, "Zhongguo mafeng shi zhong zhi mingren" (Famous People in the Chinese History of Leprosy), *Zhonghua yixue zazhi* 27, no. 9 (1941): 565–568; Yu Shenchu, *Zhongguo mafeng bingxue* (*Study on Leprosy in China*) (Shanghai: Fuxing zhongyishe, 1941), especially 2–3; You Jiajun, *Mafeng bingxue gailun* (*General Discussion on Leprosy*) (Shanghai: Huadong yiwu shenghuo she, 1953), especially 2; Yue Meizhong, "Guanyu zuguo yixue mafeng shishi ji qi zhuzuo di xushu" (On the Historical Facts of Leprosy and Its Description in Medical Texts in Our Mother Country), *Shanghai zhongyi zazhi* 9 (1956): 40–43; Xiao Yunchun, "Zuguo yixue duiyu mafeng zhi renshi" (Our Mother Country's Knowledge

on Leprosy), *Zhongyi zazhi* 4 (1956): 170–173; Liang Zhangchi, "Zhongguo gudai mafeng shishi kaobian" (Analysis of Historical Facts on Leprosy in Ancient China), *Pifu xing bing fangzhi tongxun* 2, no. 1 (1963): 51–63.

2. There are three main parts in the *Inner Canon:* "Plain Questions"(Suwen), "Divine Pivot" (Lingshu), and "Grand Basis"(Taisu), the last being less quoted in the later age. "Plain Questions" is mostly theoretical discussions on cosmology, the body, and disorders, whereas "Divine Pivot" is mostly on acupuncture. There is no agreement on the dating of the compiled text; many Chinese scholars have considered the text to have been compiled not later than the second century B.C., such as Ma Jixing, who thinks that the classic was first compiled toward the end of the Warring States period, that is, the third century B.C. (*Zhongyi wenxian xue* [*Studies on Traditional Chinese Medical Texts*] [Shanghai: Kexue jishu chubanshe, 1990], 68).

Nathan Sivin, on the other hand, dates the work, based on David Keegan's research, between the first century B.C. and the first century A.D. (*Traditional Medicine in Contemporary China* [Ann Arbor: Center for Chinese Studies, University of Michigan, 1987], 5); see also "Huang ti nei ching," in *Early Chinese Texts: A Bibliographical Guide,* ed. Michael Loewe, 196–215 [Berkeley: Society for the Study of Early China, 1993]).

3. G. D. Lu and J. Needham, "Records of Disease in Ancient China," in *Diseases in Antiquity,* ed. D. Brothwell and A. T. Sandison, 222–237 (Springfield, Ill.: Thomas, 1967).

4. S. Nakayama and N. Sivin, *Chinese Science: Explorations in an Ancient Tradition* (Cambridge, Mass.: MIT Press, 1973), 306.

5. The character *li* is now believed to have two readings in this context: *li* or *lai.* This was suggested mainly by Tang historians and philologists. In fact, texts before the fourth century mostly used the ideogram *li* and rarely that for *lai.* The glossing of *li* as identical to *lai* in pronunciation, by Sima Zhen of the Tang in his commentaries on the biography of Yu Rang in the *Shiji* somehow fixed the interchangeability of the two words. The *Huainan zi* (second century B.C.) names the illness of Boniu, Confucius's disciple, *li.* The Tang philologist Kong Yingda (574–648) replaced the character *li* with *lai* when quoting this passage in his commentaries on the *Zuo Tradition of the Spring and Autumn Annals,* clearly showing the interchangeability of the two ideograms by this time.

6. M. Porkert, *The Theoretical Foundations of Chinese Medicine: Systems of Correspondence* (Cambridge, Mass.: MIT Press, 1974), chap. 1 ("Basic Standards of Value: Yin and Yang and the Five Evolutive Phases").

7. Porkert's translation.

8. According to Fan Xingzhun, the late authority on the history of Chinese medicine, the notion of the six *qi* arose around the tenth century from the originally five atmospheric influences described in the *Inner Canon* (*Zhongguo yixue shilue* [*A Brief History of Chinese Medicine*] [Beijing: Zhongyi guji chubanshe, 1986], 127–128). The five influences described in the ancient classic did not include Summer Heat (*shu*).

9. The character *li* had multiple meanings in early texts. The three main ones of interest here are "terrifying ghost," "serious illness" or "epidemic," and "horrifying" or "ugly." The character can also be pronounced as *lai* and have the same meanings as the character *lai*, whose primary meaning is "disease with ugly sores." For a discussion of the early meanings of *li*, see Lin Fushi, "Shi shi Shuihudi Qin jian zhong di 'li' yu 'ding sha'" (Explanations of the Terms "*Li*" and "*Ding Sha*" in Qin Bamboo Strips Discovered at Shuihudi), *Shiyuan* 15 (1986): 1–38.

10. A sixth element, Summer Heat (*shu*), was added to the list of atmospheric influences around the tenth century. *Juan* 19 of the classic, believed to have been added in the tenth century, included *shu* as one of the six influences (see n. 8). The frequently quoted sentence "Wind is the origin of hundreds of disorders" appears several times in the "Plain Questions" (Suwen) section of the classic (42, *juan* 5:58). It also appears several times in other sections: section 3 ("Sheng qi tong tian lun"), section 19 ("Yuji zhen cang lun"), section 42 ("Feng lun"), and section 60 ("Gu kong lun").

11. For an analysis of Wind based on ancient literary and medical classics, see S. Kuriyama, "The Imagination of Winds and the Development of the Chinese Conception of the Body," in *Body, Subject, and Power in China*, ed. A. Zito and T. Barlow, 23–41 (Chicago: University of Chicago Press, 1994): 23–41.

12. This translation of the text is based on the interpretation of the Qing doctor Zhang Zhicong (1619–1674), who differentiated in this ancient text two types of *li*, a serious and a less-serious type. The translated part here is a description of the more serious type. For the significance of Zhang's reading of this passage in the understanding of the disease, see Zhang Zhicong, *Huangdi neijing suwen ji zhu* (*Annotated Plain Questions of the "Yellow Emperor's Inner Canon"*), vol. 1 of *Zhongguo yixue dacheng* (hereafter *YXDC*), ed. Cao Bingzhang (Shanghai: Shanghai kexue jishu chubanshe, 1990), *juan* 5:57. The constructive energy (*rong qi*) should normally flow within the channels and not digress into the flesh.

13. The term *dafeng* appears in sections 3 and 60 of "Plain Questions" of the *Inner Canon* and section 75 of "Divine Pivot," referring in all cases to a particularly noxious Wind influence and not to any specific disorder. *Efeng* appears as a pathogenic influence in section 17 of "Plain Questions," and as a symptom in sections 36 and 42. *Zeifeng* appears in sections 2, 13, and 29 of "Plain Questions" and in sections 58 and 59 of "Divine Pivot" in reference, in all cases, to a particularly bad atmospheric influence.

14. Zhang Zhicong, *Huangdi*, *juan* 6:15.

15. I am referring here to the annotated edition by Ding Guangdi, *Zhubing yuan hou lun jiaozhu* (Beijing: Renmin weisheng chubanshe, 1996).

16. The "eight Winds" constituted a cosmic notion in this text; Chao describes three different kinds of Winds from each of the eight directions, provoking different symptoms. The number of pathogenic Winds described in this text varies within the systematic numerology of ancient medicine, sometimes in accordance with the greater cosmic

order, other times corresponding to the bodily order, such as the five Winds attacking the five viscera.

17. Chao, *Zhubing yuan hou,* 2:70–71.

18. The effects of *efeng* on the viscera that produced serious symptoms were specified as type 50, "symptoms of [produced by] *efeng*" (ibid. 2:73).

19. Sun Simiao, *Beiji qianjin yaofang* (Beijing: Renmin weisheng chubanshe, 1982; repr. of the Edo igaku facs. of the Northern Song ed.).

20. Wang Tao, *Waitai miyao fang* (Osaka: Toyo ikagu, 1981).

21. Sun, *Beiji qianjin yaofang,* 8:159, 171, with recipes for disorders causing the falling out of hair, itchiness, deafness, and so on; 23:427–428, on *eji/dafeng.*

22. Ibid., 23:427; Wang Tao, *Waitai miyao fang,* 30:2. Sun provides a lengthy description of *ebing* in another work, *Qianjin yifang* (*Supplementary Recipes Worthy of a Thousand Gold Pieces*) [Beijing: Renmin weisheng chubanshe, 1955; based on a 1307 ed.], 21:250–256), in which he incorporates more details on *lai* symptoms, with relevant recipes.

23. The Qing philological scholar Duan Yucai (1735–1815) considered *li* simply an archaic term for *lai.* See his annotated edition of Xu Shen's [ca. first century A.D.] *Shuo wen jie zi* (*Etymological Dictionary*) (Shanghai: Shanghai guji chubanshe, 1988), *pian* 7b, under "*li*"; see also n. 5.

24. The story of Yu Rang in the *Zhanguo ce* (*Record of the Warring States*) is a more detailed account, where the assassin is described as having painted his body and removed his hair and eyebrows to disguise himself as a *li* sufferer ([Shanghai: Guji chubanshe, 1978], 18:591). The *Shiji* (Sima Qian, *Records of the Grand Historian*) repeats the story briefly ([Beijing: Zhonghua shuju, 1982]: 86:2520). Most of these early stories are quoted in the articles cited in n. 3.

25. For this reason, I do not support translating *li/lai* as "leprosy" in the early texts, as did Burton Watson (*Chuang Tzu: Basic Writings* [New York: Columbia University Press, 1968], 4) and Graham (as quoted in D. Bodde, "Forensic Medicine in Pre-imperial China," *Journal of the American Oriental Society* 102, no. 1 [1982]: 10). The contrast between the *li* woman and Xishi in this passage of the *Zhuangzi* is between ugliness and beauty. *Li* here can have the meaning of appalling ugliness, as that attributed to ghosts, or ugliness due to repulsive sores. Rendering the term as "leprosy" is an overtranslation. It is more appropriate to follow the glossing of Cheng Xuanying of the Tang, who rendered *li zhi ren* as an "ugly sick person." See also Lin, "Shi shi Shuihudi," 13–14.

26. These bamboo texts were excavated in Shuihudi in 1975. The translation is from K. McLeod and R.Yates, "Forms of Ch'in Law: An Annotated Translation of the *Feng-chen shih,*" *Harvard Journal of Asiatic Studies* 41, no. 1 (1981): 152–153. In his 1982 article ("Forensic Medicine in Pre-imperial China," *Journal of the American Oriental Society* 102, no. 1 [1982]: 9–14), Derk Bodde used an earlier translation, by Donald Harper (*Early China,* 1977).

27. Ma Jixing, *Mawangdui gu yishu kaoshi* (*Research and Explanations on Old Medical Texts Found in Mawangdui*) (Changsha: Hunan kexue jishu chubanshe, 1992), 162.

28. Ge Hong, *Zhou hou beiji fang* (*Handy Recipes for Urgent Use*) (Beijing: Renmin weisheng chubanshe, 1983), 5.40:105. The extant edition of this text was reedited and recompiled by a number of later authors so that descriptions and recipes are of different periods after the fourth century. For the history of this book, see Ma, *Zhongyi wenxian xue,* 159–162.

29. Recipes related to *dafeng* and anecdotes concerning famous people suffering from the disorder of the later periods, especially Sui-Tang, were added at the end of this section (Ge, *Zhou hou bieji fang,* 5.40:106–110).

30. Chao, *Zhubing yuan hou,* 2:79.

31. M. Dols, "Leprosy in Medieval Arabic Medicine," *Journal of the History of Medicine and Allied Sciences* 34, no. 3 (1979): 327.

32. This point is mentioned by J. V. Kinnier Wilson ("Leprosy in Ancient Mesopotamia," *Revue d'assyriologie* 60, no. 1 [1966]: 47–58) and also by M. Stol ("Leprosy: New Light from Greek and Babylonian Sources," *Jaarbericht Ex Oriente Lux* 30 [1987–1988]: 22–31); a more up-to-date review of the problem is presented by David Wright in his entry "Leprosy" (*Anchor Bible Dictionary,* ed. D. N. Freedman [New York: Doubleday, 1992], 277–282). These works indicate that the Old Babylonian *saharšuppû,* or the term in Leviticus, *ṣāraʿat,* or the Greek terms *elephantiasis* or *lepra* do not readily correlate to the modern concept of leprosy or Hansen's disease. There were also other words, such as the Greek *lōbè,* which may also imply some form of leprosy. The authors of the works cited agree that leprosy would be only one among many skin diseases designated by most of these ancient terms. I am grateful to Tzvi Abusch and Amneris Roselli for introducing me to these sources and deciphering the Old Babylonian and Greek texts for me.

33. *Taiping shenghui fang* (Taipei: Xinwenfeng chuban gongsi, 1969; facs. of the Japanese ms. ed., National Central Library), 24:16a. In this chapter, the *dafeng* category with the main symptom of the falling out of the eyebrows still followed closely the descriptions in the *Inner Canon,* whereas the *dafeng lai* category clearly repeats Ge Hong's descriptions.

34. Discussion of *chong* can be found in a subsequent section of the present chapter.

35. *Shengji zonglu* (Beijing: Renmin weisheng chubanshe, 1992), 18:449.

36. The *Shengji zonglu* was first published during the northern Jin dynasty in the late eleventh century and had greater influence among northern medical experts in the Jin and Yuan periods up to the fourteenth century.

37. On the importance of the Jin-Yuan masters in Chinese medical history, see A. K. C. Leung, "Medical Learning from the Song to the Ming," in *The Song-Yuan-Ming Transition in Chinese History,* ed. P. Smith and R. von Glahn, 374–398 (Cambridge, Mass.: Harvard University Press, 2003).

38. Liu Wansu, *Suwen bingji qi yi baoming ji* (*Lifesaving Book on the Pathogenesis and Qi Mechanism of "Plain Questions"*), in *Congshu jicheng xinbian* (Taipei: Xinwenfeng chuban gongsi, 1985), vol. 45, *juan* 2:42.

39. The book *Huofa jiyao* (*Essential Mechanisms of Methods That Save Lives*), attributed to Li Gao (1180–1251), is an example. There is controversy over the real author of this text, who totally agrees with Liu's position on *dafeng/lai.* See the modern edition of this work, *Dongyuan yiji* (*Medical Works of Li Gao*) (Beijing: Renmin weisheng chubanshe, 1993), 8, 345.

40. Leung, "Medical Learning."

41. Chen Yan, *San yin ji yi bingzheng fang lun* (Wenyuange Siku quanshu ed.) (Taipei: Shangwu yinshuguan, 1983), vol. 743, *juan* 15:21b.

42. Leung, "Medical Learning."

43. The Daoist compilation is attributed to Zhao Yizhen and was edited by Liu Yuanran; see K. Schipper and F. Verellen, eds., *The Taoist Canon: A Historical Companion to the "Daozang"* (Chicago: University of Chicago Press, 2004), 2: 777–779 (entry on the text by Nathan Sivin).

The author of the text on *dafeng* in chapter 11 of the compilation is given as Shuran-zi, known otherwise as the important Northern Song Daoist master Zhang Jixian. It is impossible to date this text except to say that it was already included in the fifteenth-century Ming dynasty canon, and it was probably a fourteenth-century text; see the *Xianchuan waike bifang,* in *Daozang yaoji xuankan* (*Selections of Important Texts in the Daoist Canon*), *juan* 9:589–598 (Shanghai: Shanghai guji chubanshe, 1989).

44. Leung, "Medical Learning"; on the development of diagnostic sophistication of mainstream doctors in the Song, see C. Furth, *A Flourishing Yin* (Berkeley: University of California Press, 1996), 65–66, 71–72.

45. On the popularization of medical knowledge of the late imperial period, see A. K. C. Leung, "Medical Instruction and Popularization in Ming-Qing China," *Late Imperial China* 24, no. 1 (2003): 130–152.

46. Shen Zhiwen, *Jiewei yuansou* (Shanghai: Shanghai guji chubanshe, 1997; facs. of the 1816 Wuxi ed.), 571.

47. On the life of Huang Zhong, see the preface by Gu Gao of the 1816 edition. Gu, also a Wuxi native, passed the highest grade in the civil examination and had the title of *jinshi;* see also He Shixi, *Zhongguo lidai yijia chuanlu* (*Biographies of Medical People in Chinese History*). (Beijing: Renmin weisheng chubanshe, 1991), 2:564.

48. This brief biography of Xiao Xiaoting has been constructed from the various prefaces written by himself, his son, and the publisher of the 1845 reprint (Guangdong: Jingye tang engraving) of the 1836 Wuyun lou edition. A modern edition, including all these prefaces, was published in 1999 by Zhongguo yiyao chubanshe, Beijing, as part of its Zhenben yishu jicheng series.

49. Their marginality does not mean they lacked influence. Xiao's work was quoted as an authority as early as the mid-nineteenth century, shortly after its first publication. It was quoted, for example, by Chen Huiyan in his popular collection of writings *Nanyue youji* (*Records on a Voyage in the Southern Yue Region*) (1851), 3:6a.

50. Wong Foon [Huang Kuan], "Dr. F. Wong's Memorandum on Leprosy," in "Medical Report for the Half Year ended 30th September 1873, Forwarded by the Surgeons to the Customs at the Treaty Ports in China, Being Number 6 of the Series and Forming the 6th Part of the Customs Gazette for July–September 1873" (Shanghai: Imperial Maritime Customs Statistical Department, 1874), 43–44.

51. The adding of the radical "ailment" to the character *feng* in *mafeng* in the late imperial period transformed the word into one that could have the connotation of "insanity" or "mental disorder." This sometimes causes confusion. All the more so when a late imperial doctor such as Zhang Jiebin discusses the *da mafeng* category in a chapter on "miscellaneous" disorders together with insanity (*diankuang*), dementia (*chidai*), constipation, difficulty in urination, and so forth (*Jingyue quanshu* [*The Complete Works of Zhang Jiebin*] [Shanghai: Shanghai kexue jishu chubanshe, 1991; facs. of the 1711 Kangxi ed.]), *juan* 34). Despite this confusion and sporadic comments on the possibility of insanity in *mafeng* cases, the symptom of insanity was not considered typical of *mafeng*.

52. Chen Yan, *San yin*, 15:21b.

53. C. Furth, "The Physician as Philosopher of the Way: Zhu Zhenheng (1282–1358)," *Harvard Journal of Asiatic Studies* 66, no. 2 (2006): 423–459.

54. Zhu Zhenheng, *Jingui gou xuan* (*Enlightening Comments on the "Golden Chamber Classic"*), in *Danxi yiji*, ed. Zhejiang sheng Zhongyiyao yanjiu yuan wenxian yanjiu shi (Beijing: Renmin weisheng chubanshe, 1993), 1:112.

55. Xu Chunfu, *Gujin yitong daquan* (*A Complete Book of Old and New Medical Traditions*) (Taipei: Xinwenfeng chubanshe, 1978; facs. of the 1570 Ming ed.), *juan* 9:13b.

56. Another example is the *huo* (fire) element. This external environmental factor was also gradually discussed as an internal cause of disease after the Yuan. See Li Jianmin, "Bencao gangmu huobu kaoshi" (Fire as Medicine: The "Fire" Section of the *Bencao gangmu*), *Bulletin of the Institute of History and Philology, Academia Sinica* 73, no. 3 (2002): 396–441.

57. Wu Youxing, *Wenyi lun buzheng* (*Treatise on Epidemics Caused by the Warm Factor, with Supplementary Verifications*) (Taipei: Xinwenfeng shuju, 1985; facs. of the 1895 ed. by Zheng Chongguang), *juan* 2:43.

58. On the development of such an idea in the late imperial period, see A. K. C. Leung, "Jibing yu fangtu zhi guanxi: Yuan zhi Qing jian yijie di kanfa" (The Relations Between Diseases and Locality: The Views in Medical Books from the Yuan to the Qing), in *Xingbie yu yiliao: Di san jie guoji hanxue huiyi lunwen ji* (*Gender and Medicine: Volume of the Third International Conference on Sinology*), ed. Huang Kewu, 165–212 (Taipei: Insti-

tute of Modern History, Academia Sinica, 2002); see also M. Hanson, "Robust Northerners and Delicate Southerners: The 19th-Century Invention of a Southern Medical Tradition," *Positions* 6, no. 3 (1998): 515–550.

59. He subdivided the *li* disorder into "classic symptoms," "symptoms [concurrent with other disorders]," "varied symptoms," and "pseudo-symptoms"(Xue Ji, *Liyang jiyao* [*Keys and Essentials to Skin Disorders of the* Li *Category*], in *Xue shi yi an xuan* [*Selections of Xue Ji's Medical Cases*] [Beijing: Renmin weisheng chubanshe, 1986], *juan* 1:7).

60. Dou Menglin, *Chuangyang jingyan quanshu* (Kangxi ed., Chunshun tang, 1717), 3:46a. This work was first published under the name of Dou's ancestor, Dou Muo (1196–1280); Qi Kun, *Waike dacheng* (Shanghai: Shanghai weisheng chubanshe, 1957), 314.

61. *Xianchuan waike bifang, juan* 9:589.

62. Xue, *Liyang jiyao, juan* 1:7.

63. Shen, *Jiewei yuansuo,* 1:585.

64. Xiao Xiaoting, *Fengmen quanshu, juan* 1:6a, 21a. Xiao quotes Zhu as having written, "Anesthesia [*mamu*] is the basic symptom [*ben*] of the *li* disorder." I cannot find this quote in any of Zhu's extant works, but in his *Danxi xin fa* (*Authentic Methods of Zhu Zhenheng*), he mentions at least three recipes for the *mafeng* disorder, showing that Zhu probably did use the term, as anesthesia was for him an essential symptom (in *Danxi yiji* [*Medical Works of Zhu Zhenheng*] [Beijing: Renmin weisheng chubanshe, 1993], 4:369).

The Daoist text in question is the *Xianchuan waike bifang,* and the relevant passage is attributed to a Song Daoist master of the twelfth century; see n. 43.

65. The term *mafeng* is also present sporadically in some Song poems and medical recipe books. It is uncertain if the term specifically implied *lai* disorders when used in poems, or if later editors of the Song medical texts (the earliest extant editions are of the Ming dynasty) had modified the terms. One example is the important Southern Song text *Renzhai zhizhi,* which contains at least three recipes for the *da mafeng* disorder. Since the earliest extant edition is a sixteenth-century text, we cannot be sure that the term for the disorder was not modified by Ming editors (see the 1550 edition, 24:18a–19a). We can at least say that, even if the term did appear during the Song, it was not used widely, as it was during the Ming and Qing periods.

66. Zhang Jiebin, *Jingyue quanshu, juan* 34:590.

67. Qi, *Waike dacheng,* 314.

68. Shen, *Jiewei yuansou,* 1:2b–3a.

69. Zhang Zhicong, *Huangdi, juan* 5:57.

70. Xu Dachun, *Xu ping waike zhengzong* (*Comments by Xu Dachun on Chen Shigong's "Orthodoxy of External Medicine"*), in *YXDC* (Changsha: Yuelu shushe, 1990), 5:134.

71. Wong, "Dr. F. Wong's Memorandum," 43.

72. The famous Yuan medical compilation *Lingnan weisheng fang* (*Life-Preserving Recipes for the Lingnan Region*) was a typical product of such a concept. A modern edi-

tion of the work is the 1983 (Beijing: Zhongyi guji chubanshe) facsimile of the 1841 Japanese edition.

73. Xue, *Liyang jiyao, juan* 1:7.

74. This Ming medical book is no longer extant, but the passage is quoted in the Qing book *Yifang leiju* (*A Collection of Medical Recipes*) (1861; repr. Beijing: Renmin weisheng chubanshe, 1981), 24:649. The original Tang story is in *Guoshi bu* (*Supplement to the History of the Dynasty*); in *Biji xiaoshuo daguan* (Taipei: Xinxing shuju, 1977), ser. 21, vol. 2, *juan* 1:8b.

75. Chen Shidou, *Shishi milu* (Beijing: Zhongguo zhongyiyao chubanshe, 1986), 5:211.

76. Wu Qian et al., *Yizong jinjian* (Beijing: Renmin weisheng chubanshe, 1990; based on the 1742 Wuyingdian ed.), vol. 2, *juan* 73:376–377. There is an English translation of this passage by B. A. J. Van Wettum, "A Chinese Opinion on Leprosy: Being a Translation of a Chapter from the Medical Standard Book, *Imperial Edition of the Golden Mirror for the Medical Class*," *T'oung Pao*, ser. 2, vol. 2 (1901): 256–268.

77. L. Demaître, "The Description and Diagnosis of Leprosy by 14th-Century Physicians," *Bulletin of the History of Medicine* 59, no. 3 (1985): 334. Coitus with a leprous woman was also considered in medieval Europe a likely cause of contracting the disease.

78. Shen, *Jiewei yuansou*, 1:7a–b.

79. Xiao Xiaoting, *Fengmen quanshu, juan* 1:9a.

80. This text was excavated at the famous archaeological site in Mawangdui in the 1970s. In this text, the ailment named *ming* is described as follows: "*Ming* is a kind of *chong*. The places where it chews holes . . . It does not emerge at a regular spot. Sometimes it is located at the nose, sometimes at the side of the mouth, sometimes at the teeth and gums, sometimes at the hands and fingers. . . It causes the collapse of the bridge of one's nose and the breaking off of one's fingers." My translation is based on both Ma Jixing's rendition in modern Chinese (*Mawangdui gu yishu kaoshi*, 437) and Donald Harper's English translation in *Early Chinese Medical Literature* (London: Kegan Paul, 1998), 250.

81. Chao, *Zhubing yuan hou*, 2:73.

82. Ibid.

83. Ibid.

84. Sun, *Beiji qianjin yaofang*, 18:335.

85. Li Qinpu thinks that the idea of "80,000 corpse *chong*" could have come from an early Buddhist sutra of the fifth century that mentions "eighty thousand *hu chong*" ("Bawan shi chong yu bawan hu chong," *Zhonghua yishi zazhi* 26, no. 2 [1996]: 108). K. Schipper mentions "three corpses" (corresponding to the upper, middle, and lower parts of the body) inside the human body containing "three worms" or "nine worms." If the worms could be expelled from the body by dietetic or other means, the person could become an immortal (*Le corps taoiste: Corps physique, corps social* [Paris: Fayard, 1982], 152,179, 232).

86. It is true, however, that major books like the *Taiping shenghui fang* of the early Song and the *Renzhai zhizhi* of the late Song nonetheless mention *chong* in passages devoted to *dafeng lai.* But they simply copy word for word Chao's descriptions as a required task to pay respect to earlier classics. Medical writers who critiqued the medical tradition in this period all seem to disregard the element of *chong* in the *li/lai* disorder.

87. Shen, *Jiewei yuansuo,* 1:8b.

88. For a useful explanation of *gu* magic and the long history of its practice, see H. T. Feng and J. K. Shryock, "The Black Magic in China Known as *Ku,*" *Journal of the American Oriental Society* 55, no. 1 (1935): 1–30.

89. Ge, *Zhou hou beiji fang,* all of section 63 in *juan* 7 is on recipes to combat *gu* poisoning.

90. Chao, *Zhubing yuan hou,* 24.13:702–703; 25.1:716–717.

91. Richard von Glahn mentions an incident involving *gu* witchcraft and female seduction quoted in the *Chronicles of Zuo* that took place in 541 B.C. (*Sinister Way: The Divine and the Demonic in Chinese Religious Culture* [Berkeley: University of California Press, 2004], 110).

92. Feng and Shryock, "Black Magic in China," 10.

93. Lu Shizhong, *Wushang xuanyuan santian yutang dafa* (*Great Method of the Jade Hall of the Three Heavens, of the Supreme Mysterious Origin*) (30 *juan,* ca. 1158), vol. 30 of *Zhonghua Daozang,* ed. Zhang Jiyu (Beijing: Huaxia chubanshe, 2004). For a description of the text, see Schipper and Verellen, *Taoist Canon,* 2:1070–1073. Strickmann has reminded readers that Liu Ts'un-yan was the first to bring this text to the attention of the learned world in 1971 on the question of the Daoist concept of tuberculosis in the twelfth century (*Chinese Magical Medicine* [Stanford, Calif.: Stanford University Press, 2002], 37).

94. Lin, "Shi shi Shuihudi," 15; Feng and Shryock have also postulated that *gu* became a "southern" custom during the Song ("Black Magic," 10).

95. Jihong, ed., *Lingnan weisheng fang* (Beijing: Zhongyi guji chubanshe, 1983; facs. of the 1841 Japanese ed.), 135–144 (*juan* 2:39a–45b).

96. Gong Tingxian, quoting Zhu, in *Jishi quanshu* (*A Comprehensive Work to Save the World* [1616]) (Beijing: Zhongguo zhongyiyao chubanshe, 1999), *juan* 1:875. Zhu went on to say that "on the fifth day of the fifth month, they put centipedes, vipers, and toads in the same vessel and let them devour one another. The surviving creature will be *gu.*"

97. Feng and Shryock, "Black Magic," 10. A modern study of *gu* magic in China's southwest is N. Diamond, "The Miao and Poison: Interactions on China's Southwest Frontier," *Ethnology* 27, no. 1 (1988): 1–26. The other tribe that late Ming scholars thought to be practitioners of *gu* was the Dong.

98. Zhang Jiebin, *Jingyue quanshu, juan* 34:590.

99. Chao Yuanfang, "On the Symptoms of *Lai* Disorders," in *Zhubing yuan hou,* 2:78.

100. The term *bu ren* (unkindly) is very probably a pun on a main symptom of "Wind intrusion": numbness (*bu ren*) of the skin.

101. Sun, *Beiji qianjin yaofang,* 23:427; Wang Tao, *Waitai miyao fang,* 30:2b.

102. Chen repeats the same passage from Tang medical texts; it was used almost as a formula for the moral causes of the disease (*San yin, juan* 15:21b). Another important late Song text, *Renzhai zhizhi* (*Easy and Direct Formulas by Mr. Yang Shiying*), by Yang Shiying, also records these recommendations by the Tang doctors (Siku quanshu wenyuange ed. [Taipei: Shangwu yinshuguan, 1983], vol. 744, *juan* 24:11b).

103. For a good up-to-date general description of this important text, see Schipper and Verellen, *Taoist Canon,* 277–280.

104. Yang Lien-sheng, "The Concept of 'Pao' as a Basis for Social Relations in China," in *Chinese Thought and Institutions,* ed. J. K. Fairbank (Chicago: University of Chicago Press, 1957), especially 298–299; Li Jianmin, "Xian Qin liang Han bingyin guan ji qi bianqian: Yi xin chutu wenwu wei zhongxin" (The Etiological Concepts and Their Changes in the Qin and Han Periods: Based on Recent Archaeological Findings) (unpublished document, 2006). See also Li Jianmin, "Contagion and Its Consequences: The Problem of Death Pollution in Ancient China," in *Medicine and the History of the Body: Proceedings of the 20th, 21st and 22nd Iternational Symposia on the Comparative History of—East and West* (Ishiyaku EuroAmerica, 1999), especially 203. I thank Li Jianmin for sharing his thoughts on this point with me.

105. The term *chuanran* did not exist in Chao's time; Chao used mostly terms like *xiangran* (mutual contamination) and *ranyi* (contamination mutation) to describe the spread of diseases.

106. When explaining the infectious epidemic *qi,* Chao specified at one point that the *qi* of the sick (*bingqi*) was transmitted from one to another (*zhuanxiang ranyi*), "until it annihilated the entire household, and was extended to outside people [*wairen*]" (*Zhubing yuan hou,* 10:333–334).

107. *Xianchuan waike bifang, juan* 9:589–598; see also n. 43.

108. Shen, *Jiewei yuansuo,* 1:4b–6b.

109. Gong, *Jishi quanshu,* 8:1066.

110. A. K. C. Leung, "Evolution of the Idea of *Chuanran* Contagion in Imperial China," in *Health and Hygiene in Modern Chinese East Asia,* ed. A. K. C. Leung and C. Furth (Durham, N.C.: Duke University Press, forthcoming).

111. Chen Yan, *San yin, juan* 15:21b.

112. Lu Shizhong, *Wushang xuanyuan,* 24:470.

113. Strickmann, *Chinese Magical Medicine,* 35–38; for a detailed description of the Daoist text, see n. 93.

114. Xu repeats Chen Yan's text on *lifeng,* mentioning the term *chuanran* without giving any comment.

115. Liu Chun, ed., *Yuji weiyi* (*The Subtle Meanings of the Precious Machine* [1396]), by Xu Yanchun, in *Liu Chun yixue quanshu* (Beijing: Zhongguo zhongyiyao chubanshe, 1999; based on the 1439 ed.), 40:389.

116. Shen, *Jiewei yuansuo,* 1:6b–7a.

117. Ibid., 1:7a–b.

118. Ibid., 1:8a–b.

119. Ibid., 1:6b, 8b. The idea of *zhu* transmission is an old one; see Li Jianmin, "Contagion and Its Consequences," 201–222.

120. Gong, *Jishi quanshu,* 8:1066.

121. He added, for example, the danger of smoking: "One should avoid a patient who smokes, and a healthy person who smokes should also avoid being near a patient. The urine of a patient should not be used to irrigate tobacco plants. Those who smoke the grass irrigated by such urine will develop leprosy" (Xiao Xiaoting, *Fengmen quanshu, juan* 1:9b).

122. Ibid.

123. Yu Bin, *Xu yishuo* (*Sequel to "On Medicine"*) (Shanghai: Shanghai kexue jishu chubanshe, 1984; repr. of the 1598 Japanese ed.), 10:13b, under the heading of the herb *bixie* (*Rhizoma dioscoreae septemlobae* or *Rhizoma septemlobae*), a yam plant known for its antirheumatic qualities. This herb was recommended by Yu for curing Guangdong sores, the mercurous derivatives *qingfen* being too aggressive. (The *Yishuo* was a Song work [1224] by Zhang Gao.)

124. Li Shizhen, *Bencao gangmu* (Taipei: Wenguang tushu gongsi, 1955; facs. of the 1885 Guangxu ed.), 18:36.

125. It is worth noting that sixteenth-century doctors did not consider this new disease to have been brought into China by European "barbarians." I have found no such mention in medical texts. Yu Bin's 1522 text and his observation that the ailment appeared in the Hongzhi period seem to rule out the possibility of contamination by European travelers, who arrived in southeast China later on in the sixteenth century.

126. Chen Sicheng, *Meichuang milu* (Beijing: Xueyuan chubanshe, 1994; based on the 1885 ed), "Zongshuo" (General Descriptions), 6, "Meichuang huowen" (Questions and Answers on Rotting Sores), 10–11.

127. Shen, *Jiewei yuansuo,* 1:3a.

128. "*Iyang,*" referring to the warmth during the transition between spring and summer.

129. Chen Sicheng, *Meichuang milu,* "Meichuang huowen," 10.

130. Wu Qian et al., *Yizong jinjian,* vol. 2, *juan* 73:376–396.

131. Liu Hengrui [Jiren], *Fuxie xinshu,* in *YXDC* (Changsha: Yuelu, 1990), 3:781. There is no date to the text and we know little about the author. The text was first collected in the famous medical anthology *San san yishu* (*Three Three Medical Books*), edited by Qiu Qingyuan in 1925, and it is clearly a later Qing text.

132. On the diagnostic strategy that Charlotte Furth has called pattern diagnosis (*bianzheng*), see Furth, *Flourishing Yin,* 65–66, 71–72.

133. Leung, "Medical Learning," 383–386. The modern authority on the history of traditional Chinese medicine, Xie Guan (1885–1950), in his influential book, describes the development of *waike* since the Song as a particularly problematic one, with simplistic, often dangerous therapeutic principles (attacking the *du* [toxin] of the body) and only a few reputed specialists learned in theoretical diagnosis (*Zhongguo yixue yuanliu lun* [*On the Traditions of Chinese Medicine*] [Taipei: Guting shuwu, 1970], 43–44).

134. Xiao Xiaoting, *Fengmen quanshu,* 2b–3a.

135. Zhang Zhicong, *Huangdi, juan* 6:15.

136. Guo Aichun, ed., *Huangdi neijing lingshu* (*The Yellow Emperor's Inner Canon: Celestial Lancets*) (Tianjin: Tianjin kexue chubanshe, 1992), sect. 19, "*Qi* of the Four Seasons," 185.

137. Liu Wansu, *Suwen, juan* 2:42.

138. Wang Tao, *Waitai miyao fang,* 30:4.

139. Chen Yan, *San yin , juan* 15:22b–23a. The treatment was to be repeated after five days.

140. Zhang Congzheng, *Rumen shiqin* (*How Confucian Scholars Should Care for Their Parents*), in *Zihe yiji,* ed. Deng Tietao et al. (Beijing: Renmin weisheng chubanshe, 1994), *juan* 6:162–163.

141. Frédéric Obringer has pointed out this important evolution in drug use from the ancient to medieval periods (*Aconit et l'orpiment: Drogues et poisons en Chine ancienne et médiévale* [Paris: Fayard, 1997], 42–51).

142. *Wuwei Handai yijian* (*Medical Texts in Bamboo Strips of the Han Period Discovered in Wuwei*), in *Zhongguo xibei wenxian congshu: Xibei kaogu wenxian,* ed. Wu Jian et al. (Lanzhou: Lanzhou guji shudian, 1990), ser. 7, vol. 6:383. Realgar is a mineral composed of arsenic disulfide used externally for sores and scabies; cinnabar is a mineral composed of red mercuric sulfide and is a detoxicant for sores and furuncles. Both were frequently used in later recipes for skin disorders. Other, lesser-known minerals included *xuanshi* (magnetite) and *xiaoshi* (niter).

143. Sun, *Beiji qianjin yaofang,* 8:159. *Duhuo* is a dried root, typically used as an antirheumatic. *Fangfeng* is also a root, used as a diaphoretic for an affection due to Wind and Cold. *Mahuang* is also known for its qualities as a diaphoretic for an affection due to Wind and Cold, or as a diuretic for edema caused by Wind.

144. *Kushen* was later used often externally as a parasitide and antipruritic for skin diseases like eczema, and for ringworm with pruritus.

145. This recipe, named after a certain Yao, was probably one copied from the sixth-century *Jiyan fang* (*Collected Effective Recipes*) by a Yao of the sixth century. See Ma, *Zhongyi wenxian xue,* 160.

146. Ge, *Zhou hou beiji fang,* 5:38b.

147. Dols, “Leprosy,” 316, n.10; A. Roselli, “Les maladies d’Arétée de Cappadoce” (unpublished document, 2004), especially 8–9, where Roselli writes that folk stories concerning various therapeutics such as the viper wine circulated widely in Asia Minor during the time of the youth of Aretaeus of Cappadocia.

148. A. Tsukimoto, “By the Hand of Madi-Dagan, the Scribe and *Apkallu*-Priest: A Medical Text from the Middle Euphrates Region,” in *Priests and Officials in the Ancient Near East,* ed. K. Watanabe (Heidelberg: Universitätsverlag C. Winter, 1999), 196–197.

149. Chen Bosheng, “Mafeng yu she lei di guanxi” (Relationship Between Leprosy and Snakes) *Leper Quarterly* 4, no. 2 (1930): 36–38, in which the author claims that a leper was cured using a viper; in a 1938 issue of the same journal (12, no. 3), there appears a history of the use of viper wine in treating leprosy.

150. Chao, *Zhubing yuan hou,* 2:79; Li Shizhen, *Bencao gangmu,* 3:7–8. For a modern definition of the drug, see Li Yongchun, *Shiyong zhongyi cidian* (*A Practical Dictionary of Chinese Medicine*) (Taipei: Zhiyin chubanshe, 1992), 772.

151. Sun, *Qianjin yifang,* 21:251.

152. Li Shizhen, *Bencao gangmu,* 34:35. Li Shizhen explains the “barbarian” origin of the herb *awei,* which gave a bad smell, indicating the Indian, Persian, and Mongolian pronunciations of the word. Song Xian, using Arabic medical texts, explained that *awei* was a typical Persian drug that was introduced to Tang China (*Gudai Posi yixue yu Zhongguo* [*Ancient Persian Medicine and China*] [Beijing: Jingji ribao chubanshe, 2001], 31–32).

153. Sun, *Qianjin yifang,* 21:250–251; Wang Tao, *Waitai miyao fang,* 30:4.

154. *Taiping shenghui fang,* 24:1a–22b.

155. Chen Yan, *San yin juan* 15:23a–27a.

156. Xiao Xiaoting, *Fengmen quanshu, juan* 1:11a.

157. Though in modern Western medicine, arsenic and mercury compounds were still used to treat leprosy, and they were proved to be efficient in alleviating some of the external symptoms.

158. *Gengdao ji,* in *Daozang yaoji xuankan,* vol. 9, *juan* 9:134; *Xianchuan waike bifang,* vol. 9, *juan* 11:590. For descriptions of these two Daoist texts, see Schipper and Verellen, *Taoist Canon,* 777–779, 867.

159. *Lingnan weisheng fang, juan* 2:48a. It is unclear what *yangmei chuan* means here. It is too early for the same ailment described in sixteenth-century medical texts, and there is no description of the sores in this Song-Yuan text. The passage could have been added later.

160. Li Shizhen, *Bencao gangmu,* 35:49. Zhu’s comment is said to appear in a text entitled *Danxi xiansheng yishu zhuanyao* (*Esssentials of Mr. Zhu Zhenheng’s Medical Texts*), which I have never succeeded in locating. The source is quoted in Liu Muzhi, “Mafeng bing zai Zhongguo yixue ji lishi shang de jizai” (Records of Leprosy in Chinese History and Medical Works), *Zhonghua pifuke zazhi* 4, no. 1 (1956): 4.

161. Zhu Xiu, *Puji fang* (*Recipes for General Relief*) (Taipei : Taiwan shangwu yinshuguan, 1983), *juan* 109:13a, 15b; *juan* 110:6a, 15a, 22b, 27a.

162. Chao, *Zhubing yuan hou,* 2:80.

163. Sun, *Qianjin yifang,* 21:252.

164. Sun, *Beiji quanjin yaofang,* 23:427.

165. Ibid.; Sun, *Qianjin yifang,* 21:251; Wang Tao, *Waitai miyao fang,* 30:2.

166. Zhang Jiebin, of the late Ming, warned that if a patient did not abstain, he would be "incurable" (*Jingyue quanshu, juan* 34:594).

167. *Xianchuan waike bifang, juan* 11:589.

168. It is interesting to note that an old Greek recipe also included cedar resin. See the one recorded by Oribasius (ca. 325–400) from a third-century text by Philumenus, in U. C. Bussemaker and C. Daremberg, eds., *Oeuvres d'Oribase* (Paris: Imprimerie impériale, 1862), 80–82. I thank Amneris Roselli for informing me of this text.

169. This story is quoted as an annex in Ge, *Zhou hou beiji fang,* 5:40b.

170. Sun, *Beiji qianjin yaofang,* 23:428.

171. This was written by Yuan Shixi, the publisher of Xiao Xiaoting's text and also author of the preface of *Fengmen quanshu* (Yuan's preface, 5a).

2. A CURSED BUT REDEEMABLE BODY

1. This social rejection owes much to the restrictions in regard to what was believed to be the leper in Leviticus, "He is unclean: he shall dwell alone; without the camp shall his habitation be" (13:46). The Third Lateran Council (1179) ordered that lepers should be cut off from the rest of society. In France, a leper was declared by the priest as "dead to the world," and to "be reborn to God." See R. Palmer, "The Church, Leprosy and Plague in Medieval and Early Modern Europe," in *The Church and Healing,* ed. W. J. Sheils (Oxford: Basil Blackwell, 1982) 81; V. Nutton, "Medicine in Medieval Western Europe, 1000–1500," in *The Western Medical Tradition 800BC–AD 1800* (Cambridge: Cambridge University Press, 1995), 187–189. Olivier Touati and Luke Demaître have provided nuanced studies on medieval leprosaria in Europe (see chap. 3). A more recent study, by Carole Rawcliffe, on medieval segregation of lepers "reflects a combination of motives from compassion to fear and self-promotion to humility" (*Leprosy in Medieval England* [Suffolk, U.K.: Boydell Press, 2006], 357).

2. M. Dols, "The Leper in Medieval Islamic Society," *Speculum* 58, no. 4 (1983): 891–916.

3. The fear of the contagiousness of *li*/*lai* was as great as that of epidemics. The latter seemed to be great even in the medieval period. One of the main tasks of officials and mainstream doctors was to dissuade people from abandoning their family and relatives when they had serious diseases or during epidemics. Li Deyu, of the Tang, was said

to have "transformed" such customs by asking respected local elders to persuade people to be filial and stay behind to take care of their sick parents. (*Xin Tangshi* [*New History of the Tang*], *juan* 180, biography no. 105, on Li Deyu). Cheng Jiong, the famous doctor of the Song, wrote his famous anticontagion essay on similar grounds, arguing that kindness and filial piety would overcome all kinds of pollution and disease transmission. Such "anticontagion" ideas and acts, in fact, showed the popularity of beliefs in disease transmission.

4. The late historian of medicine, Fan Xingzhun, called the Buddhist and Daoist doctors of this period "doctors of the mountains and forest" (*shan lin di yijia*) who exerted great influence on medical thought in the medieval period (Fan Xingzhun, *Zhongguo yixue shilue* [*A Brief History of Chinese Medicine*] [Beijing: Zhongyi guji chubanshe, 1986], especially 64–67). For more recent and detailed studies, see Ge Jianmin, *Daojiao yixue* (*Daoist Medicine*) (Beijing: Zongjiao wenhua chubanshe, 2001); M. Strickmann, *Chinese Magical Medicine* (Stanford, Calif.: Stanford University Press, 2002).

5. Strickmann, *Chinese Magical Medicine*, 26–32.

6. Scholars have different interpretations of the text. Derk Bodde prefers to use "shore execution" for the Chinese term *ding sha*, though he admits that he is not sure of this interpretation (D. Bodde, "Forensic Medicine in Pre-imperial China," *Journal of the American Oriental Society* 102, no. 1 [1982]: 11). I choose the interpretation of Lin Fushi ("Shi shi Shuihudi Qin jian zhong di 'li' yu 'ding sha'" [Explanations of the Terms "*Li*" and "*Ding Sha*" in Qin Bamboo Strips Discovered at Shuihudi] *Shiyuan* 15 [1986], especially 15–18).

7. Lin Fushi, "Shi shi Shuihudi," 2–38. According to Lin, drowning in still water in a particular locale was a customary punishment for *gu* witches or important political traitors in ancient times. This amplifies the ritual significance of the punishment.

8. Bodde, "Forensic Medicine," 11; Yu Zongfa, *Yunmeng Qinjian zhong sixiang yu zhidu gouzhi* (*Thought and Institution Revealed in the Qin Bamboo Strips Excavated in Yunmeng*) (Taipei: Wenjin chubanshe, 1992), 132. I avoid translating *li* categorically as "leprosy" or *mafeng* illness, as do Bodde and Yu, as explained in chapter 1. In these early texts, it is clear that the term *li* has a broader and much more complex meaning than simply "leprosy" as we understand it today.

9. In the early medieval period, charitable acts toward victims of *li* were also accompanied by occasional collective violence against them. The last emperor Youzhu of the Northern Qi (577) was said to have massacred groups of victims of *li* that he encountered during one of his trips. Some of these victims could have been those kept by the charitable asylum sponsored by his predecessor some two decades earlier (see chap. 3) (Tang Changru, *Wei-Jin Nan-Bei Chao shi lun shiyi* [*Miscellaneous Writings on the History of the Wei-Jin Nan-Bei Dynasties*] [Beijing: Xinhua shuju, 1983], 275 [quoting the *Bei Qi shu* (*History of the Northern Qi*) (Taipei: Dingwen shuju, 1980), *juan* 8, "Chronicle of Youzhu"]).

10. On the historical development of the glossing of *li* and *lai,* see chapter 1, n. 5. I believe that the interchangeability of the two characters was possible only after the fourth

century, when *lai* became a popular character. *Lai* was rarely used in texts earlier than the fourth century.

11. *Da Dai liji* (*Book of Rites by Elder Dai*) (Shanghai: Shanghai shudian, 1989) (Sibu congkan ed.), sect. 80, "Benming," 509.

12. Ibid.; *Yili zhushu* (*Annotations of Etiquette and Ceremonies*) (Taipei: Yiwen yinshuju, 1955; based on the 1815 ed.), quoting the *Kongzi jiayu* on the seven legitimate reasons for divorcing a wife, one of which was that she had a malignant disease ("Shi li" 2, *juan* 5:49); *Hanshi waizhuan,* quoted in a note in the *Hou Hanshu* (*Book of the Later Han*) (Taipei: Dingwen shuju, 1979), *juan* 48:1609, cited in Sima Guang, *Zizhi tongjian* (*Comprehensive Mirror to Aid in Government*) (Beijing: Guji chubanshe, 1956; based on the thirteenth-century annotated Yuan ed.), *juan* 55:1783.

In an annotation of the Gongyang tradition of the *Spring and Autumn Annals, eji* is explained as follows: dumbness, deafness, blindness, *li,* baldness, lameness, hunchback, barrenness. Twentieth year of the reign of Zhao Gong, *Chunqiu Gongyang zhuan jiaokan ji* (*Corrected Edition of the Gongyang Tradition of the "Spring and Autumn Annals"*), ed. Ruan Yuan (Taipei: Yiwen yinshuju, 1959): 293.

13. Changsun Wuji et al., *Tang lü shuyi* (*Interpretations of the Tang Code*) (Taipei: Xinwenfeng shuju, 1986), *juan* 14:267; Li Jing et al., trans., *Tangling shiyi* (*Supplementary Amplifications of the Tang Code*), by Niida Noboru (Changchun: Changchun chubanshe, 1989; based on the 1983 Japanese ed.): 163–164. People with *duji* usually had special legal status as defendants or victims.

14. Xu Yuanrui, *Lixue zhinan* (*Instructions to Bureaucrats*), *juan* 15 of *Jujia biyong shilei* (*Necessary Things in Daily Life*) (Taipei: Zhongwen chubanshe, 1984; facs. of the 1673 Japanese print of the 1560 Ming ed.), "Weizheng" (Policies), 4, "Zhenghun" (On Marriage), 74a.

15. *Tian paochuang* was a common term in the Ming-Qing period for ugly sores on the skin as symptoms of either Guangdong sores (syphilis) or *mafeng.*

16. Pu Songling, *Xingshi yinyuan* (*Marital Relations Awakening the World*) (Taipei: Lianjing chubanshe, 1986), chap. 95, 1155.

17. A Ming doctor, Li Lian (1488–1566), recorded that a Yuan doctor, Lü Fu, had treated a woman afflicted with *lifeng* who had been divorced by her husband (Li Lian, *Yi shi* [*History of Medicine*] [Xiamen: Xiamen daxue chubanshe, 1992]: 178–179 [originally published in 1515]).

18. "Wife of [the Man of] Cai," in Liu Xiang, *Lienü zhuan* (*Biographies of Virtuous Women*) (1591; repr., Taipei: Guangwen shuju, 1981), 4:8b–9a.

19. Zhang Tingyu, ed., *Ming shi* (*History of the Ming Dynasty*) (Taipei: Dingwen shuju, 1979), *juan* 303:7741.

20. The sick husband turned out to be bad tempered, frivolous, and an addicted

gambler. He spent all her dowry, and, on top of that, he beat her up. Yuan returned home to serve her mother and cried her heart out on learning of the death of her husband. She died one year after his death (Zhao Erxun et al., eds., *Qing shi gao* [*Draft of the History of the Qing Dynasty*] [Taipei: Hongshi chubanshe, 1981], "Liezhuan" [Biographies], *juan* 509:14089). Stories of this kind were not rare in the Qing. There is another, the story of Shen of the Qing, the wife of Lu Tinghua. Shen was neglected and alienated by her husband, who left her to live elsewhere. Shen was then badly treated by her mother-in-law, even though she was an obedient daughter-in-law. But Shen never complained. She even went to care for Tinghua after he had contracted *eji*. She eventually died as a virtuous widow after he had died from the ailment (ibid., 2:14074).

21. This is taken from one of the reports of the cases that had to be read and approved by the emperor for the capital punishment to be implemented. There are two major collections of such documents, one at the No. 1 Archives in Beijing, *Xingke tiben* (*Documents of the Ministry of Punishment*), and the other in the Ming-Qing Archives at the Institute of History and Philology, Academia Sinica, Taipei. The former collection is partially reproduced in microfilms purchased by Academia Sinica. The latter collection, Archives of the Grand Secretariat (Neige daku [NGDK]), is largely online. I have so far located ten cases that involve *mafeng* patients in the NGDK collection, and four in the microfilms purchased from the Number 1 Archives. This particular case is no. 147 in the Beijing collection.

22. NGDK, A101-082, no. 013555.

23. NGDK, A170-038, no. 015790.

24. Ishikawa Rikizan, "Xuansha sanshu byōnin kō" (Study on the Three Kinds of Xuansha Patients), in *Kamada Shigeo hakase kanreki kinen ronshū: Chūgoku no bukkyō to bunka* (Tokyo: Ōkura shuppan kabushiki kaisha, 1988), 440–444.

25. *Gao seng zhuan, Zhu Daosheng zhuan: Fo shuo zuiye baoying jiaohua diyu jing* (*Sutra on Sin, Retribution, Moral Transformation, and Hell, as Spoken by the Buddha*), trans. An Shigao [148–170], quoted in Fan Jiawei, "Han-Tang jian fojiao yu yiliao jiuji: Yi laibing wei zhongxi" (Medical Relief in the Han-Tang Periods, with Special Emphasis on the *Lai* Ailment) (unpublished document), 4, 5.

26. "I heard that he who assassinates the emperor will have the *lai* ailment" (*Beishi* [*History of the Northern Dynasties*] [Taipei: Dingwen shuju, 1980], *juan* 19:690–691, "Prince Xi of Xianyang"; *Zizhi tongjian, juan* 144, "Chronicles of the Qi," 10:4487).

27. Lin Guang, a famous general, was said to have fatally contracted the "malignant ailment" because he had executed barbarian enemies who had surrendered upon his order (Tuotuo, *Songshi* [*History of the Song Dynasty*] [Taipei: Dingwen shuju, 1979], *juan* 334:10739).

28. "If one has vicious sores of the *lai* ailment that cannot be cured despite medi-

cation, causing unbearable pain, it is because in one's former life, one took pleasure in whipping all other living things" (*Fayuan zhulin* [*Forest of Gems in the Garden of Law*], in *Taishō shinshū daizōkyō* [*The Tripitaka in Chinese*], ed. Takakusu Junjirō and Watanabe Kaigyoku [Tokyo: Taishō issaikyō kankōkai, 1924–1934] [hereafter *TD*], vol. 53, no. 2122, *juan* 68:805b).

29. A magistrate of the southern Liang dynasty (502–557) was said to have laughed at the killing of a buffalo for sacrifice. After wakening from his drunkenness, he felt an itchiness on his body and he began to scratch. He soon developed *lai* and died within a year (Yan Zhitui [530–ca. 590], *Yanshi jiaxun* [*Family Precepts of the Yan Lineage*] [Shanghai: Guji chubanshe, 1980], 369). The narrator of this story was aware of the medical discourse on *lai,* for the magistrate was said to have slept under the eaves after getting drunk. In medical terms, vicious Wind and Dampness must have entered his body.

30. See, for example, the *Taishang dongyuan shenzhou jing* (*Scriptures of Divine Incantations of the Abyssal Caverns*), fourth to fifth centuries, edited by Du Guangting (855–933). In the *Daozang* edition, there are long passages in *juan* 20 on the various types of disease demons that cause ugly and painful diseases with skin symptoms, such as white *lai,* to sinners of the world (*Zhengtong Daozang* [*Orthodox Daoist Canon*] [Taipei: Xinwenfeng chubanshe, 1985; repr. of the 1607 long ed., based on the 1445 ed.] [hereafter *DZ*], vol. 10, *juan* 4:9, *juan* 16:3). See the description of this text in K. Schipper and F. Verellen, eds., *The Taoist Canon: A Historical Companion to the "Daozang"* (Chicago: University of Chicago Press, 2004), 269–272.

31. Strickmann, *Chinese Magical Medicine* 14.

32. See n. 30 and also *Zhengyi fawen jingzhang guanpin* (*Chapter on Petitions and Officials of the Zhengyi Canon*), in *DZ,* vol. 48, *juan* 4:1–12.

33. *Fayuan zhulin,* in *TD,* vol. 53, no. 2122, *juan* 70:822b–c, the story of Du Tongda, in the Zhengguan reign of the Tang.

34. In medieval Christianity, lepers were declared dead to the world, but "reborn to God." The Christian church often quoted Luke (16:19–25) on how the leper rested on Abraham's bosom in Paradise. St. Lazarus was the performer of miracles on lepers, as well as the creator of "lazaretto," charity hospitals for patients. See R. Palmer, "Church, Leprosy and Plague," 81; V. Nutton, "Medicine in Medieval Western Europe," 188.

35. On miracle healing in the Old Testament, see Y. Zakovitch, "Miracles (Old Testament)," in *The Anchor Bible Dictionary,* ed. by D. N. Freedman (New York: Doubleday, 1992), 852. Zakovitch quotes in particular two examples: the example of Miriam, who is punished with leprosy for not acknowledging Moses' authority and for her rebellious speech to him, but who is healed after Moses' prayer, and, second, that of Naaman, cured of his leprosy but whose servant falls victim to the disease because he showed disrespect to his master.

36. This idea comes from Étienne Lamotte, quoted in B. Faure, *The Red Thread: Buddhist Approaches to Sexuality* (Princeton, N.J.: Princeton University Press, 1998), 55.

37. According to the Buddhist classics, the reason for forbidding ordination was that, since Jīvaka treated only Buddhas and monks with any of the five diseases, most laypersons with the diseases asked to be ordained only for the purpose of being treated by her. Once cured, these latter left the Buddhist community. The Buddhist community thus refused to ordain people with any of the five diseases. See *Si fen lü* (*The Four-Part Regulations*), in *TD*, vol. 22, no. 1428, *juan* 34:808c; *juan* 57:989c; *juan* 59:1003b. I thank Liu Shu-fen for drawing my attention to this text. However, there should be a deeper reason for why these five diseases stood out as "difficult" diseases.

38. For the Hindu tradition, see J. Buckingham, *Leprosy in Colonial South India: Medicine and Confinement* (New York: Palgrave, 2002), 31.

39. B. Faure, *The Power of Denial: Buddhism, Purity, and Gender.* (Princeton, N.J.: Princeton University Press, 2003), 238.

40. Fan Jiawei, *Liu Chao Sui-Tang yixue zhi chuancheng yu zhenghe* (*Heritage and Consolidation of Medicine from the Six Dynasties to the Sui-Tang Periods*) (Hong Kong: Chinese University Press, 2004), 177–179; Stanley Weinstein, *Buddhism under the Tang* (Cambridge: Cambridge University Press, 1987), 3–11.

41. *Fozu tongji* (*General Biographies of Buddhas*), in *TD*, vol. 49, no. 2035, *juan* 38:354c, on Emperor Taiwu of the Northern Wei; *juan* 42:392c, on Emperor Shizong of the Zhou; *Xu gao seng zhuan* (*Further Biographies of Eminent Monks*), in *TD*, vol. 50, no. 2060, *juan* 1:428a; vol. 49, no. 2035, *juan* 34:354c, on Emperor Taiwu of the Northern Wei.

42. *Fozu lidai tongzai* (*Records of Buddhas Throughout History*), in *TD*, vol. 49, no. 2036, *juan* 8:537a–538a; *Fozu tongji*, in *TD*, vol. 49, no. 2035, *juan* 38:354b; *Xu gao seng zhuan*, in *TD*, vol. 50, no. 2060, *juan* 1:427c.

43. *Fozu lidai tongzai*, in *TD*, vol. 49, no. 2036, *juan* 10:555b.

44. *Nanshi* (*History of the Southern Dynasties*) (Taipei: Dingwen shuju, 1980), "Liezhuan," *juan* 52, *liezhuan* 42:1291

45. *Guang hong ming ji* (*The Enlarged Hong Ming Collection*), in *TD*, vol. 52, no. 2103, *juan* 12:170c–171a.

46. Fan Jiawei, *Liu Chao Sui-Tang*, 178–180.

47. Other examples: Emperor Wu of the Northern Zhou dynasty (557–581) was also known to have persecuted Buddhism, burning Buddhist sutras and statues, destroying monasteries and pagodas. He also ended up dying of *eji* and had *lai* sores (*Guang hong ming ji*, in *TD*, vol. 52, no. 2103, *juan* 12:174c). Li Deyu, of the Tang, also famous for his hostility to Buddhism, in the mid-ninth century, was said to have died from *eji* (*Fozu tongji*, in *TD*, vol. 49, no. 2035, *juan* 42:386c); see also n. 28.

48. This held true also in medieval Japan; see S. Burns, "From 'Leper Villages' to Lep-

rosaria': Public Health, Nationalism and the Culture of Exclusion in Japan," in *Isolation: Places and Practices of Exclusion,* ed. C. Strange and A. Bashford (London: Routledge, 2003), 105–106: "the sufferer of leprosy was an ambivalent figure in medieval culture—seemingly the physical manifestation of sin, but also potentially capable of bringing salvation to one who offered compassion."

49. *Xu gao seng zhuan, juan* 2, quoted in Tang, *Wei-Jin Nan-Bei Chao,* 275.

50. *Xu gao seng zhuan, juan* 18, "Shi Daoxun," quoted in Tang, *Wei-Jin Nan-Bei Chao,* 275; see also *Xu gao seng zhuan,* in *TD,* vol. 50, no. 2060, *juan* 20:602c.

51. *Xu gao seng zhuan, juan* 16, "Shi Seng Chou," quoted in Tang, *Wei-Jin Nan-Bei Chao,* 275.

52. *Xu gao seng zhuan, juan* 28, "Shi Daoji," quoted in Tang, *Wei-Jin Nan-Bei Chao,* 276.

53. *Xu gao seng zhuan,* in *TD,* vol. 50, no. 2060, *juan* 20:602c; also quoted in Tang, *Wei-Jin Nan-Bei Chao,* 276.

54. *Jingde chuan deng lu* (*The Transmission of the Lamp of the Jingde Era*), in *TD,* vol. 51, no. 2076, *juan* 20:366c.

55. *Bei Qi shu, juan* 32:428.

56. Fan Jiawei, *Liu Chao Sui-Tang,* 180–182.

57. Ibid., 182; *Lingnan weisheng fang* (*Life-Preserving Recipes for the Lingnan Region*) (Beijing: Zhongyi guji chubanshe, 1983; facs. of the 1841 Japanese ed.), *juan* 2:43a, records several so-called Buddhist incantations that travelers were to recite several times before taking their food and drink on the road in order to avoid poisoning by *gu.*

58. See the story of Jiang Tengsheng in the *Fayuan zhulin,* in *TD,* vol. 53, no. 2122, *juan* 79:877b.

59. Weinstein, *Buddhism under the Tang,* 114–136; Kenneth Chen, *Buddhism in China: A Historical Survey* (Princeton, N.J.: Princeton University Press, 1964), 225–233.

60. Buddhist texts after the Song dynasty mention *lai* and other monstrous skin diseases mostly in the context of retribution for sins and healing by incantation; one no longer finds stories of famous sinners having contracted the malignant ailment or of monks healing such ailments.

61. *Taiping jing hejiao* (*Collated Edition of the Taiping Canon*) (Beijing: Zhonghua shuju, 1960), 744.

62. *Yunji qiqian* (*Bookcase of the Clouds with the Seven Labels*), in *DZ,* vol. 38, *juan* 119:7. For a description of the *Yunji qiqian,* see Schipper and Verellen, *Taoist Canon,* 27–28.

63. *Xianju xianzhi* (*Gazetteer of Xianju County*), quoted in Ren Linhao, *Liang Song shiqi di Taizhou daojiao* (*Taizhou Daoism Under the Song*), http://www.lhinfo.net/minren/rlh/taizhoudaojiao3.htm, 3 (accessed September 10, 2006).

64. *Songshi, juan* 461:13513.

65. For a description of elixirs and healing in the early medieval period, especially of *lai,* see F. Pregadio, *Great Clarity: Daoism and Alchemy in Early Medieval China* (Stanford, Calif.: Stanford University Press, 2006).

66. Sun Simiao, *Beiji qianjin yaofang* (*Essential Recipes for Urgent Use Worthy of a Thousand Gold Pieces*) (Beijing: Renmin weisheng chubanshe, 1982; repr. of the Edo igaku facs. of the Northern Song ed.), 23:427.

67. For a general discussion of illness and attaining sainthood in the Daoist tradition, see Lin Fushi, "Jibing yu xiudao: Zhongguo zaoqi daoshi xiudao yinyuan kaoshi zhiyi" (Illness and Practicing the Dao: Analysis of the Causes Behind the Practice of the Dao in Early China), *Hanxue yanjiu* 19, no. 1 (2001): 137–166.

68. Su Che [1039–1112], *Longchuan lue zhi* (*A Brief History of Longchuan*) (Beijing: Zhonghua shuju, 1982), 1:4.

69. *Xianyuan bianzhu* (*Garden of Immortals: A Pearl Treasury* [ca. 960]), in *DZ,* vol. 18, *juan* 3:427.

70. Ge Hong, *Shenxian zhuan, juan* 3, "Zhao Qu," quoted in Lin Fu-shi, "Jibing yu xiudao," 144. The Siku quanshu edition of the *Shenxian zhuan* records the story in *juan* 7:4a–b. The text is simpler in the latter edition, but the idea of *zhu* is in both versions. The original text, written by Ge Hong, was likely lost and extant editions were compiled in later periods. It is uncertain if the idea of the fear of transmission by *zhu* to one's posterity was present in Ge's original fourth-century text.

71. Pine trees, a symbol of longevity and immortality, occupied a special position in Daoist thought. Sun Simiao, the most important Daoist doctor of the medieval period, wrote, "I, during the reign of Zhenguang [627–649], sent a sick literatus into the mountain, and told him to eat pine resin. A hundred days later, his hair and eyebrows grew again. This shows that [healing] depends essentially on [how] the patient [behaves], and one cannot rely entirely on medicines" (*Beiji qianjin yaofang,* 23:427). For Sun, willingly leading a genuinely reclusive life was the essential cure, and consuming pine resin was secondary but also important.

72. Ge, *Shenxian zhuan* quoted in Lin, "Jibing yu xiudao," 144. This story is repeated many times in Ge's other writings and in later texts like the *Taiping yulan* (*Imperial Overview of the Era of Great Peace*) (Taipei: Shangwu yinshuguan, 1975; facs. of the Sibu congkan ed.), *juan* 670:3118a. Similar stories of immortals can be found in other Daoist texts, such as the twelfth-century *Hunyuan shengji* (*Annals of the Sage of Undifferentiated Beginning*), in *DZ,* vol. 30, *juan* 9:156, which recounts the similar fate of a peasant of the Tang period, although in this case, the patient's savior was the Daoist supreme being Taishang Laojun, appearing as a holy man with white hair riding a white horse, who cured him with chants and bathing. For a description of this text, see Schipper and Verellen, *Taoist Canon,* 872–874.

73. See note 168 in chapter 1.

74. For a description of the uses of alchemical and herbal drugs in the early Daoist tradition for healing and longevity, see Pregadio, *Great Clarity,* 132–139.

75. A fine description of the development of Daoist therapeutic rituals can be found in E. Davis, *Society and the Supernatural in Song China* (Honolulu: University of Hawai'i Press, 2001), especially chaps. 2 and 3. See also R. Hymes, *Way and Byway: Taoism, Local Religion, and Models of Divinity in Sung and Modern China* (Berkeley: University of California Press, 2002).

76. "Laozi shi shi lantai zhong zhi lai fu," in Wei Zheng, *Suishu* (*Book of the Sui Dynasty*) (Taipei: Dingwen shuju, 1980), *juan* 34:1047.

77. Schipper and Verellen, *Taoist Canon,* 28; Strickmann, *Chinese Magical Medicine,* 34; Davis, *Society and the Supernatural in Song China,* chap. 2, especially from p. 32 onward; Vincent Goossaert also points out that the Daoist Zhang Heavenly Master Institution that became increasingly influential in the late imperial period owed much of its success to court patronage from the Southern Song period on ("Bureaucratic Charisma: The Zhang Heavenly Master Institution and Court Taoists in Late-Qing China," *Asia Major,* ser. 3, vol. 17, no. 2 [2004]: 122).

78. Davis, *Society and the Supernatural in Song China,* 41–42.

79. Strickmann, *Chinese Magical Medicine,* 14.

80. Ibid., 34; Goossaert, "Bureaucratic Charisma," 134.

81. One important twelfth-century text in this tradition, the *Taishang zhuguo jiumin zongzhen biyao* (*Secret Essentials of the Highest Zhenren Assisting the Country and Saving the People*), describes talismans and rituals to stop *chuanran* contagion related to *wen* epidemics and poisonous *qi* (see the *DZ,* vol. 54). Robert Hymes also emphasizes the therapeutic uses of rituals of this tradition (*Way and Byway,* 27–28).

82. Strickmann, *Chinese Magical Medicine,* 35–36. For a description of this text, see Schipper and Verellen, *Taoist Canon,* 1071–1073. *Juan* 13, 23, and 25 of this interesting Daoist text contain details on expelling disease demons.

83. Strickmann, *Chinese Magical Medicine,* 38.

84. *Wuxi Jingui xian zhi* (*Gazetteer of Wuxi and Jingui*) (1813), 40:20a–b.

85. This virtue was central in Confucian ethics, but it was also important in the Daoist and Buddhist traditions in China.

86. Song Lian, *Yuanshi* (*History of the Yuan Dynasty*) (Taipei: Dingwen shuju, 1980), *juan* 200:4487.

87. Huang Zhangjian, ed., *Ming shilu* (*A Veritable Record of the Ming*) (Taipei: Institute of History and Philology, Academia Sinica, 1984), 166:3214.

88. Liang Gongchen, *Beidong yuan bilu* (*Notes of the Northeastern Garden*) (Kaifeng: Xu Yi wenzhai, 1866; preface dated 1848), ser. 4, vol. 8:16b–17b. Xie Lansheng was a *jinshi* (successful candidate of the imperial examination) in 1802 and was entrusted with the important task of compiling the Guangdong gazetteer by Ruan Yuan, the governor general.

89. Xu Hao, *Fuzhai riji* (*Diary of Xu Hao*), in *Ming-Qing shiliao huikan* (Taipei: Wenhai shuju, 1967–1969), ser. 8, vol. 4, *juan* 1:4a.

90. There are at least two English translations of the story: Chau-mun Lau, *The Everlasting Couple* (Taipei: Liberal Arts Press, 1975), and H. Acton and Lee Yi-hsieh, trans., "The Predestined Couple," in *Glue and Lacquer* (London: Golden Cockerel Press, 1941).

91. Wang Jimin, "Zhongguo mafeng shi zhong zhi mingren"(Famous People in the Chinese History of Leprosy), *Zhonghua yixue zazhi* 27, no. 9 (1941): 565–568. An earlier version of this paper was published in *Mafeng jikan* (*Leper Quarterly*) 4, no. 4 (1930): 12–16. The quarterly was the organ of the Chinese Mission to Lepers. The 1941 version presents a more researched article.

92. Wang notably mentions Boniu, of the sixth century B.C., Cao Shi, of the Han, Wang Can (177–217), Zhou Xingsi (?–521), Cui Shen (550–577), Lu Zhaolin (ca. 550), Cui Yanyue (n.d.), Liu Ban (1022–1088), and Zu Ke (Song). Besides Wang Jimin, many of his contemporaries also quoted the same historical examples to show the long history of leprosy in China. They include the famous Chinese leprologist Yu Shenchu (1915–?), *Zhongguo mafeng bingxue* (*Study on Leprosy in China*) (Shanghai: Fuxing zhongyishe, 1941), especially 9–10; Xiao Yunchun, "Zuguo yixue duiyu mafeng zhi renshi" (Our Mother Country's Knowledge on Leprosy), *Zhongyi zazhi* 4 (1956): 170–173; Xiao Xi, "Boniu you ji kao" (A Philological Study on the Ailment of Boniu), *Guangdong zhongyi* 1 (1958): 25–28; Yue Meizhong (another famous leprosy specialist, 1900–1982), "Zuguo yixue dui dafeng bing di renshi ji qi zhiliao bing ji xiandai yixue duiyu mafeng bing di zhishi" (Knowledge and Therapeutics of Leprosy in Our Country and Modern Medical Understanding of the Disease), *Xin zhongyi yao* 8, nos. 3–4 (1957): 5–16; Liang Zhangchi, "Zhongguo gudai mafeng shishi kaobian" (Analysis of Historical Facts on Leprosy in Ancient China), *Pifu xing bing fangzhi tongxun* 2, no. 1 (1963): 51–63.

93. Wang, "Zhongguo mafeng shi," 568.

94. A. Waley, trans., *The Analects of Confucius* (London: Allen and Unwin, 1938; repr., Taipei: Jinshan tushu chubanshe, 1970), 117.

95. Zhu Xi, the influential Song Confucian master, glosses Boniu's malignant ailment as *lai* in his commentaries on the *Analects*.

96. Yao Silian, *Liangshu* (*Book of the Liang Dynasty*) (Taipei: Dingwen shuju, 1980), *juan* 49:697–698.

97. Mao Qiling was a scholar from Zhejiang province. An erudite involved in the compilation of the official history of the Ming in the early Qing period, he was considered one of the most influential scholars of the Qing dynasty. See A. Hummel, *Eminent Chinese of the Ch'ing Period* (Taipei: Ch'eng-wen, 1970), 563–565.

98. Lu Yitian, *Lenglu yihua* (*Medical Talks by Lu Yitian*) (Taiyuan: Shanxi kexue jishu chubanshe, 1993), 103–104.

99. Wang Pizhi, *Mianshui yangtan lu* (1095), quoted in He Shixi, ed., *Lidai wuming yijia yan'an* (*Cases Showing Medical Efficacy of Unnamed Doctors in Past Dynasties*) (Shanghai: Xuelin chubanshe, 1983), 205; He Wei [Yuan] [1077–1145], *Chun zhu jiwen* (*Records of Things Heard on a Spring Islet*) (Shanghai: Shanghai shudian, 1990), 6:7b.

100. Sun, *Beiji qianjin yaofang*, 23:427.

101. Lu Zhaolin, considered one of the four talents of the early Tang, was said to have been treated by Sun Simiao. See *Jiu Tang shu* (*Old Book on the Tang Dynasty*) (Taipei: Wending shuju, 1979), *juan* 191:1389.

3. THE DANGEROUSLY CONTAGIOUS BODY

1. Chen Yan, *San yin ji yi bingzheng fang lun* (*A Treatise on the Three Categories of Pathogenic Factors of Disorders*), Wenyuange Siku quanshu ed. (Taipei: Shangwu yinshuguan, 1983), 15:21b. See also chap. 1, p. 40.

2. See the section entitled "Daoist Redemption" in chap. 2.

3. See chap. 1, p. 45.

4. This was a recurring theme in many Ming-Qing writings. The important Qing scholar Ji Yun (1724–1805) wrote that children of managers of private brothels often fell victim to malignant ailments. He quoted the example of Ruan Ji, the famous decadent of the third century, whose two sons, Ji said, were infected by *li* by going to brothels and consequently were without posterity (*Yueweicao tang biji* [*Notes on the "Yueweicao" Study*] [Chengdu: Bashu shushe, 1995], 13:308).

5. Interestingly, such an image also existed in late medieval Western Europe, where leprosy was explained at the same time in terms of Galenic humoral theory (melancholy was the main cause) and contagion, under the influence of Arabic medicine from the thirteenth century onward. See L. Demaître, "The Description and Diagnosis of Leprosy by 14th-Century Physicians," *Bulletin of the History of Medicine* 59, no. 3 (1985): 327–344. Demaître indicates that such negative traits of the leper's character could be traced back at least to Avicenna. For Olivier Touati, the notion of contagion of leprosy was introduced to Europe only in the thirteenth century from Arabic medicine ("Historiciser la notion de contagion: L'exemple de la lèpre dans les sociétés médiévales," in *Airs, miasmes et contagion: Les épidémies dans l'Antiquité et au Moyen Age*, ed. S. Bazin-Tacchella, D. Quéruel, and É. Samama [Langres, Fr.: Guéniot, 2001], 175).

6. Here I have consulted judicial cases involving capital punishment committed in the provinces (see also chap. 2, n. 21). I have so far located ten cases involving *mafeng* patients in the NGDK collection in Taipei, and four in the Number 1 Archives in Beijing. Ding Yizhuang, of the Institute of History, Academy of Social Sciences, in Beijing, has pointed out to me another case in the Number 1 Archives in Beijing, for which I am

grateful. There are probably many more cases that involved *mafeng* patients, but it is quite difficult to locate them as there is not yet a reliable index.

7. NGDK, case A114-111, no. 013956.

8. Ibid., case A093-102, no. 014931. As punishment, the cousin was beaten and exiled.

9. Ibid., no. 070804.

10. *Xingke tiben* (*Documents of the Ministry of Punishment*), Number 1 Archives (Ming-Qing dynasties), Beijing, case 1033.

11. S. Ell, "Blood and Sexuality in Medieval Leprosy," *Janus: Revue internationale de l'histoire des sciences, de la médicine et de la technique* 71 (1984): 153–164.

12. *Jiangxi tongzhi* (*General Gazetteer of Jiangxi*) (Taipei: Shangwu yinshuguan, 1983; Siku quanshu ed., based on the 1732 ed.), 69:40a.

13. Wang Zhi, *Changshi yu* (*Pronouncements on Things Tried*), 1762 preface, "Da an" (Important Judicial Cases), 71a–b. I thank Pierre-Etienne Will for making this interesting text known to me.

14. *Xingke tiben,* case 269.

15. Ibid., case 907.

16. NGDK, case A108-41, no. 013675.

17. Ibid., case A107-094, no. 013025.

18. Ibid., case A101-082, no. 013555.

19. Ibid., case A170-038, no. 015790.

20. The descriptions come from NGDK, case A141-052, no. 044300.

21. The account from this point has been reconstructed from the formal depositions and confessions recorded by the *yamen* (local government) clerks; they are not spontaneous narratives iterated by the witnesses.

22. This was a common practice for men from modest families, as marrying into their wife's family and changing their family name saved them all the costs of marriage and assured them a livelihood after marriage.

23. There were quarantine measures in place against two epidemic diseases: smallpox and plague. Some kind of quarantine against smallpox was established in Beijing in the seventeenth century by the Manchus, who were susceptible to smallpox and were conquering China. Toward the end of the imperial period, an epidemic of bubonic plague also generated the first "modern" quarantine measures in Manchuria, managed by Wu Lien-teh, whom we will meet again in chap. 4. See Liang Qizi, "Ming-Qing yufang tianhua cuoshi zhi yanbian" (History of Measures to Prevent Smallpox in the Ming-Qing Period), in *Guoshi shilun,* ed. Yang Liansheng et al. (Taipei: Shihuo chubanshe, 1987), 246–247; see also Chang Chia-feng's [Zhang Jiafeng] article on the question of smallpox segregation, "Qingchu di bidou yu chadou zhidu" (The Institutions of Smallpox Avoidance and Inspection in the Early Qing), *Hanxue yanjiu* vol. 14, no. 1 (27) (1996): 135–156. On

quarantine measures during the late Qing plague, see C. Benedict, *Bubonic Plague in 19th-Century China* (Stanford, Calif.: Stanford University Press, 1996).

24. There are also two mentions in the Zhejiang and Hunan gazetteers.

25. See my book on Ming-Qing philanthropy: Liang Qizi, *Shishan yu jiaohua* (*Philanthropy and Moral Transformation*) (Taipei: Lianjing chubanshe, 1997), 32–33.

26. For such support to charitable institutions, see Liang Qizi, *Shishan yu jiaohua*, 62–70, 123–127.

27. *Fujian tongzhi* (*General Gazetteer of Fujian* [1737]), *juan* 13:36b.

28. Ibid., *juan* 13:41a; *Jinjiang xian zhi* (*Gazetteer of Jinjiang* [1765]), *juan* 2:37a; Wang Daokun, [1525–1593], "Epitaph of Hu Cheng'an," in *Taihan ji* (*Collection of Writings by Wang Daokun*) (1591 Wanli ed.), *juan* 48:14a–18a. The *cunxu yuan* in other districts in the same period, such as Tongan and Huian, might also have been *mafeng* asylums, though sources do not specify (*Fujian tongzhi* [1868], *juan* 52:20b).

29. *Fujian tongzhi* (1868), *juan* 52:20b–21a. This leper house was said to have been established by the prefect of the Hongzhi period, and it was one of three branches of the local *yangjiyuan* (*Fujian tongzhi* [1737], *juan* 13:42a).

30. *Fujian tongzhi* (1868), *juan* 52:38b, 39b, 40a, 40b; *Fujian tongzhi* (1737), *juan* 13:37b, 43a, 44a, 45a, 46a, 47a; *Shaowu fu zhi* (*Gazetteer of Shaowu Prefecture* [1900]), 17:1b; *Liancheng xian zhi* (*Gazetteer of Liancheng* [1938]), 18:10a.

31. *Liancheng xian zhi* (1938), 18:10a; *Zhanghua xian zhi* (*Gazetteer of Zhanghua*) (Daoguan ed.), in *Taiwan wenxian congkan*, no. 156 (Taipei: Taiwan yinhang jingji yanjiushi, 1962), 61–62.

32. J. Gray, *Walks in the City of Canton* (Hong Kong: De Souza, 1875), 689. The date of 1380 was probably the year of the establishment of the general poorhouse, which was turned into a leper asylum in 1573.

33. Qu Dajun, *Guangdong xinyu* (*New Stories on Guangdong Province*) (Beijing: Zhongguo shuju, 1985), *juan* 7:245. An early-nineteenth-century quota was given by Chou Juchuan, *Yangcheng guchao* (*Old Manuscript of Canton City* [1806]) (Guangzhou: Guangdong renmin chubanshe, 1993), 3:283. This information was confirmed by the Swedish observer Anders Ljungstedt (*An Historical Sketch of the Portuguese Settlements in China: And of the Roman Catholic Church and Mission in China* [Hong Kong: Viking, 1992; repr. of the 1836 ed.], 216).

34. *Chinese Repository* (Canton: Printed for the proprietors, 1832–1851), vol. 16 (1847): 27.

35. Gray, *Walks in the City of Canton*, 690.

36. Both Nanhai and Dongguan counties each had two *yangjiyuan*, one of which in both cases was built outside the city gate in the sixteenth century (*Xinhui xian zhi* [*Gazet-*

teer of Xinhui (1690)]), 4:10b–11a; *Nanhai xian zhi* (*Gazetteer of Nanhai* [1609]), 3; *Nanhai xian zhi* (1691), 2:21a; *Dongguan xian zhi* (*Gazetteer of Dongguan* [1639]), 2:87.

Similarly, in Leizhou prefecture, *lai* patients and the other poor were originally accommodated together in the same *yangjiyuan,* but the former were later, in the early seventeenth century, moved and interned separately (*Leizhou xian zhi* [*Gazetteer of Leizhou* (1614)], 8:17a).

37. *Jingning xian zhi* (*Gazetteer of Jingning* [1872]), 2:6a.

38. Liang Qizi, *Shishan yu jiaohua,* 103.

39. *Longxi xian zhi* (*Gazetteer of Longxi* [1762]), 9:3b. The same likely happened in Nanjing, in the same prefecture, where a *pujitang* was built outside the northern city gate, with *mafeng* victims dwelling in a separate wing from the other poor and sick (*Fujian tongzhi* [1868], *juan* 52:39b, 40a; *Fujian tongzhi* [1737], *juan* 13:45a, 46a, 47a).

Other districts in Fujian that kept *mafeng* patients apart from the other poor and sick residents of their poorhouses include Nanping, Sha, and Jianyang (*Fujian tongzhi* [1868], *juan* 52:39b, 40a; *Fujian tongzhi* [1737], *juan* 13:45a, 46a, 47a).

40. Zhenghe, Jiangle, Shaowu, Liancheng, and even Zhanghua, Taiwan, had their asylums enlarged during this period (*Fujian tongzhi* [1868], *juan* 52:39b, 40b; *Shaowu xian zhi* [*Gazetteer of Shaowu* (1900)], 17:1b; *Liancheng xian zhi* [1938], 18:10a; *Zhanghua xian zhi,* 61–62).

41. *Fengxin xian zhi* (*Gazetteer of Fengxin* [1824]), 3:16a; *Nanchang fu zhi* (*Gazetteer of Nanchang Prefecture* [1873]), 12:21a; *Nan'an fu zhi buzheng* (*Supplementary Gazetteer of Nan'an Prefecture* [1875]), 3:37b.

42. *Jingning xian zhi* (1872), 2:6a; *Hanyang xian zhi* (*Gazetteer of Hanyang* [1868]), 12:8b.

43. The poem, entitled "*Mafeng* Asylums," is collected in Zhang Yingchang [1790–1874], ed., *Qing shiduo* (*Collection of Qing Poems*) (Beijing: Zhonghua shuju, 1960), 2.23:869.

44. Liang Shaoren, *Liangban qiuyu an suibi* (*Random Notes in the Autumn Rain Study*) (1837; repr. Shanghai: Guji chubanshe, 1982, based on the 1895 ed.), *juan* 4:197.

45. The same was true for asylums in Changle during in the 1560s, Sha county in the 1580s (where the move was carried out under the magistrate Yuan Yingwen, appointed in 1583 for six years), and Leizhou, Guangdong, before 1614 (*Fujian tongzhi* [1737], *juan* 13:37b, 46a; *Sha xian zhi* [*Gazetteer of Sha* (1928)], 6:18a; *Leizhou xian zhi* [1614], 8:17a).

46. *Zengcheng xian zhi* (*Gazetteer of Zengcheng* [1801]), 6:28a. Similarly, in Zhenghe, Jianning prefecture, besides the original asylum three *li* away from the western city gate, a second asylum was built "in an isolated spot far from the town" in 1735 (*Fujian tongzhi* [1868], *juan* 52:40a).

47. Yongna Jushi, *Zhiwen lu* (*Records of Things Heard from Near and from Afar*), in

Biji xiaoshuo daguan, ser. 2, vol. 6 (1817; repr. Taipei: Xinxing shuju, 1978, based on the 1817 ed.): *juan* 8:7a–b (3490–3491).

48. M. Foucault, *Les anormaux: Cours au Collège de France (1974–1975)* (Paris: Gallimard/Seuil, 1999), 41–43.

49. Touati, "Historiciser la notion de contagion," especially 160–175, where the author points out that, in Europe before the thirteenth century, contagion was not considered a main cause of leprosy, and leprosaria were not established for the purpose of stopping contagion.

50. Like charitable hospices for the elderly, some *mafeng* asylums provided stipends to registered patients who did not live inside the institution. Probably these nonresidents were more mobile and could make extra money by begging or doing other odd jobs in the area.

51. Chou, *Yangcheng guchao,* 3:283; *Chaozhou fu zhi* (*Gazetteer of Chaozhou Prefecture* [1893 (1762)]), 15:17a–b; *Guangdong tongzhi* (*General Gazetteer of Guangdong* [1864]), 164:24a, 25b, 26a; *Zengcheng xian zhi* (1801), 6:28a; *Dongguan xian zhi* (1921), 19; *Gaoyao xian zhi* (*Gazetteer of Gaoyao* [1826]), 9:18b.

52. *Chaozhou fu zhi* (1893 [1762]), 15:17a–b.

53. Qu, *Guangdong xinyu, juan* 7:245.

54. *Chaozhou fu zhi* (1893 [1762]), 15:17b.

55. Ibid., 15:17a–b.

56. Choosing a headman to supervise was also the typical way of controlling the local beggar population (Xu Dong, ed., *Muling shu* [*Collected Writings by Magistrates*] [1838], 15:20a).

57. "Medical Reports for the Half Year Ended 30th September 1873, Forwarded by the Surgeons to the Customs at the Treaty Ports of China: Being No. 6 of the Series and Forming the Sixth Part of the Customs Gazette for July-September 1873" (Shanghai: Imperial Maritime Customs Statistical Department, 1874), 41, 43.

58. J. Doolittle, *Social Life of the Chinese: With Some Account of Their Religious, Governmental, Educational, and Business Customs and Opinions; With Special but Not Exclusive Reference to Fuhchau* (New York: Harper, 1865; repr., Taipei: Cheng-wen, 1966), 2:254.

59. Ibid., 2:255–256. Doolittle writes here that twenty years before his visit, a rich man had bribed the headman with a thousand taels of silver to allow him to stay in his own house.

60. J. Cantlie, "Report on the Conditions under Which Leprosy Occurs in China, Indo-China, Malaya, the Archipelago, and Oceana: Compiled Chiefly during 1894," in *Prize Essays on Leprosy,* 239–413 (London: New Sydenham Society, 1897), 303. Cantlie's conclusion from observation of the headman was that good food and clothing would be

the correct treatment for lepers. John Gray, who visited the asylum in eastern Canton City also reported that the two superintendents received a fee from each resident (Gray, *Walks in the City of Canton*, 689).

61. *Leizhou xian zhi* (1614), 8:17a.

62. *Chenghai xian zhi* (*Gazetteer of Chenghai* [1815]), 9:9b–10b.

63. *Shaowu xian zhi* (1900), 17:1b.

64. *Xinhui xian zhi* (1690), 4:10b–11a; *Fengxin xian zhi* (1824), 3:16a.

65. *Leizhou xian zhi* (1614), 8:17a: "Shimin kuai zhi"(The citizens were very happy with this).

66. The rhetoric of the *mafeng* patients being "abandoned by men" refers to the ancient concept that women from a family with criminal records should not be taken as wives since they have been "abandoned by men." As we have seen, people with critical diseases were conceived to be "abandoned by heaven." *Mafeng* patients thus came to be described as being abandoned not only by heaven but also by human society (*Da Dai liji* [*Book of Rites by Elder Dai*] [Shanghai: Shanghai shudian, 1989] [Sibu congkan ed.], sect. 80, "Benming," 509).

67. *Dayu xian zhi* (*Gazetteer of Dayu* [1748]), 19:2a–3a.

68. Quoted in Dai Wenfeng, "'*Haiguan yibao' yu Qing mo Taiwan kaigang diqu di jibing*" ("Medical Reports of the Chinese Imperial Maritime Customs Service" and Diseases in Developed Regions in Taiwan During the Latter Part of the Qing), *Si yu yan* 33, no. 2 (1995): 185.

69. Liang Qizi, *Shishan yu jiaohua*, 103–128.

70. They were Chengdu, Chongqing, Guizhou, Xuzhou, Ningyuan, and Baoning.

71. Li Rulan, *Junjichu lu fu zouzhe* (*Copy Record of Memorial to the Emperor Kept by the Grand Secretariat*), nineteenth day, ninth month, seventh year of Qianlong, Number 1 Archives, Beijing, no. 335-27, microfilm no. 022-1525. I thank Zhang Li, of the Number 1 Archives, for informing me of this interesting document.

72. Qu, *Guangdong xinyu, juan* 7:245.

73. J. Gray, *China: A History of the Laws, Manners and Customs of the People* (London: Macmillan, 1878; repr., New York: AMS Press, 1974), 52–53.

74. *Chinese Repository* (Canton: Printed for the proprietors, 1832–1851), vol. 16 (1847): 494.

75. Warren Winter, "The Gospel Boat for Lepers," *Leper Quarterly* 1, no. 1 (1927): 32–33.

76. K. Schipper, "Seigneurs royaux, dieux des épidémies," *Archives de sciences sociales des religions* 59, no. 1 (1985): 33; P. Katz, *Demon Hordes and Burning Boats: The Cult of Marshal Wen in Late Imperial Chekiang* (Albany: SUNY Press, 1995), 153–156; M. Szonyi, "The Illusion of Standardizing the Gods: The Cult of the Five Emperors in Late Imperial

China," *Journal of Asian Studies* 56, no. 1 (1997): 118–120. For a more general discussion of early Daoist liturgical texts on the "expulsion of pestilent gods," see Li Fengmao, "*Daozang* suo shou zaoqi daoshu di wenyi guan" (Views on Epidemics as Shown by Early Daoist Texts in the *Daoist Canon*), *Zhongguo wenzhe yanjiu jikan* 3 (1993): 448–451.

77. A similar report was made by S. Johnson (*Chinese Repository* [Canton: Printed for the proprietors, 1832–1851], vol. 16 [1847]: 494).

78. Some of the rituals surrounding the death of someone who had died of *eji* or in an epidemic were also telling of the fear of pollution: the clothes and bedding of the dead and of those who had cared for him were to be smoked with *Atractylodes* rhizome and frankincense (Yan Yuan, *Yan Yuan ji* [*Collected Writings of Yan Yuan*] [Beijing: Zhonghua shuju, 1987], "Liwen shouchao" [Writings on Rituals], 4, "Sang li [Death Rituals]," 361–362). Recall the ancient punishment by drowning of a criminal diagnosed to have *li*, revealing the dread of the disease. See chap. 2, p. 62, and n. 6 of the present chapter.

Violent deaths of lepers were recorded numerous times even in the modern period, showing the weight of tradition. Many were buried alive, some were massacred collectively with machine guns, others were abandoned in the mountains to starve to death, many more were burned to death; see chap. 4, and also a more recent record of violent killings of patients in post-1949 PRC, in *Fujian sheng weisheng zhi* (*Gazetteer on Hygiene of Fujiang Province*) (Fuzhou, 1989), 207. These include burying victims alive and burning them to death, even by family members. Similar happenings, in Guangdong province, are recorded in O. K. Skinsnes, "Leprosy in Society," *Leprosy Review* 35 (1964): 31.

79. The association of lepers with beggars seems to be common to many cultures. The study by Navon in modern Thailand confirms the negative image of lepers in that country (L. Navon, "Beggars, Metaphors, and Stigma: A Missing Link in the Social History of Leprosy," *Social History of Medicine* 11, no. 1 [1998]: 89–105).

80. Qu, *Guangdong xinyu, juan* 7:245–246.

81. Xu Ke, *Qing bai lei chao* (*Collection of Popular Customs of the Qing*) (1917; repr., Beijing: Zhonghua shuju, 1984), 5476.

82. Gray, *China,* 52.

83. Qu, *Guangdong xinyu, juan* 7:245.

84. There was a judicial case involving a group of leper-beggars committing petty crimes (NGDK, case A088-006, no. 017308). Such crimes were apparently a rather widespread phenomenon in late imperial China.

85. Tan Dihua, ed., *Guangdong beike ji* (*Texts on Steles in Guangdong Province*) (Guangzhou: Guangdong gaodeng jiaoyu chubanshe, 2001). A stele in Dapu district dated 1772 (894), one in Haifeng district dated 1790 (840–841), and two in Wuhua dated 1796 and 1803 (905–906) contained such public announcements.

86. Wu Zhenfang [*jinshi* 1679], *Lingnan zaji* (*Miscellaneous Records on the Ling-*

nan Region), in *Biji xiaoshuo daguan,* ser. 3, vol. 10 (Taipei: Xinxing shuju, 1974), *juan* 1:34b–35a.

87. Liang Shaoren, *Liangban qiuyu an suibi, juan* 4:197.

88. Chen Huiyan, *Nanyue youji* (*Records on a Voyage in the Southern Yue Region*) (1851), 1:17a–b.

89. Qu, *Guangdong xinyu, juan* 7:246.

90. Gray observed that patients' descendants who had no sign of the disease regarded the asylum as their home and were "most reluctant to leave it" (Gray, *Walks in the City of Canton,* 690).

91. Doolittle, *Social Life of the Chinese,* 254–255.

92. Sakura Magozou, *Minfeng zaji* (*Miscellaneous Records of Fujian Customs*) (Fuzhou: Meihua shuju, 1904), 3b. I thank Lin Mei-rong for providing me with this information.

93. *Shaowu xian zhi* (1900), 17:1b.

94. *Chaozhou fu zhi* (1893 [1762]), 15:17a–b. Finally, the magistrate had to check their registration (to make sure that they had the right to dwell in the district) and ask local constables to forbid their entering the town. The gazetteer did not seem optimistic, however, about the effectiveness of such measures.

95. *Fujian tongzhi* (1737), *juan* 13:44a.

96. Gu Zhentao, *Wumen biao yin* (*Record of Obscure Things in the Wu Area*) (Nanjing: Jiangsu guji chubanshe, 1999), 4:45.

97. Wu Zhenfang, *Lingnan zaji,* 1:35a.

98. Jiang Cheng, "Mafeng bingren chuangban di zazhi: 'Chenguang jikan'" (A Journal Created by Patients of Leprosy: *Morning Light Quarterly*), *Zhongguo mafeng zazhi* 8, no. 1 (1992): 44–45. Although written only partly by patients, this journal preceded that (*The Star*) created by inmates of America's Carville (Louisiana) Leprosarium's by one year.

99. Susan Burns uses such materials to look at the "leper" identity in modern Japan ("From 'Leper Villages' to Leprosaria,'"114–118).

100. The idea that the deep south was dominated by lascivious women was mentioned as early as the *Han shu* (*Book of the Han Dynasty*): "There are many women in the country of Yue. They bathe in the same river with men. They are mostly lascivious women born of perverse *qi*" (quoted in Xiao Fan, "Han-Song jian wenxian suojian gudai Zhongguo nanfang di dili huanjing yu difang bing ji qi yingxiang" [Geographic Environment, Endemic Diseases of China's South as Described in Texts from the Han to the Song, and Their Influences], *Bulletin of the Institute of History and Philology, Academia Sinica* 63, no. 1 [1993]: 84). This idea was elaborated by Zhou Qufei, of the Southern Song, who wrote in a text published in 1178, "The south is extremely hot and is not suitable for men but for women. It is because yang clashes with yang, but when combined with yin, things will thrive. I notice that women in the Guangdong region are numerous and strong, while men are thin

and short with a dismal complexion" (*Lingwai daida* [*Answers to Questions on the Deep South*] [Shanghai: Gushu liutong chu, 1921; repr., Taipei: Xingzhong shuju, 1964], 10:15a).

101. For an analysis of the "civilizing process" in Guangdong province since the early Ming through the household registration and tax system, see Liu Zhiwei, *Zai guojia yu shehui zhijian: Ming-Qing lijia fuyi zhidu yanjiu* (*Between State and Society: The Study of the Household Registration and Tax System in Guangdong of the Ming-Qing Period*) (Guangzhou: Zhongshan daxue chubanshe, 1997), 17–32, 35–43, 64–66.

102. On the question of state penetration and ethnic identities of southern China, see David Faure, *Emperor and Ancestor: State and Lineage in South China* (Stanford, Calif.: Stanford University Press, 2007), especially 38–50, on the discourse that opposed the cultured "we" to the semibarbarian "they" in the Pearl River delta region. See also P. K. Crossley, H. F. Siu, and D. S. Sutton, eds., *Empire at the Margins: Culture, Ethnicity, and Frontier in Early Modern China* (Berkeley: University of California Press, 2006).

On the question of cultural identity of the Lingnan region in the late imperial period, see Cheng Meibao, *Diyu wenhua yu guojia rentong: Wan Qing yilai Guangdong wenhuaguan di xingcheng* (*Regional Culture and National Identity: The Construct of the Concept of Guangdong Culture Since the Late Qing*) (Beijing: Sanlian shudian, 2006).

103. Many, but not all, of the firsthand historical sources cited in this section are quoted in Jiang Zhushan, "Ming-Qing huanan diqu youguan mafeng bing di minjian liaofa" (Popular Healing of Leprosy in Southeastern China in the Ming and Qing Periods), *Dalu zazhi* (April 1995): 182–192.

104. Zhou Mi, *Guixin zashi* (*Miscellaneous Writings in the Guixin Neighborhood*) (Beijing: Zhonghua shuju, 1988), 81.

105. Shen Zhiwen, *Jiewei yuansuo* (*Sources of Relief*) (Shanghai: Shanghai guji chubanshe, 1997; facs. of the 1816 Wuxi ed.), 1:7a–b.

106. The use of the verb *sell* here implies prostitution: the *mafeng* poison of female prostitutes was transferred to male clients. See the discussion on p. 121 of the link between prostitution in Guangdong province and the spread of *mafeng* as described by the seventeenth-century Cantonese scholar Qu Dajun.

107. Xiao Xiaoting, *Fengmen quanshu* (*A Complete Work on the Feng Disorder*) (Guangzhou: Jingye tang, 1845 engraving of the 1836 Wu Yunlou ed.), 1:9a. The hepatic orb (*gan jing*) is responsible for producing and regulating blood.

108. By the early twentieth century, the *guolai* custom seems to have further transformed so that not only women but men could also pass the disease on to their sexual partners (see chap. 4).

109. Several famous leprologists of the early Communist regime in the 1950s warned against the practice. Yue Meizhong (1900–1982), a doctor specializing in leprosy in the 1950s, wrote several articles in medical journals warning against the custom ("Zuguo yixue dui dafeng bing di renshi ji qi zhiliao bing ji xiandai yixue duiyu mafeng bing di

zhishe" [Knowledge and Therapeutics of Leprosy in Our Country and Modern Medical Understanding of the Disease], *Xin zhongyi yao* 8, nos. 3–4 [1957]: 13, quoting the findings of Liu Muzhi, a surgeon of Western training; "Guanyu zuguo yixue mafeng shishi ji qi zhuzuo di xushu" [On the Historical Facts of Leprosy and Its Description in Medical Texts in Our Mother Country], *Shanghai zhongyi zazhi* 9 [1956]: 41). See also Xiao Yunchun, "Zuguo yixue duiyu mafeng zhi renshi" (Our Mother Country's Knowledge on Leprosy), *Zhongyi zazhi* 4 (1956): 172).

110. Shen, *Jiewei yuansou,* 1:3a–b.

111. Wang Linheng, *Yue jian lu* (*Records on Guangdong*) (Beijing: Zhonghua shuju, 1987; based on the 1601Wanli ed.), *juan* 2:76.

112. *Shouyu shenfang* (*Miraculous Recipes for Achieving Longevity*), in *Yifang leiju* (*Compilation of Medical Recipes by Kind*) (Beijing: Renmin weisheng chubanshe, 1981; based on the 1852 Japanese ed.), 649.

113. The author gives another example to illustrate the different body types of central and southern China: a northerner contracted the disease in Guangdong and, on the advice of the local people, took viper wine as a remedy. His body melted into water as a result. The author commented that this strong remedy was suitable only for the barbaric southern body and too strong for the body type from central China. In fact, in saying the man got the disease and died in Guangdong, the author reveals he was perverting an old Tang tale. The idea of fundamentally different southern and northern bodies was obviously a construct of the late imperial period (*Shouyu shenfang,* 649).

114. M. Hanson, "Northern Purgatives, Southern Restoratives: Ming Medical Regionalism," *Asian Medicine: Tradition and Modernity* 2, no. 2 (2006): 115–170; Liang Qizi [Leung, A. K. C.], "Jibing yu fangtu zhi guanxi: Yuan zhi Qing jian yijie di kanfa" (The Relations Between Diseases and Locality: The Views in Medical Books from the Yuan to the Qing), in *Xingbie yu yiliao: Di san jie guoji hanxue huiyi lunwen ji* (*Gender and Medicine: Volume of the Third International Conference on Sinology*), 165–212 (Taipei: Institute of Modern History, Academia Sinica, 2002).

115. Qingchengzi, *Zhiyi xubian* (*Sequel to the Account of Extraordinary Things*), early Qing facs. in *Biji xiaoshuo daguan,* ser. 1, vol. 6 (Taipei: Xinxing shuju, 1962), *juan* 2:6a–b (5755).

116. Wu Qian et al., *Yizong jinjian* (*Golden Mirror of Medical Orthodoxy*) (Beijing: Renmin weisheng chubanshe, 1990; based on the 1742 Wuyingdian ed.), 73:1a (371).

117. Yongna jushi, *Zhiwen lu,* 8:7b–8a (3490–3491). The term *waijiang* is a general one used by the Cantonese to designate people from more northern regions. According to early Qing writings by non-Cantonese, *waijiang* referred to people outside Guangdong province but not to those from Fujian and Guangxi provinces. Guangdong inhabitants thus seemed to consider Fujian and Guangxi people as insiders having a similar culture. See Zhang Qu [?–1740, qualified as tribute student 1711, prefect of Huizhou, Guangdong

province, 1730, died as provincial governor of Hubei], *Yuedong wenjian lu* (*A Record of Things Heard and Seen in Eastern Guangdong* [preface, 1739]) (Guangzhou: Guangdong gaodeng jiaoyu chubanshe, 1990), *juan* 1:59.

The expression "One should not enter Guangdong when one is young" seems to have been a popular saying. It is mentioned also in a Qing popular novel, Zuohua san ren, *Feng liu wu* (*Reflections After Amorous Encounters*) (Shanghai: Shanghai guji chubanshe, 1990; facs. of a ca. mid-eighteenth century ed.), 105–106.

118. Wu Chichang, *Xu kechuang xianhua* (*Sequel to "Miscellaneous Stories Told by Guests"*) (Beijing: Wenhua yishu chubanshe, 1988), 354–355.

119. Qu, *Guangdong xinyu, juan* 7:244–245.

120. Fan Duan'ang, *Yue zhong jianwen* (*Things Seen and Heard in Guangdong*) (1730; repr., Guangzhou: Guangdong gaodeng jiaoyu, 1988), 20:233.

121. Liang Tingnan, *Yifen wenji* (*Records of Things Heard in an Atmosphere of Barbarism*) (Beijing: Zhonghua shuju, 1959), 3:72–73. Liang was a collaborator of Lin Zexu's, the Chinese official who fought the so-called Opium War with the British in the mid-nineteenth century.

122. The episode was rewritten by another Cantonese writer of a decade later to express the Cantonese hatred toward the Hunanese soldiers, described as particularly cruel and barbaric. Young women with *mafeng* were deliberately sent out to seduce them in order to contaminate them, so that more than half died of the disease (Chen Huiyan, *Nanyue youji*, 1:17a–b).

123. Wu Jianren, *Ershi nian mudu zhi guai xianzhuang* (*Strange Phenomena Observed During the Past Twenty Years*) (Taipei: Guangya chuban youxian gongsi, 1984; based on the 1909 ed.), 60:547–549.

124. R. Edmond, *Leprosy and Empire: A Medical and Cultural Study* (Cambridge: Cambridge University Press, 2006), 10.

125. Recent historical and anthropological studies on the ethnic identities of the Lingnan region also show the ambiguities of such boundaries; see, for example the works by D. Faure, D. Sutton, H. Siu, and Liu Zhiwei on the questions of the Yao, Miao, and Dan in the south and the history of their cultural identities (D. Faure, "The Yao Wars in the Mid-Ming and Their Impact on Yao Ethnicity"; D. S. Sutton, "Ethnicity and the Miao Frontier in the Eighteenth Century"; Siu and Liu, "Lineage, Market, Pirate, and Dan: Ethnicity in the Pearl River Delta," all in Crossley, Siu and Sutton, *Empire at the Margins*).

126. Liang Shaoren, *Liangban qiuyu an suibi, juan* 4:197–198; the poem, with the story, and with other aspects of the *guolai* phenomenon in Guangdong, were also recorded in Chen Kun, *Lingnan zashi shi chao* (*Poems Related to Miscellaneous Matters in Guangdong Province*) (Guangzhou: Yiyuanlou, 1876), *juan* 5:23b–26a.

127. Wu Chichang, *Xu kechuang xianhua*, 355–356.

128. Xuan Ding, *Yeyu qiudeng lu* (*Records of Night Rain and Autumn Lamp*), re-

printed in the drama *Bing yu yuan chuanqi* (Shanghai: Zhonghua shuju, 1932) (first ed., 1907), with a 1913 preface by the author. The first printing of Xuan Ding's work is probably the 1877 Shenbao edition.

129. One recent discussion on a performance can be found at http://www.xiqu.org/forums/thread/158/8267/ (accessed March 16, 2008). The discussions dated from 2005 to 2007.

130. The reference here is to the 1913 printing, based on the first 1907 edition, by Zhonghua shuju, Shanghai.

131. "Modengxian" (Nonidling) is from a famous poem, "Man jiang hong" (River Red with Blood), attributed to the patriotic general Yue Fei, of the Song dynasty, who lost his life fighting the northern "barbarians." Yue became a symbol of Chinese patriotism, and this poem became extremely popular in modern China when it was threatened by Western "barbarians."

132. Chen's lineage can be seen at http://www.bbs.chens.org.cn. See also http://baike.baidu.com/view/929688.html (accessed March 16, 2008).

133. *Bing yu yuan chuanqi,* 19, 37.

134. Ibid., 224, 230.

135. Ibid., 13.

136. Ibid., 66–69, 141, 257.

137. Ibid., 38, 55.

138. Ibid., 75, 78, 89, 199.

139. Ibid., 75, 251.

140. Many northern visitors to Guangdong in the late imperial period remarked on the fact that many women had large feet; the early Qing Zhejiang scholar Wu Zhenfang, for example, wrote that, except for a few women of very wealthy families, most Lingnan women did not bind their feet (*Lingnan zaji,* 1:14b–15a [6287]).

141. *Bing yu yuan chuanqi,* 30–31.

142. Ibid., 101.

143. For the modern meaning of the term *weisheng,* see R. Rogaski, *Hygienic Modernity: Meanings of Health and Disease in Treaty-Port China* (Berkeley: University of California Press, 2004).

144. For the comic role of medical doctors in novels and plays, see W. Idema, "Diseases and Doctors, Drugs and Cures: A Very Preliminary List of Passages of Medical Interest in a Number of Traditional Chinese Novels and Related Plays," *Chinese Science* 2 (1977): 37–63.

145. *Bing yu yuan chuanqi,* 137.

146. Ibid., 138.

147. Ibid., 146.

148. Ibid., 231, 232, 246, 258.

4. THE CHINESE LEPER AND THE MODERN WORLD

1. The most recent study on the renewed interest in leprosy in the imperialist age of the nineteenth century is R. Edmond, *Leprosy and Empire: A Medical and Cultural Study* (Cambridge: Cambridge University Press, 2006).

2. H. P. Wright, *Leprosy: An Imperial Danger* (London: Churchill, 1889), 1.

3. Edmond devotes an entire chapter to this development (*Leprosy and Empire,* chap. 2).

4. Among the many published observations on leprosy in nineteenth-century India, an early synthesis is T. R. Lewis and D. D. Cunningham, *Leprosy in India: A Report* (Calcutta: Office of the Superintendent of Government Printing, 1877); the report is based on census reports of 1872 and highlights the noncontagiousness of the disease and its heredity (71–72).

5. D. Arnold, *Science, Technology and Medicine in Colonial India* (Cambridge: Cambridge University Press, 2000), 211.

6. H. Lamson, *Social Pathology in China: A Source Book for the Study of Problems of Livelihood, Health, and the Family* (Shanghai: Commercial Press, 1935; repr., Taipei: Cheng-wen, 1974). Besides leprosy, the section on health discusses tuberculosis, venereal diseases, mental deficiency, mental disease, and the public health movement in general. Leprosy was obviously considered a major health concern in China in the 1930s.

7. C. A. Gordon, comp., *An Epitome of the Reports of the Medical Officers to the Chinese Imperial Maritime Customs Service, from 1871 to 1882: With Chapters on the History of Medicine in China; Materia Medica; Epidemics; Famine; Ethnology; and Chronology in Relation to Medicine and Public Health* (London: Baillière, Tindell, and Cox, 1884), 153.

8. Chen Yuan, *Chen Yuan zaonian wenji* (*Early Writings of Chen Yuan*) (Taipei: Institute of Chinese Literature and Philosophy, Academia Sinica, 1992), 301, 322, 323.

9. See chap. 1, n. 1.

10. S. Burns, "From 'Leper Villages' to Leprosaria': Public Health, Nationalism and the Culture of Exclusion in Japan." In *Isolation: Places and Practices of Exclusion,* ed. C. Strange and A. Bashford (London: Routledge 2003), 108.

11. Most of the metaphors of AIDS described by Susan Sontag are those that have been associated with leprosy (*AIDS and Its Metaphors* [New York: Farrar, Straus and Giroux, 1988]).

12. S. S. Pandya, "Anti-contagionism in Leprosy, 1844–1897," *International Journal of Leprosy and Other Mycobacterial Diseases* 66, no. 3 (1998): 377–380.

13. Ibid., 377, 379; M. Worboys, *Spreading Germs: Disease Theories and Medical Practice in Britain, 1865–1900* (Cambridge: Cambridge University Press, 2000), 42. For a similar view in relation to the situation in India, see the *Report on Leprosy by the Royal College of Physicians* (London: George Edward Eyre and William Spottiswoode, 1867), and

S. Kakar "Leprosy in British India, 1860–1940: Colonial Politics and Missionary Medicine," *Medical History* 40 (1996): 215.

14. Li Shang-jen has recently done a comprehensive study on the various views of leprosy held by British doctors in late-nineteenth-century China ("Shijiu shiji houqi Yingguo yixue jie dui Zhongguo mafeng bing qing di diaocha yanjiu" [British Medical Research on Leprosy in Late Nineteenth-Century China], *Bulletin of the Institute of History and Philology, Academia Sinica* 74, no. 3 [2003]: 445–506).

15. For Hobson's role in introducing Western medical science into China, see B. Elman, *On Their Own Terms: Science in China, 1550–1900.* (Cambridge, Mass.: Harvard University Press, 2005), 287–296.

16. B. Hobson, "On the Leprosy of the Chinese: Letter from Dr. Hobson," *Medical Times and Gazette* (London) 1 (June 2, 1860): 558–559 (I thank Li Shang-jen for copying this article for me). In an 1842 report on Macao Hospital, Hobson wrote, "Want of time forbids me to compare the leprosy of the Chinese with that of the Jews, Arabs and Hindoos. Beyond them this disease does not appear to extend" (*Chinese Repository* [Canton: Printed for the proprietors, 1832–1851], vol. XX [1842]: 664).

17. Li Shang-jen, "Shijiu shiji houqi," 455.

18. W. H. Jefferys and J. L. Maxwell, *The Diseases of China: Including Formosa and Korea* (Philadelphia: Blakiston's, 1911), 96.

19. Edmond, *Leprosy and Empire,* 20.

20. P. Manson, *Tropical Diseases: A Manual of the Diseases of Warm Climates,* 6th ed. (1898; repr., London: Cassell, 1918), 639. Manson's view was directly influenced by Jonathan Hutchinson, who later published his famous thesis on the relation between leprosy and fish eating (*On Leprosy and Fish-Eating: A Statement of Facts and Explanations* [London: Archibald Constable, 1906]).

21. Gordon, *Epitome of the Reports,* 309.

22. Hobson, *Chinese Repository* [Canton: Printed for the proprietors, 1832–1851], vol. 11 (1842): 664.

23. Gordon, *Epitome of the Reports,* 151.

24. A. W. Douthwaite, "Leprosy," *Chinese Medical Missionary Journal* (*CMMJ*) 4 (1892): 253.

25. J. Edkins, "Leprosy," *CMMJ* 1 (1891): 23–24. Edkins quotes the episode in the *Analects,* also mentioned by J. Needham and G.-D. Lu ("Records of Diseases in Ancient China," in *Diseases in Antiquity: A Survey of the Diseases, Injuries and Surgery of Early Populations,* ed. D. Brothwell and A. T. Sandison [Springfield, Ill.: Charles Thomas, 1967], 236), to show the long existence of the disease.

26. J. Cantlie, "Report on the Conditions under Which Leprosy Occurs in China, Indo-China, Malaya, the Archipelago, and Oceania: Compiled Chiefly during 1894," in

Prize Essays on Leprosy (London: New Sydenham Society, 1897), 269. Cantlie thought that north China would soon be uninhabitable.

27. This was the view of the French doctor Max Durand-Fardel, who wrote that "le caractère le plus spécial et le plus frappant de la nation chinoise est l'uniformité," which led him to ask if this trait explained the pathology all over China ("Pathologie médicale: La lèpre en Chine," *Gazette médicale de Paris* 33 [1877]: 403).

28. "Weisheng bu diaocha mafeng ling" (Order to Conduct Surveys on Leprosy, Issued by the Ministry of Pubic Health), *Mafeng jikan* 3, nos. 2, 3 (1929): 50.

29. Li Zuwei, "Laibing yange shuo lue" (Brief History of Leprosy), *Xin yiyao,* 4, no. 7 (1934): 1010. The article otherwise conformed to most contemporary Western views on leprosy.

30. See chap. 3, p. 111.

31. Wong Foon [Huang Kuan], "Dr. F. Wong's Memorandum on Leprosy," in "Medical Reports for the Half Year Ended 30th September 1873, Forwarded by the Surgeons to the Customs at the Treaty Ports of China: Being No. 6 of the Series and Forming the Sixth Part of the Customs Gazette for July-September 1873" (Shanghai: Imperial Maritime Customs Statistical Department, 1874), 45.

32. Hobson, *Chinese Repository* [Canton: Printed for the proprietors, 1832–1851], vol. 11 (1842): 664; Hobson, *Medical Times and Gazette,* 558.

33. Ibid.; Durand-Fardel, "Le caractère le plus spécial," 404.

34. *Report on Leprosy by the Royal College of Physicians* (London: George Edward Eyre and William Spottiswoode, 1867), lxvii-lxviii. This conclusion was apparently based on the report on Hong Kong by Dr. Dickson, who wrote that the disease "is considered hereditary in China, but all agree in saying that it dies out in the third generation" (sect. 34, "China, Japan, &c.," 73); the one on Canton by Dr. Hobson: "Leprosy is undoubtedly a hereditary disease. It is said to become mild in the third generation, and to run itself out in the fourth. . . . Their progeny is considered free from taint, and need no longer be secluded from society"; and that from Consul Robertson: "The disease is often hereditary. It is believed in most cases to run through four generations, after which the virus becomes exhausted" (sects. 76–77).

35. Most of the medical missionaries in both India and China shared the belief that what they observed personally in those countries on the nature of leprosy applied only to those places. On India, see Pandya, "Anti-contagionism in Leprosy," 382.

36. For instance, doctors of the Chinese Imperial Maritime Customs reported with interest the Chinese classification of the subtypes of leprosy. What Hobson and Dr. Meadows reported, in 1842 and 1871, respectively, was a mixture of local beliefs and old theories such as those of Chao Yuanfang; both showed a keen curiosity toward the natives' description of the disease. Similarly, Dr. Dudgeon, reporting in 1875 from Beijing, also provided an objective account of the Chinese views of the disease and the various drugs

used by Chinese. He added, "The hereditary and infectious nature of leprosy is noticed" (Gordon, *Epitome of the Reports,* no. 20, "Leprosy," 150, appendix 28, "Leprosy," 310). Hobson also described the Chinese popular methods of leprosy diagnosis: "A suspected person is placed in a dark room where some nitre is burning; if the complexion changes to light blue it is not leprosy, if it remain unchanged of a reddish hue it is. Another mode is to take the person to a shop and expose the face or diseased part to the large blaze of a refining furnace, when if it remains a dullish red, it is the leprosy" (*Chinese Repository* [Canton: Printed for the proprietors, 1832–1851], vol. 11 [1842]: 664). Hobson seems to have been greatly interested in the Chinese views on leprosy in 1842, and, other than his reservations on the contagiousness of the disease, did not challenge the other views.

37. N. Shah, *Contagious Divides: Epidemics and Race in San Francisco's Chinatown* (Berkeley: University of California Press, 2001), 99, quoting American writings on the subject from 1869 to 1876. Dr. Foye, of the City and County Small-Pox Hospital of San Francisco, made a statement in 1884 to the Board of Supervisors of the City and County of San Francisco that the Chinese leper admitted to the hospital in 1871 was indeed the first one. Seventy-eight cases were subsequently admitted (W. Farwell, *The Chinese at Home and Abroad* [San Francisco: Bancroft, 1885], 105).

38. Shah, *Contagious Divides,* 100.

39. Farwell, *Chinese at Home and Abroad,* 111.

40. Farwell, quoting Foye's statement of 1884 (ibid., 109).

41. H. P. Wright (1889) did a comprehensive history and geography of leprosy, including the European origin of the disease in North America. But his balanced account was eclipsed by the alarmist view apparent in the title, which many scholars too quickly labeled as racist. In fact his stance, European centrist, was much less racist than the average contemporary writings. Another late but objective account of the American situation published in China was that by Dr. O. E. Denny, "The Leprosy Problem in the United States," *National Medical Journal* (The English part of the *Zhonghua yixue zazhi*) 30, no. 5 (1927): 391–398.

42. P. Moblo, "Blessed Damien of Moloka'i: The Critical Analysis of Contemporary Myth," *Ethnohistory* 44, no. 4 (1997): 697.

43. A. A. Mouritz, *The Path of the Destroyer: A History of Leprosy in the Hawaiian Islands and Thirty Years Research into the Means by Which It Has Been Spread* (Honolulu: Honolulu Star-Bulletin, 1916), 29–30.

44. S. Parry, "Of Vital Importance to the Community: The Control of Leprosy in the Northern Territory," *Health and History* 5, no. 1 (2003): 2.

45. A. Bashford, *Imperial Hygiene: A Critical History of Colonialism, Nationalism and Public Health* (New York: Palgrave Macmillan, 2004), 88–89, 103, 143.

46. Burns, "From 'Leper Villages' to Leprosaria,'"108–109.

47. Mitsuda Kensuke, the leading twentieth-century Japanese leprologist, active

during the colonial period, wrote numerous papers on the topic. He wanted the colonial government in Taiwan to build a colony on the Culion model and declared a "sacred war" against leprosy in the East Asian region (*Mitsuda Kensuke to Nihon no rai yobō jigyū—Rai yobōhō gojūshūnen kinen* [*Mitsuda Kensuke and Japan's Leprosy Prevention Enterprise: Fiftieth Anniversary of the Leprosy Prevention Law*] [Tokyo: Tōfū kyōkai, 1958], 145–148; 527–530).

48. Ichiro Kikkuchi, "Hansen's Disease Patients: Responses to Stigma and Segregation in Kumamoto, Japan," *International Journal of Dermatology* 33, no. 2 (1994): 142–145.

49. Mouritz observed: "The true duration of his disease was between ten and eleven years, for during the summer of the year 1878 . . . true prodromal symptoms of leprosy manifested themselves. . . . After about five years of intimate contact with lepers (from the year 1873 to year 1878), he suffered the before mentioned symptoms" (*Path of the Destroyer*, 234–235). Mouritz examined Damien for the first time in 1885 (235–236).

50. Z. Gussow, *Leprosy, Racism, and Public Health: Social Policy in Chronic Disease Control* (Boulder, Colo.: Westview Press, 1989), 116, 123–124.

51. Z. Gussow and G. Tracy, "Stigma and the Leprosy Phenomenon: The Social History of a Disease in the 19th and 20th Centuries," *Bulletin of the History of Medicine* 44, no. 5 (1970) : 425–449; D. Obregon, "La construction sociale de la lèpre en Colombie, 1884–1959," in *Les sciences hors d'Occident au XXe siècle*, ed. A.-M. Moulin (Paris: Orstom, 1996), 4:161–162, 166.

52. Cantlie was famous for getting Sun Yat-sen out of captivity of the Qing embassy in London before the Republican Revolution.

53. Cantlie, "Report," 361; Gussow, *Leprosy, Racism, and Public Health*, 126. The "three centers" here mean Hawaii, Fiji, and New Caledonia.

54. Weisheng bu (Ministry of Health), "Fangyi" (Disease Prevention) (Taipei: Guoshi guan [Academia Historica]), 112/4:11793, July 11, 1948. The man was a Cantonese working for the Inland Water Transport Organization during the war and was diagnosed with the disease in 1945 at the Kondhwar Leper Hospital in Poona, which requested his repatriation. I thank Chang Chia-feng for providing me with this document.

55. For example, Patrick Manson's discoveries on filarial worms were recorded in the 1880s as contributions to germ theory, since parasitic worms were then considered as germs (Worboys, *Spreading Germs*, 15; D. Haynes, *Imperial Medicine: Patrick Manson and the Conquest of Tropical Disease* [Philadelphia: University of Pennsylvania Press, 2001]).

56. Worboys, *Spreading Germs*, 176, 193, 206.

57. Gordon, *Epitome of the Reports*, 151.

58. Li Shang-jen, "Shijiu shiji houqi," 456.

59. Gordon, *Epitome of the Reports*, 152.

60. *Report on Leprosy*, xli–xliii. The quote is from a Dr. Fleming of Murshidabad. The question was one among seventeen. The conclusion of the report was that leprosy was a

disease sui generis, independent of any other disease. The survey results show, however, the discrepancy between such a conclusion and the beliefs of many British doctors working in various parts of the world at the time.

61. Mouritz, *Path of the Destroyer*, 54–55.

62. Arthur Mouritz explained to readers of the Hawaiian press that the specific features of syphilis in its tertiary stage were nonexistent in leprosy, and that Fitch was considered by his colleagues to be a "charlatan, quack, and a knave" (ibid., 55–56). Dr. George Newman also wrote a short notice, in 1895, refuting the popular belief that leprosy and syphilis were related (G. Newman, E. Ehlers, and S. Impey, *Prize Essays on Leprsoy* [London: New Sydenham Society, 1895], 4–5).

63. *Report on Leprosy*, 74–75, 77.

64. Cantlie, "Report," 249, 259–261.

65. A. K. C. Leung, "The Business of Vaccination in 19th-Century Canton," *Late Imperial China* 29, no. 1, supplement (2008): 7–39.

66. Hobson, *Chinese Repository* [Canton: Printed for the proprietors, 1832–1851], vol. 11 (1842): 664.

67. Cantlie, "Report," 308, 375–376; Mouritz, *Path of the Destroyer*, 95–96. J. Ashburton Thompson (1846–1915), an Australian medical officer who visited Hawaii in 1896 and wrote on the history of leprosy on the islands, also discussed the alleged relation between vaccination and the spread of the disease, which he considered also to be unproven (Thompson, "Leprosy in Hawaii: A Critical Enquiry," in *Mittheilungen und Verhandlungen der internationalen wissenschaftlichen Lepra-Conferenz zu Berlin im October 1897* [Berlin, 1897–1898], part 2:289–290).

68. Douthwaite, "Leprosy," 252–253.

69. The 1865 act isolating all patients of leprosy in Hawaii ended only in 1969, when admission to Kalaupapa stopped. With a dozen elderly patients still living on the peninsula, Molokai was declared a national historical park in 1980. My account here has been constructed from the following works: Moblo, "Blessed Damien of Moloka'i," 692–726; Thompson, "Leprosy in Hawaii," 274–281; Gussow, *Leprosy, Racism, and Public Health*, 91–107; R. D. K. Herman, "Out of Sight, out of Mind, out of Power: Leprosy, Race and Colonization in Hawai'i," *Journal of Historical Geography* 27, no. 3 (2001): 319–337. A recent popular work on the Molokai colony is J. Tayman, *The Colony: The Harrowing True Story of the Exiles of Molokai* (New York: Scribner, 2006).

70. There is a long history of failed inoculation of leprous blood and the bacillus by leprologists. It began in 1844 with the Norwegian Danielssen, who inoculated himself and others with leprous blood and serum. Dr. Mouritz also inoculated a leprous serum to willing natives of Molokai in the 1880s (natives in Hawaii often wanted to be lepers in order to be maintained at public expense), essentially without success. A famous successful case was the inoculation of Keanu, a native prisoner in Hawaii condemned to death,

in 1884 by Dr. E. Arning. Keanu was a confirmed leper three years later. However, it was disclosed later that Keanu was born into a family of lepers, and the question whether he was a leper previous to his inoculation was raised. Mouritz's conclusion was that leprosy could not be inoculated on any dermal surface in man or animals (*Path of the Destroyer,* 138–156). Hansen also tried to inoculate the bacillus into an uninformed patient, again in vain, and for which he was punished by a demotion in 1880 (Li Shang-jen, "Shijiu shiji houqi," 468, n. 86). Manson also tried to cultivate the bacillus outside the human body using an egg, without success (ibid., 459).

71. Jefferys and Maxwell, *Diseases of China,* 95.

72. L. Huizenga, "Fourth International Leprosy Congress," *Leper Quarterly* 12, no. 2 (1938): 82–83.

73. Hobson, *Chinese Repository* [Canton: Printed for the proprietors, 1832–1851], vol. 11 (1842): 664.

74. Hobson, "On the Leprosy of the Chinese," 558. Hobson's observations were echoed by T. C. Wu, of the Chinese Mission to Lepers, in an address entitled "Fighting Leprosy in China" (Annual Meeting of the American Mission to Lepers, New York City, October 18, 1934), 2; there is a 1935 copy in the Shanghai Municipal Archives, U1-16-4854.

75. Jefferys and Maxwell, *Diseases of China,* 95–96. Although other missionaries observed that in some parts of China populations did not seem to dread mingling with lepers, they admitted that such behavior was contradictory to the Chinese belief in contagion (Durand-Fardel, "Le caractère le plus spécial," 403). Such observations were also made in Jiangsu province, where the local population did not seem to fear lepers as much as in the south ("Reports from the Provinces," *China Medical Journal* [1930], 795).

76. Xu Ke, *Qing bai lei chao* (*Collection of Popular Customs of the Qing*) (1917; repr., Beijing: Zhonghua shuju, 1984), 5476.

77. Wong Foon, "Dr. F. Wong's Memorandum on Leprosy," 45–46.

78. Li Shang-jen, "Shijiu shiji houqi," 464–466; Wong's account is reported in some detail in Durand-Fardel, "Le caractère le plus spécial," 404.

79. Li Shang-jen, "Shijiu shiji houqi,"464.

80. See p. 145.

81. Liu Botang and Liu Zhongru, "Mafeng zheng gailun"(A General Discussion on Leprosy), *Guangdong yiyao yuebao* 1, no. 2 (1929): 8.

82. J. Maxwell, "Ridding China of Leprosy," *China Medical Journal* 44 (1930): 760.

83. "Sihui fangjun qiangjue da bang fengji nan nü" (Army Defending Sihui Executed Male and Female Patients of Leprosy), *MFJK* 11, no. 1 (1937): 44, report on Sihui, Guangdong province. Other reports in the same journal indicated that suicides often followed rapes by lepers. The prominent literatus Zhou Zuoren (1885–1967) wrote on April 29, 1937, quoting a news clipping dated April 27, that in Guangdong province, some recommended the ex-

ecution of lepers on the model of "some Western countries that execute people of inferior races." (Zhou Zuoren, "Tan guolai" [On the Custom of Passing on *Lai*], in *Bing zhu ye tan* [*Night Talks in Front of a Lit Candle*] [Shijiazhuang: Hebei jiaoyu chubanshe, 2002], 89).

84. Chen Tongchang, magistrate of Shunde county, suggested, in January 1936, that patients should be sterilized the same way as Hitler sterilized patients of TB, syphilis, and madness in order to improve the national race. His proposal apparently obtained much support among the political elite but was not implemented due to practical difficulties and doubt about its effectiveness in stopping contagion (*Guangdong sheng zhengfu gongbao* [*Public Announcements of the Guangdong Provincial Government*], Municipal Archives of Guangzhou, zi zheng 139, no. 321, "Minzheng" [Civic Affairs] [1936], 35–38). A regulation passed in 1935 by the central government was specific on the punishment against rapists with leprosy: under some circumstances, they were punishable by death; in general they were punished more severely than rapists without the disease (*Guangdong sheng zhengfu gongbao,* Municipal Archives of Guangzhou, zi zheng 601, no. 489, "Zhongyang faling" [Central Regulations] [1935], 1–3).

85. The "lascivious" sexual relations between Chinese women and white men in Hong Kong leading to the spread of leprosy after it became a British colony constituted a popular topic also in Chinese journalism. For instance, the *Shen pao* quoted, on May 16, 1873, widespread rumors in Hong Kong of the spread of the disease by a beautiful "boat girl" (prostitute working on a boat) much visited by Western men.

Cantlie's observation of "cohabitation" in Hong Kong was in fact a general phenomenon in the British colonies in the nineteenth century. On the question of sexuality, colonialism, and race, see A. Stoler, *Carnal Knowledge and Imperial Power: Race and the Intimate in Colonial Rule* (Berkeley: University of California Press, 2002), especially 48: "Nearly half of the Indies' European male population in the 1880s were unmarried and living with Asian women." Such domestic arrangements were condemned by the religious authorities but especially by medical ones later on, as they were perceived to be a cause of degeneration or infertility.

86. Cantlie, "Report," 254–255.

87. Ibid., 309.

88. For the establishment of the mission, see the previous discussion of segregation in the present chapter.

89. Wang Yogan, chairman of the board of the Taikam leprosarium, was the author ("Zhonghua mafeng jiujihui jikan chuban congci" [Eulogy for the Publication of the Quarterly of the Chinese Mission to Lepers] *MFJK* 1, no. 1 [1927]).

90. The translator of a speech by V. G. Heiser used the title "Down with the Leprosy Devil" for the Chinese translation in the *MFJK* (1, no. 3 [1927]: 26). The term *mamo* appeared time and time again in the journal.

91. Liu Botang and Liu Zhongru, "Mafeng zheng gailun," 8–9, echoing the advice of Ming-Qing doctors, advised against any mingling with lepers. Some articles, translated from Japanese, adopted a similarly alarmist attitude as the Japanese (Nagamata Yoshirō, trans., "Mafeng" [Leprosy] *Yiyao pinglun* 84 [1932]: 19–30). A similarly alarmist attitude was taken by Li Zuwei, who recommended strict and total isolation of patients ("Laibing yange shuo lue," especially 1018–1019).

92. *Leper Quarterly* 1, no. 3 (1927): 2. The Chinese version of the editorial appeared on page 3 of the *MFJK*, the Chinese section of the issue.

93. J. Maxwell, "Leprosy in China," *Chinese Recorder* 64 (1933): 544. Another doctor, William Cadbury, of Lingnan University, estimated that there were 1 to 1.5 million lepers in China, and "one half the people of China live in areas where they are exposed to infection" ("China Mobilizes Against Leprosy," *Leper Quarterly* 11, no. 2 [1937]: 55–58).

94. J. Maxwell, "Zhongguo mafeng yu yimin wenti" (Leprosy in China and the Question of Emigration), trans. Hong Zhongdao, *MFJK* 4, no. 2 (1930): 2–4.

95. Apparently the 1897 conference did not have delegations from India and China, where medical missionaries were still skeptical about the contagion theory. The conference was initiated by "alarmists" who considered segregation and an interventionist policy of governments necessary for putting leprosy under control (S. S. Pandya, "The First International Leprosy Conference, Berlin, 1897," *História, Ciências, Saúde: Manguinhos* 10, suppl. no. 1 [2003]: 161–177).

96. Manson, *Tropical Diseases*, 642.

97. D. Arnold, *Colonizing the Body: State Medicine and Epidemic Disease in Nineteenth-Century India* (Berkeley: University of California Press, 1993), 293.

98. W. H. P. Anderson, "The World Leprosy Situation," *Chinese Medical Journal* 47 (1933): 225.

99. Jiang Cheng, "Sun zhongshan xiansheng guanxin mafeng" (Mr. Sun Yat-sen Was Concerned About Leprosy), *Manxing bing fangzhi tongxun* 2 (1985): 48, quoting an article in the *Zhonghua yixue zazhi* 28, no. 6 (1942): 209–216. Cantlie also recalled the visit with Sun in his famous 1897 report ("Report," 302).

100. John Fitzgerald quotes at length Sun's lectures of 1924 on the unhygienic behavior of his countrymen and thus the necessity to "remake" the "Chinaman" (*Awakening China: Politics, Culture, and Class in the Nationalist Revolution* [Stanford, Calif.: Stanford University Press, 1996], 9–12).

101. Ibid., 12.

102. T. C. Wu, "Wei shenme women yao jiuji mafeng" (Why Should We Provide Relief for Patients of Leprosy) *MFJK* 1, no. 3 (1927): 2. Wu was a Christian doctor and, as a child, a classmate of Chiang Kai-shek. He obtained from Chiang in 1927 the privilege of visiting a remote leper colony in the Canton area by riding on a warship in order to avoid

pirates and rebels ("Min-Yue youji" [An Account of My Tour in Fujian and Guangdong], *MFJK* 1, no. 1 [1927]: 12–14).

103. Foucault thought that the exclusion of lepers from the medieval period to the seventeenth century and the inclusion of victims of the plague thereafter were two major models of control of the individual in the West. While the former was to purify the community, the latter, the modern model, was intended to maximize health and longevity (M. Foucault, *Les anormaux: Cours au Collège de France (1974–1975)* [Paris: Gallimard/Seuil,1999]: 41–43).

104. On the concern for the improvement of the Chinese race and eugenics, see F. Dikotter, *The Discourse of Race in Modern China* (London: Hurst, 1992),167–173.

105. Whereas nineteenth-century Western medical missionaries observed that the use of chaulmoogra had been traditionally "kept secret" in China while it was used openly in missionary hospitals (W. Lockhart, *Medical Missionary in China* [London: Hurst and Blackett, 1861], 184–185).

106. A. H. Smith, "A Centennial of Protestant Missions in China," *Chinese Recorder* 38 (1907): 486.

107. Chen Yuan, "Song Zheng xueshi zhi Bai Er Gen wanguo mafeng hui xu" (Preface to Bid Bon Voyage to Bachelor Zheng, Who Is Attending the International Conference on Leprosy in Bergen), in *Chen Yuan zaonian wenji* (*Early Writings by Chen Yuan*) (1909; repr., Taipei: Academia Sinica, 1992), 300–301.

108. T. C. Wu, "Zhongguo di mafeng wenti yu benhui jinhou zhi jihua" (The Leprosy Problem in China and the Mission's Plan for the Future), *MFJK* 1, no. 2 (1927): 7.

109. Chen Yuan, "Mafeng zhongwai gujin jie you" (Leprosy Exists in All Times, in China and Elsewhere), in *Guanghua yishi weisheng zazhi* 2, quoted in Chen, "Song Zheng xueshi," 343.

110. T. C. Wu, "What the Chinese Are Doing to Rid China of Leprosy," *Chinese Recorder* 58 (1927): 257.

111. Burns, "From 'Leper Villages' to Leprosaria,'"109–110. The quote is from Sawa Riichirō in a 1902 article published in the *Kyōto iji eisei shimbun* (*Kyoto Newspaper of Medicine and Public Health*) on traditional shelters for lepers in premodern Japan.

112. J. Doolittle, *Social Life of the Chinese: With Some Account of Their Religious, Governmental, Educational, and Business Customs and Opinions; With Special but Not Exclusive Reference to Fuhchau* (New York: Harper, 1865; repr., Taipei: Cheng-wen, 1966), 2:254–257. Later readers sometimes took the asylums described to be in Tientsin, as it was the last city mentioned in the book before the passage on leprosy, but as there were no major leper asylums recorded in Tientsin, it is more likely that these were institutions in Fuzhou, where Doolittle was stationed most of the time (he was a member of the American board of the Fuzhou Mission).

113. S. Johnson, *Chinese Repository* [Canton: Printed for the proprietors, 1832–1851], vol. 16 (1847): 494.

114. Wong Foon, "Dr. F. Wong's Memorandum on Leprosy," 41, 43.

115. W. Milne, *Chinese Repository* [Canton: Printed for the proprietors, 1832–1851], vol. 2 (1832): 364, and vol. 16 (1847): 27 both mention the leper asylum at Canton, "where leprosy of a most hideous, disgusting, and incurable form has too many victims. In 1832 the number of patients in it was 341, who were supported at an expense of 300 taels per annum or 100 [English pounds]."

116. As Fitzgerald points out, these middlemen were considered feudal remnants and enemies of the new Chinese nation (*Awakening China,* 14).

117. For a brief history of the relation between China and Christianity in the nineteenth century, see P. Cohen, *China and Christianity: The Missionary Movement and the Growth of Chinese Antiforeignism, 1860–1870* (Cambridge, Mass.: Harvard University Press, 1963), especially part 2, chap. 2.

118. G. B. Souza, *The Survival of Empire: Portuguese Trade and Society in China and the South China Sea, 1630–1754* (Cambridge: Cambridge University Press, 1986), 27. According to Souza, the first Santa Casa da Misericórdia in Asia was established at Cochin in 1505, and the second at Goa in the period 1515–1518.

119. F. Guerra, *El hospital en Hispanoamérica y Filipinas, 1492–1898* (Madrid: Ministerio de Sanidad y Consumo, 1994), 580–581. I thank Li Yu-chung for providing me with this interesting source.

120. An eighteenth-century Chinese source records that this hospital accommodated foreign lepers (Yin Guangren and Zhang Rulin, *Aomen jilue* [*A Sketch of the History of Macao*] [1751; repr., Guangzhou: Guangdong gaodeng jiaoyu chubanshe, 1988], 63).

121. A recent doctoral dissertation by Dong Shaoxin, of Zhongshan University in Canton, also shows fairly active Catholic missionary activities among Chinese *mafeng/lai* patients in southeastern China in the seventeenth and early eighteenth centuries. Dong based his research on mainly Portuguese archival sources ("Xiyang chuanjiaoshi zai Hua zaoqi xingyi shiji kaoshu" [Study on the Medical Activities of Western Missionaries in China in the Early Period] [Ph.D. diss., Guangzhou Sun Yat-sen University, 2004]).

122. I make this conjecture from the two tables in the appendix and from information in Yu Shenchu, *Zhongguo mafeng bingxue* (*Study on Leprosy in China*) (Shanghai: Fuxing zhongyishe, 1941). Yu indicates that, in 1925 in Guangdong province, Shilong was one of the places where there was a leper asylum (11).

123. Guerra, *El hospital,* 582–584. There are a few descriptions of Franciscan missionaries doing evangelical work outside the city walls of Guangzhou and in another southern town in the late seventeenth century (A. van den Wyngaert, ed., *Sinica Franciscana: Relationes et Epistolas Fratrum Minorum Saeculi XVII et XVIII* [Florence: Collegium S. Bonaventurae, 1942], 4:167–168, 8:131–132). I thank Ronnie Hsia for indicating these to me.

124. Guerra, *El hospital*, 581–584. The effect of the 1732 edict was mentioned in the cases of Nangang and Chao Cheu. In fact, both emperors Kangxi and Yongzheng had published edicts prohibiting missionary activities outside the capital and Macao. Emperor Kangxi had announced such orders in 1669 and 1717; Emperor Yongzheng in 1724 and finally in 1732 (*Shengzu Ren Huangdi [Kangxi] shilu* [*Veritable Records of the Reign of Emperor Kangxi*] [Taipei: Huawen yinshuguan, 1969], 277:20b–21b; *Qingchao wenxian tongkao* [*Official Documents of the Qing Dynasty*] [1936; repr., Taipei: Shangwu yinshuguan, 1987], 298:4/6/6; *Shizong Xian Huangdi [Yongzheng] shilu* [*Veritable Records of the Reign of Emperor Yongzheng*] [Taipei: Huawen yinshuguan, 1969], 14:14a–b).

125. Notably in (Fogan) Fu'an, where a Father Garcia was reported to have visited regularly, between 1642 and 1644, a leper hospital, where he baptized a few among its residents (J. M. González, *Historia de las misiones dominicanas de China* [Madrid: Ediciones Studium, 1964], 1:172).

126. One of the two leper houses in Fu'an cared for thirteen lepers, the other served thirty-eight Christian lepers and other non-Christians before 1723 (Eugenio Menegon, pers. comm. to author, August 2001).

127. C. R. Boxer, *Dutch Merchants and Mariners in Asia, 1602–1795* (London: Variorum Reprints, 1988), 60.

128. A. J. R. Russell-Wood, *The Portuguese Empire, 1415–1808: A World on the Move* (Baltimore: Johns Hopkins University Press, 1998), 106.

129. Guerra, *El hospital*, 580–581. The lazar house in Macao continued to accommodate Chinese and European lepers in the nineteenth century, as indicated in an 1817 official document by the Chinese magistrate on the destruction of leper houses in Macao: "Because of Westerners' sense of justice and their heart of charity, lepers, handicapped, the poor and the abandoned, be they Chinese or foreign, whenever they ask to enter the hospice [would be taken in], and given means of living" (Document 14, "Aomen tongzhi Zhong Ying wei pi fu yuan bing Qianshanying youji chaihui Fafengsi shanpo fangwu shi," 1817 [To Answer the Query on the Destruction of Houses Belonging to the Leper Asylum by the Soldiers of Qianshanying, by Magistrate Zhong Ying of Aomen], in *Qingdai Aomen zhongwen dang'an huibian* [Collection of Chinese Archival Materials on Macao in the Qing Period] [Macao: Aomen jijin hui, 1999], 9).

130. L. Guiot, *La mission du Su-Tchuen au 18e siècle* (*The Mission in Sichuan Province in the Eighteenth Century*) (Paris: Téqui, 1892), 252–254.

131. For example, Pierre Foucard was said to have erected a chapel in a village for lepers where he worked in the first years of the 1860s, in a place called Si-Kiang in Guangxi province (E. Jarossay, *Une âme d'apôtre, Mgr Foucard, du diocèse d'Orléans, premier évêque de Kouang-si'(Chine), 1830–1889* [Orléans: Séjourné, 1907], 78; "Notice biographique de Foucard: Notice nécrologique de Foucard," Archives des Missions Etrangères de Paris [hereafter MEP]). Another missionary working in Guangxi, by the name of Jolly, was

found to have been infected with leprosy in 1875, indicating that he also could have been working closely with lepers in the preceding decades in Guangxi ("Nécrologie de M. Jolly," in *Comptes rendus* [MEP], 1878, 73). In fact, quite a few Catholic missionaries working in China and Indochina in the nineteenth and early twentieth centuries were infected with leprosy, and many went to the Sanatorium de Béthanie in Hong Kong for treatment and to die. Lambert Conrardy, founder of the Sheklong leprosaria in 1907, Joseph-Marie Lavest, and Louis-Eugène Louvet all worked in China and died of leprosy. See their biographies at the MEP.

132. A recent account of the history of the Mission to Lepers and its work in India is G. Joseph, "Essentially Christian, Eminently Philanthropic: The Mission to Lepers in British India," *História, Ciências, Saúde: Manguinhos* 10, suppl. no. 1 (2003): 247–275, especially 253–258. See also S. Kakar, "Medical Developments and Patient Unrest in the Leprosy Asylum, 1860–1940," in *Health, Medicine and Empire: Perspectives on Colonial India*, ed. B. Pati and M. Harrison (London: Sangam Books, 2000), 201. Huizenga gave an account of Bailey's setting up the mission and his emphasis on evangelical work in leper asylums ("Wellesley C. Bailey—An Appreciation—1846–1937," *Leper Quarterly* 12, no. 1 [1938]: 2–5).

133. Kakar, "Leprosy in British India," 215.

134. "Editorial," *Chinese Recorder* 48 (1917): 690; M. W. Danner, "The Mission to Lepers," *Chinese Recorder* 49 (1918): 110; Gussow, *Leprosy, Racism, and Public Health*, 146. On Carville, see M. Gaudet, *Carville: Remembering Leprosy in America* (Jackson: University Press of Mississippi, 2004). On the development of the Mission in the twentieth century, see Leprosy Mission, *This Spreading Tree: The Story of the Leprosy Mission from 1918 to 1970* (London: Leprosy Mission, 1974).

135. Including its president, Li Yuanxin (William Yinson Lee), general secretary Rev. T. C. Wu , vice presidents Kuang Fuzhuo (Fong F. See) and Diao Xinde (F. S. Tyau), and its vice president Wu Liande.

136. C. M. Wong and L. T. Wu, *History of Chinese Medicine* (1932; repr., Taipei: Southern Materials Center, 1985), 666, quoting the *China Medical Journal* (1930), 746.

137. There is a first list, by Dr. J. L Maxwell, established in 1935 (quoted by Wong and Wu, *History of Chinese Medicine*, 759–761), according to which there were a total of twenty-three leprosaria. According to Maxwell, the earliest ones were set up in 1887, in Pakhoi (Beihai, Guangdong province) by the Church Missionary Society, and in Hangzhou by Duncan Main of the International Mission to Lepers. A more complete list published by the *Leper Quarterly* (March 1940) and quoted in the *Chinese Recorder* (71 [1940]: 465–471) records fifty-one leprosaria and clinics in China. The earliest ones were, according to this list, also considered to be the one at Beihai and that at Hangzhou, though the year of establishment is recorded as one year earlier than that in the Maxwell list.

138. The Catholic leper colony in Moximian in Kangding (present-day Ganzi in Sichuan province), established in 1930, for instance, was not recorded. From 1930 to 1951, this

asylum accommodated 921 patients (Xiong Dongliang [director of the asylum], "Tianzhujiao Kangding jiaoqu Moximian mafeng yuan shilue ji qi jiefang hou jianzhi yange" [The History of the Leper Asylum in Moximian of the Kangding Diocese and Its Reforms After the Liberation], unpublished document, June 1995).

139. Wong and Wu, *History of Chinese Medicine,* 499.

140. Shen Yongnian, "Puren yiyuan fushe zhi mafeng yuan xuanyan" (Manifesto of the Xuanren Leper House), *MFJK* 2, no. 2 (1928): 17–19; T. C. Wu, "Ershi-wu nian lai zhi jiuji mafeng yundong" (Movement to Save Lepers During the Past Twenty-five Years), *MFJK* 1, no. 4 (1927): 4.

141. H. Fowler, "Medical and Construction Page," *Leper Quarterly* 1, no. 3 (1927): 19.

142. On the evangelical uses of segregation of lepers, see, with particular reference to Sumatra, R. Kipp, "The Evangelical Uses of Leprosy," *Social Science and Medicine* 39, no. 2 (1944):165–178.

143. *CMMJ* 8, no. 4 (1894): 212; *Chinese Recorder* 47 (1916): 133–135; *Chinese Recorder* 35 (1904): 41.

144. Joseph, "Essentially Christian"; Dr. William Gauld, who established the Swatow leper asylum, also believed the disease to be "incurable by remedies at command." But missionaries greatly treasured the "value of the hospital as an evangelistic agency" (*Chinese Recorder* 1 [1868]: 74–75; E. Band, *Working His Purpose Out: The History of the English Presbyterian Mission, 1847–1947* [1947; repr., Taipei: Ch'eng Wen, 1972], 204). P. B. Cousland, from India, made the same observation on the Swatow institution in 1894, that it should alleviate suffering and bring "the comforts of the gospel to these sad-hearted and despairing ones" ("Leprosy in China," *CMMJ* 1 [1892]: 8).

Records of medical treatment or experiments on lepers by missionaries in this period often show uncertainty and frustration. Dr. Douthwaite, working in Shandong province, tried creolin on his patients. "Unfortuantely, most of the lepers who come to me are from distant parts of the province, and are too poor to pay even the 70 cash a day charged for their food. . . . I am compelled to send them away" ("Leprosy," *CMMJ* 1 [1891]: 24). Another doctor, by the name of Razlag, of Vienna University, also tested his treatment on four inmates from a Cantonese asylum for several months. Even though the patients claimed they felt better, the complicated and costly treatment, involving regular medical baths, did not seem to be maintained after this doctor left China at the end of the experiment (J. M. Swan, "Treatment of Leprosy as Conducted by Dr. Adolph Razlag, of Vienna University, in Canton," *CMMJ* 4 [1902]: 159–162).

145. On the problem of the Hangzhou asylum, see the following section of the present chapter. The local authorities of Kangding in 1944 accused the Moximian asylum of not strictly keeping its inmates inside (Xiong, "Tianzhujiao Kangding," 9).

146. *Missions Catholiques* (MEP), 1913, 49–50.

147. Wong and Wu, *History of Chinese Medicine,* 423; "A Report of My Trip to South

China," *Leper Quarterly* 1, no. 14 (1927): 13–14. Inmates received weekly injections of gynocardia oil, probably esters of chaulmoogra and other oils commonly used at this time to relieve suffering of the patients. The official of public health of the Swatow municipality, Lin Zuze, stated in 1928 that the Swatow government had the intention of enlarging the institution by increasing local taxes and by making inmates take part in production ("Shantou shi shili mafeng yiyuan lueli ji jianglai" [Brief History of the Municipal Leprosarium of Swatow and Its Future], *MFJK* 2, no. 1 [1928]: 7–11).

148. "The Hangchow Leper Hospital After Being Nationalized," *Leper Quarterly* 1, no. 3 (1927): 26; "The Nationalization of Hangchow Leper Hospital: The Hangchow Leper Hospital of the Church Missionary Society Was Taken Over by the Provincial Government of Chekiang in March 1927," *Chinese Recorder* 58 (1927): 810–811.

149. Phyllis Haddow's report on "Hangchow," in "Reports from the Provinces," *China Medical Journal* 44 (1930): 789–792.

150. S. D. Sturton, "The Problem of Leprosy in Hangchow," *Chinese Medical Journal* 47 (1933): 263–264.

151. Ibid., 265–266.

152. *Annales de la Société des Missionnaires Étrangères (AME)* (MEP), 1928, 134, n. 182.

153. *Missions Catholiques* (MEP), 1915, 84.

154. *Comptes rendus* (MEP), 1910, 134.

155. Lagarde, "Lettre de M. Lagarde, conseiller de la Légation de France en Chine, à M. Wilden, ministre, Canton, le 17 juillet, 1932 , sur la léproserie de Chéklong" (Letter from Mr. Lagarde, Adviser of the French Embassy in China, to Mr. Wilden, Minister in Canton, on the Leprosarium in Sheklong, July 17, 1932), Archives du Ministère des Affaires Étrangères, France, série SND, vol. 1583:116.

156. T. C. Wu, "Min-Yue you ji" (An Account of My Tour in Fujian and Guangdong), *MFJK* 1, no. 1 (1927): 15–16; T. C. Wu, "Hua'nan ji Feilibin you ji" (An Account of My Tour in Southern China and the Philippines), *MFJK* 4, no. 2 (1930): 26. According to the Catholic fathers running the colony, this sum was trivial, as it was but about one-twentieth of the budget of the American Molokai colony (*Annales de la Société des Missionnaires Étrangères* [MEP], 1926, 8).

157. *Comptes rendus* (MEP), 1913, 170–171. Until 1950, the Hong Kong government routinely ordered all Chinese immigrants into the colony found to have leprosy to be repatriated to China, and Sheklong was the main place where they were shipped (Mission to Lepers Hong Kong Auxiliary, *Annual Report* [London: Mission to Lepers, 1951], 3).

158. *Annales de la Société des Missionnaires Étrangères* (MEP), 1926, 7.

159. The exact figure was 888 (*Bulletin des Missions Étrangères de Paris [BME]*, vol. 19 [1940]: 389).

160. The deterioration of the political situation in Canton consisted of Chen Jiongming's revolt against Sun Yat-sen and the rising leftist movements in the region. Gustave

Deswazière claimed, in 1932, that the Chinese government owed the colony a total of $150 million (probably Chinese yuan) (Lagarde, "Lettre de M. Lagarde," 115).

161. After the death of Father Conrardy, whose loyalty to France had been questioned, it was possible again for the French Catholic Church to build a dream leprosarium on the Molokai model in Sheklong. In this connection, the colony obtained, in 1921, the prix Buisson, of the Académie française, of 2,000 francs (*Annales de la Société des Missionnaires Étrangères* [MEP], 1921, 197). However, the French Foreign Ministry was reluctant to support Deswazières in his request of retrieving the money owed the colony by the Canton government in the 1920s. It also decided not to give a big subsidy ($10,000) to the colony for the renovation of buildings on the islands, as priority was being given to other projects in China (Lagarde, "Lettre de M. Lagarde," 112).

162. T. C. Wu, "Min-Yue you ji," 16.

163. Lin Bingliang, "Ji Shilong Guowuzhou mafeng yuan shimuo" (The History of the Leper Asylum at Guowuzhou of Shilong), *Guangdong wenshi ziliao* 57 (1988): 145–147. Lin was in fact one of the Chinese Catholic fathers stationed at the asylum, from 1943 until 1946 (*Annales de la Société des Missionnaires Étrangères* [MEP], 1928, 137–138).

164. The missionaries jeered that it was a mere one-twentieth of what the Molokai managers got from the U.S. government, all else being equal. Moreover, they had, at one point, to turn away some of the patients that came to them for help (*Annales de la Société des Missionnaires Étrangères* [MEP], 1926, 8; 1928, 135–136).

165. Lin Bingliang, "Ji Shilong Guowuzhou," 146; Lagarde, "Lettre de M. Lagarde," 113.

166. The subsidies apparently became regular again in the 1930s (Lagarde, "Lettre de M. Lagarde," 113–116).

167. This arrangement was pointed out by James Maxwell in 1928 ("The Cure of Leprosy in China," *Leper Quarterly* 2, no. 2 [1928]: 8).

168. The establishment of the leprosarium, probably inspired by the American example at Carville, attracted a great deal of publicity. From the start, the mission again pressed the national government to contribute more to the institution ("The First Annual Report of the National Leprosarium of Shanghai for the Year 1936," Shanghai Municipal Archives, no. U1-16-4853).

On the request of donations for poor patients, see the 1936 report and documents sent to the Shanghai Municipal Council, U1-16-759(1).

169. The Shanghai Municipal Archives contains a letter dated June 1945 and signed by T. C. Wu begging the city government for money to finance the institution (U1-16-753).

170. Weisheng bu (Ministry of Health), "Fangyi" (Disease Prevention) (Taipei: Guoshi guan [Academia Historica]), 112/4:0873, 6199, May 27, 1947; 112/4:11325–11326, June 24, 1948; 112/4:8993, May 15, 1948. Documents in the Yunnan Provincial Archives also reveal similar information on the Kunming asylum (21-3-199, June 20, 1947) and a few other leper colonies in the province, such as in Zhaotong county, where the Catholic asy-

lum signed an agreement with the local government on January 1, 1948, for cooperation in running the asylum (21-3-200).

171. Qingdao Municipal Archives, 28-1-733, November 4, 1946.

172. Jefferys and Maxwell, *Diseases of China,* 102–103.

173. Maxwell published frequently on these questions from 1928 onward and until the outbreak of the Sino-Japanese War in 1937 ("Leprosy: The Problem of Its Eradication from China," *China Medical Journal* 42 [1928]: 869–879; "The Cure of Leprosy in China," *Leper Quarterly* 2, no. 2 [1928]: 1–11; "Two Divergent Views on Segregation of Lepers: Gushe-Taylor and Maxwell," *Leper Quarterly* 3, nos. 2–3:36–41; "The Outlook for China," *Leper Quarterly* 2, no. 4 [1928]: 3–6; "The Leprosy Problem in China" [with Wu Lien-teh], *Leper Quarterly* 4, no. 4 [1930]: 4–12; "Leprosy in India," "Ridding China of Leprosy," *China Medical Journal* 44 [1930]: 37–45, 759–767; "The Public Health Problem of Leprosy and Its Solution," *Leper Quarterly* 12, no. 4 [1938]: 156–164).

174. F. Reiss, "Leprosy," *China Medical Journal* 43 (1929): 479–484. An article by F. Muir, who had worked in India supporting the position of loosening segregation, was translated into Chinese and published in the *MFJK* ("Yizhi mafeng di xin jian" [New Views on Treating Leprosy], *MFJK* 1, no. 3 [1927]: 31–34). C. M. Galt, who was responsible for the Kiulungkiang (Jiulongjiang) colony in Yunnan, loosened the rules of segregation, allowing patients to go home for short visits and married couples to live together, in the hope that more patients would be willing to come for treatment ("Kiulungkiang Leper Colony," *Chinese Medical Journal* 47 [1933]: 284–286).

175. C. M. Hasselmann, "Problems of Segregation and Care for the Arrested, Negative Cases of Leprosy," *Chinese Medical Journal* 47 (1933): 270–282.

176. H. W. Wade, "Segregation in the Antileprosy in the Philippines," *Leper Quarterly* 3, no. 4 (1929): 28–32; *China Medical Journal* 45 (1931): 870–872.

177. G. Gushue-Taylor, "Segregation of Lepers: Mackay Memorial Hospital, Taihoku, Formosa," *China Medical Journal* 43 (1929): 312; G. Gushue-Taylor and J. Maxwell, "The Divergent Views on Segregation of Lepers," *Leper Quarterly* 2, no. 3 (1929): 36–39.

178. G. Gushue-Taylor, "Leprosy in Formosa," *China Medical Journal* 43 (1929): 6–12. By that time, Gushue-Taylor had obtained from the Japanese colonial government on Formosa permission to build a colony for 200 inmates in Taipei that would be called Happy Mount Leper Colony. See also C. Roland, "George Gushue-Taylor and the Medical Missions of Formosa," *Journal of Medical Biography* 4, no. 2 (1996), especially 87–89, on leprosy. For a brief history of this leper asylum on Formosa, see Wang Wenji, "Laibing yuan li de yixiangren" (Strangers in the Leprosy Colony), *Gujin lunheng* (*Disquisitions on the Past and Present*), 116–124 (Taipei: Academia Sinica, 2003). See also Lai Shanghe, *Zhongguo laibing shi* (*The History of the* Lai *Disease in China*) (Taipei, 1952), 37–38; Lai was an important leprologist in Taiwan.

179. T. C. Wu, "Fighting Leprosy in China."

180. Wu announced, in the *Leper Quarterly,* that he would visit Culion, "that world-famous leprosarium, with a view to making a first hand study of its management and treatment for the benefit of the leper work in this country" (3, no. 4 [1929]: 36). After his return, an entire issue of the quarterly was devoted to the Culion colony, describing it as an example to the world of how leprosy should be treated. Wu wrote in that issue, "The high percentage of cure in Culion is, to my mind, the most hopeful thing for the whole movement—ridding the world of leprosy" (*Leper Quarterly* 4, no. 1 [1930]: 7).

181. Wu stated that "China is doing the least in tackling the problem of leprosy in comparison with the rest of the civilized world" (*Leper Quarterly* 2, no. 3 [1928]: 3).

182. T. C. Wu, "What I Hope the Nationalist Government Would Do Towards the Problem of Leprosy," *Leper Quarterly* 2, no. 3 (1928): 3. Wu's view was representative of the Chinese Mission to Lepers in the 1920s and 1930s. Jonas Lee, another activist, wrote along the same lines, urging the central government to set up more asylums (J. Lee, "The Elimination of Leprosy," *Leper Quarterly* 2, no. 3 [1928]: 19).

183. J. Maxwell, "The Public Health Problem of Leprosy and Its Solution," *Leper Quarterly* 12, no. 4 (1938): 160–164.

184. "The First National Conference on Leprosy," *Chinese Medical Journal* 47 (1933): 297–306.

185. Burns, "From 'Leper Villages' to 'Leprosaria,'" 114. On Formosa, the colonial asylum in Taipei set up its first regulations in 1931, and in 1934 a law regulating the disease was applied in the whole of Formosa that was abrogated only in 1949, after the Kuomintang takeover of Taiwan. See Lai, *Zhongguo laibing shi,* 88. Similar laws were passed in this period in Australia, where nearly all people with leprosy were removed and detained, sometimes for their whole life. Such measures were loosened only in the 1950s (Bashford, *Imperial Hygiene,* 98, 103).

5. LEPROSY IN THE PRC

1. Professor Li Bozhong, of the History Department of Tsinghua University, Beijing, told me of an episode in Yunnan that he witnessed in the 1970s: a powerful, high cadre much feared by the population, as soon as he was diagnosed with leprosy, fled with his family to the nearest leper village, for fear of being burned to death by villagers. Such treatment was apparently still common in Yunnan (pers. comm. to author, August 27, 2005).

2. O. Skinsnes, "Leprosy in Society," *Leprosy Review* 35 (1964): 21–35.

3. Jiang Cheng, "Zhongguo mafeng fangzhi wushi nian hui mou" (Looking Back on the Half Century of Leprosy Control in China), *Zhongguo mafeng pifu bing zazhi* 15, no. 3 (1999): 85. The figure can be broken down to fifty-two hospitals and 117 leper villages established between 1949 and 1956, plus 157 outpatient clinics, which were mostly mobile

units that toured rural villages with segregated leprosy patients (Chen Xianyi, Li Wenzhong, Chen Jiakun, eds., *Mafeng bing fangzhi shouce* [*Handbook for the Prevention and Treatment of Leprosy*] [Beijing: Kexue chubanshe 2002], 6).

4. Hatem's Chinese name, Ma Haide, was a household name in China. He was a member of the Communist Party of China and remained in China until his death. He gave the number of 500,000 in 1980 (*Renmin ribao,* February 1, 1980, 24, and January 28, 1991, 3). WHO stated in a report published in 2003 that in 1950 there were an estimated 500,000 cases of leprosy (WHO Regional Office for the Western Pacific, *Overview and Epidemiological Review of Leprosy in the WHO Western Pacific Region, 1991–2001* [Manila, 2003], 28).

You Jiajun, a prominent expert and activist in the 1950s in China, even claimed, in 1953, a number of 1 million, but his estimate was done before any systematic survey had been taken (You Jiajun, *Mafeng bingxue gailun* [*General Discussion on Leprosy*] [Shanghai: Huadong yiwu shenghuo she, 1953], 20).

5. This public announcement was apparently a result of the first professional meeting on the prevention and cure of leprosy, organized by the Ministry of Health, in Jinan, Shandong province, earlier in that year (Jiang Cheng, "Zhongguo mafeng fangzhi," 85).

6. You Jiajun, "Wunian lai mafeng fangzhi gongzuo di fazhang" (Growth of the Work on Leprosy Control During the Past Five Years), *Zhonghua pifu ke zazhi* 4, no. 1 (1956): 9. You, in this article, contested the figure of 1 million that he had given three years previously in his book on leprosy, saying that the figure had been made up by foreign missionaries to give China a bad name. The national figure he gave in this article was a low 280,000, which simply does not match some of the provincial figures he provided. If Guangdong was found to have more than 140,000, and Shandong more than 37,000, the national figure should be higher.

7. Jiangsu Provincial Archives, doc. nos. 3119-2-214 (October 20, 1956), 3119-3-125 (1955), 3119-3-391 (November 20, 1957). There are some differences in the figures: the *Fujian sheng weisheng zhi* (*Gazetteer on Public Health in Fujian Province*) (Fuzhou: Fujian sheng weisheng zhi bianzhuan weiyuanhui, 1989) recorded 10,029 new patients identified in 1959 in the province, with a morbidity of 0.64 (211).

8. *Guangxi tongzhi: Yiliao weisheng zhi* (*General History of Guangxi Province: On Medicine and Public Health*) (Nanning: Guangxi renmin chubanshe, 1999), 138.

9. There was a cumulative number of 14,872 patients in Hunan from 1952 to 1985; 17,232 in Jiangxi between the 1950s and 1992; and 13,746 in Hubei between 1949 and 1986 (*Hunan sheng zhi: Yiyao weisheng zhi* [*Gazetteer on Medicine and Public Health of Hunan Province*] [Changsha: Hunan renmin chubanshe, 1988], *juan* 21:183; *Jiangxi sheng zhi: Jiangxi sheng weisheng zhi* [*Gazetteer of Public Health of Jiangxi Province*] [Hefei: Huangshan shushe, 1997]: 183; *Hubei sheng zhi: Weisheng zhi xia* [*Gazetteer of Hubei Province: On Public Health*] [Wuhan: Hubei renmin chubanshe, 2000], 408).

10. This distribution of leprosy is presented in You, *Mafeng bingxue gailun,* 24–25.

11. WHO, *Overview,* 28.

12. The definition of elimination of leprosy from a country, established by WHO, is that at least 95 percent of the country should have a morbidity below 0.1 per 10,000 (*Renmin ribao,* January 27, 1987, 3; *Renmin ribao,* February 16, 1988, 3). In fact, in 1981 the PRC set the goal of eliminating leprosy by the end of the twentieth century, and by 1988, experts believed that this could be achieved by 1997 (Jiang Cheng, "Zhongguo mafeng fangzhi," 86).

13. X. Chen, W. Li, C. Jiang, and G. Ye, "Leprosy in China: Epidemiological Trends between 1949 and 1998," *Bulletin of the WHO* 79, no. 4 (2001): 306.

14. Jiang Cheng, "Zhongguo mafeng fangzhi," 85–86.

15. The drugs that You wanted to reproduce in China were the Swiss T.B.A. and German tebethion (You, "Wunian lai," 9).

16. Xinhua Agency, "Guoying zhiyaochang jihua zengchan shiji zhong yaowu" (National Drug Companies Plan to Increase the Production of a Dozen Drugs). Besides leprosy, diseases targeted were schistosomiasis, kala-azar, malaria, and filariasis (*Renmin ribao,* January 13, 1956, 2). The first issue, in 1956, of the medical journal *Zhonghua pifu ke zazhi* (*Chinese Journal of Dermatology*) was devoted entirely to discussions of Western treatment approaches to leprosy. Such doctors as You Jiajun, Liu Muzhi, and dermatologists in Shandong and Qinghai provinces published some thirty articles on the treatment of patients in China using Western drugs, in particular DDS (diaminodiphenylsulfone) and thiacetazone, produced nationally and used experimentally in major hospitals treating leprosy

17. WHO, *Overview,* 28. The national decision was made in a meeting at Chengdu in November 1986 (*Mafeng bing fangzhi shouce,* 7).

18. In PRC propaganda, leprosy and VD were often put together as targeted diseases. The belief that leprosy was transmitted sexually and its external symptoms similar to those of syphilis probably explains their being targeted together. He Biao, vice minister of health in the late 1950s, wrote an article on the combat of VD and leprosy in 1959 (He Biao, "Jixu guzhu ganjing wei quan jian xing bing, kongzhi mafeng er douzheng" [Continue to Strive in Order to Eliminate Venereal Disease, and to Control Leprosy], *Renmin baojian* 3 [1959]: 199–210).

Common targeted diseases included chronic and acute infectious diseases such as cholera, plague, smallpox, TB, leprosy, VD; parasitic diseases such as schistosomiasis, kala-azar (leischmaniasis), filariasis; and endemic diseases such as malaria, goiter, Keshan disease (*Dangdai Zhongguo di weisheng shiye* [*Enterprises of Public Health in Contemporary China*] [Beijing: Zhongguo shehui kexue, 1986], 1:2). There were local variations in the number and types of targeted diseases: in Sanshui, Guangdong province, the three diseases of interest in 1959 were leprosy, VD, and favus of the scalp (*Sanshui xian weisheng zhi* [*Gazetteer on Public Health in Sanshui*] [Sanshui: Sanshui xian weisheng ju xiuzhi bangongshi, 1989], 288–291); in Jiangsu province, schistosomiasis, filariasis, hookworm, kala-azar, and leprosy were targeted in 1955 (Jiangsu Provincial Archives, doc. no. 3119-3-381 [November 20, 1957]); in Nanning, Guangxi, the so-called seven diseases were VD, TB, leprosy, malaria, hookworm, filariasis, and trachoma in 1958 (*Nanning shi weisheng zhi* [*Gazetteer on Public Health in Nanning City*] [Nanning: Nanning shi weisheng ju, 1996], 71 [internal document]).

19. Jiangsu province, for instance, sent two doctors as trainees at the beginning of the course. Between 1951 and 1983, the province sent thirty-four sets of medical trainees for leprosy in various training programs, with a total of seventy specialists. By 1956, the province's Taizhou Hospital was able to provide a first training class (*Jiangsu sheng zhi weisheng zhi* [*Gazetteer of Jiangsu Province: On Public Health*] [Nanjing: Jiangsu guji chubanshe, 1999], 320). See also "Quan guo mafeng bing fangzhi guihua" (National Plan for Leprosy Control), 1957, in Zhejiang Provincial Archives, doc. no. 101-6-80: 6.

20. According to You Jiajun, training classes were held not only in the capital but also in different provinces, including Shandong, Gansu, Xinjiang, Hubei, Jiangxi, Fujian, and Guangdong, between 1950 and 1956, and trained personnel would carry out prevention and treatment in their own provinces. There were altogether seven training courses organized by the ministry for experts, which had created a core of more than 200 leprologists, who in turn trained almost 85,000 local workers during the thirty-five years following 1951 (Yang Lihe, "Zhongguo mafeng fangzhi sanshiwu nian ji jianwang" [Thirty-five Years of Leprosy Control in China and Future Prospects], *Zhongguo mafeng zazhi* 2, no. 1 [1986]: 13–14).

21. According to Jiang Cheng, there were at all times around 10,000 specialists throughout the country in the first decades of leprosy control (e-mail message to author, February 22, 2005).

22. A copy of a circular from the ministry, of October 27, 1952, is kept in the Zhejiang Provincial Archives (doc. no. J176-1-32). In 1955, Zhejiang claimed a serious lack of personnel, including cadres, for its leprosy hospitals and clinics, in particular the Hangzhou hospital, one of the most important of the time (Zhejiang Provincial Archives, doc. nos. J176-1-257, J176-1-258).

23. Jiang Cheng, "Zhongguo mafeng fangzhi," 85.

24. The central directive of 1957 specified that, except for a few provinces like Jilin and Liaoning, where cases of leprosy were few and where all contagious patients could be concentrated in leprosy hospitals, other provinces were to establish leper villages to immediately segregate patients (*Quanguo mafeng bing fangzhi guihua* [*National Plan for Leprosy Control*], 1957, Zhejiang Provincial Archives, doc. no. 101-6-80).

25. In Guangdong, Shaoguan district had set up a committee on leprosy control as early as 1956, before the announcement of the national plan (Jiang Cheng, "Zhongguo mafeng fangzhi," 85; Huang Huakai, "Shaoguan mafeng fangzhi shi ji" [On the History

of Leprosy Control in Shaoguan], in *Shaoguan wenxian ziliao* [*Historical Materials on Shaoguan*], nos. 1–2 [1983]: 60–61, 131).

26. *Quanguo mafeng bing fangzhi guihua,* Zhejiang Provincial Archives, doc. no. 101-6-80:11.

27. Jiang Cheng, "Zhongguo mafeng fangzhi," 85–86.

28. Jiang Cheng, pers. comm. to author, August 2005.

29. *Guangxi tongzhi,* 138.

30. In Hubei in the 1960s and 1970s, the amount was from seven to nine yuan, plus half of the amount as medical aid. In Gansu, the stipend was fifteen yuan in the 1970s. In Wuxian, Jiangsu province, hospitalized patients received six yuan a month in 1976 (*Wuxian weisheng zhi* [*Materials on Public Health in Wuxian*] [Shanghai: Shanghai shehui kexue yuan chubanshe, 1992], 101).

31. *Kaiping xian weisheng zhi, 1885–1985* (*Materials on Public Health in Kaiping, 1885–1985*), 1988, 266.

32. Ibid., 266.

33. *Sanshui xian weisheng zhi,* 288–291.

34. Patients in Hubei received thirteen to twenty-five yuan in the 1980s; those in Gansu, fifteen to twenty yuan; in Nantong, Jiangsu province, twenty yuan was given monthly to each of the sixty-five inmates of the "leper village for the elderly and crippled" (*mafeng bing ren can lao cun*), one-fifth (four yuan) of which was provided by the district financial bureau, three-fifths (twelve yuan) from the civil affair bureau, and one-fifth (four yuan) from the production team (*Nantong xian weisheng zhi* [*Materials on Public Health in Nantong*], 1988, 117–118).

35. *Kaiping xian weisheng zhi,* 266.

36. In Guangxi province, for instance, from 1956 to 1985, seventeen such courses were organized, producing 718 specialized workers, out of whom some 300 were medical experts (*Guangxi tongzhi,* 138–139).

37. *Anhui sheng zhi weisheng zhi* (*Gazetteer of Anhui Province: On Public Health*) (Hefei: Anhui renmin chubanshe, 1996), 53.

38. Zeng Huichou,"Wo wanquan tongyi dongyuan rucun buyao kuada xuanchuan" (I Totally Agree That We Should Not Exaggerate the Propaganda to Mobilize Patients to Enter [Leper] Villages), *Mafeng bing fangzhi jianbao* 2, no. 3 (1958): 73. The report was written in Haifeng, Guangdong province.

39. "Weisheng gongzuo dayaojin quanmin juban mafeng cun" (Great Leap Forward in Public Health: The Entire People Organize Leper Villages), *Mafeng bing fangzhi jianbao* (*Bulletin of Leprosy Control*) 9–10 (1958): 7–10, especially 8–9. The report came from Shandong province.

40. In Gansu province, for instance, despite the early efforts to set up hospitals and villages in 1953, many leper villages were abandoned or forced to regroup into fewer units

as early as 1960 as a result of the lack of funding, and some of the more important hospitals also underwent reduction of personnel in the 1970s (*Gansu sheng zhi* [*Gazetteer of Gansu Province*], vol. 67, *Yiyao weisheng zhi* [*On Medicine and Public Health*] [Lanzhou: Gansu wenhua chubanshe, 1999], 465–467). Though Gansu may not be a representative case, it at least reveals the general problem of this unpopular yet "necessary" social measure to isolate patients of leprosy.

41. Jiangsu Provincial Archives, doc. no. C36-1-39 (March 17, 1966).

42. M. Rosenthal, *Health Care in the People's Republic of China: Moving toward Modernization* (Boulder, Colo.: Westview Press, 1987), 79–81; S. Rifkin, "Health Care for Rural Areas," in *Medicine and Public Health in the People's Republic of China,* ed. J. Quinn (Washington, D.C.: U.S. Department of Health, Education, and Welfare, National Institutes of Health, 1973), 143–150.

43. Leading experts in leprosy control in China reported that, over the period 1981–1998, less than 1 percent of all registered cases were not treated (Chen, Li, Jiang, and Ye, "Leprosy in China," 309).

44. Chen Yongfa, *Zhongguo gongchandang geming qishi nian* (*Seventy Years of Revolution of the Chinese Communist Party*) (Taipei: Lianjing chubanshe, 1998), 552.

45. Li Wenzhong, ed., *Xiandai mafeng bing xue* (*Modern Leprology*) (Shanghai: Shanghai kexue chubanshe, 2006), 13. In Guangxi province, where missionary institutions were widespread before 1949, a Christian leprosy asylum at Suilu was taken over by the provincial authorities in 1951, the same time as the takeover of the famous Beihai (Pakhoi) asylum, established by French missionaries. It is recorded that, after the takeover, inmates of the two institutions were each given a monthly stipend of four yuan (*Guangxi tongzhi,* 138).

Yunnan is another province where missionary activities had been widespread. It is reported that all foreign missionaries left in 1952, leaving behind in leprosy clinics only one microscope, a few pairs of tweezers, a dozen injection needles, a small amount of chaulmoogra compounds, and some dozen doses of other ordinary medicines (*Kunming weisheng zhi* [*Gazetteer of Public Health of Kunming*] [Kunming: Yunnan renmin chubanshe, 1998], 262).

In northern China, the famous Qilu leprosy hospital had been established by British missionaries and was taken over by the Shandong provincial authorities as early as 1950 (*Zhongguo yiyuan daquan: Shandong fence* [*Volume on Shandong Province of the Encyclopedia of Hospitals in China*] [Beijing: Guangming Ribao chubanshe, 1989], 44).

46. Guangdong sheng weisheng ting manxing bing fangzhi chu (Chronic Disease Control Unit of the Public Health Department of Guangdong Province), "Guangdong mafeng fangzhi shinian licheng, 1951–1962" (Ten Years of Leprosy Control in Guangdong Province), *Pifu xing bing fangzhi tongxun* 2, no. 2 (1963): 1.

47. Jiang Cheng, pers. comm. to author, August 2005.

48. R. Rogaski, "Nature, Annihilation, and Modernity: China's Korean War Germ-Warfare Experience Reconsidered," *Journal of Asian Studies* 61, no. 2 (2002): 381–415, especially 382.

49. From 1953 to late 1956, almost all peasants were involved in various levels of collective rural production units, from mutual aid teams to communes (Chen Yongfa, *Zhongguo gongchandang,* 590–603).

50. *Dangdai Zhongguo di weisheng shiye,* 1:59.

51. The 1957 plan is kept in many provincial archives, for example Zhejiang Provincial Archives, doc. no. 101-6-80; Jiangsu Provincial Archives, doc. no. 3119-2-277.

52. M. Durand-Fardel, "Pathologie médicale: La lèpre en Chine," *Gazette médicale de Paris* 26 (1877): 318.

53. J. Cantlie, "Report on the Conditions under Which Leprosy Occurs in China, Indo-China, Malaya, the Archipelago, and Oceana: Compiled Chiefly during 1894," in *Prize Essays on Leprosy* (London: New Sydenham Society, 1897), 301.

54. Li Junchang strongly advocated for this kind of institution in China to uplift the spiritual life of Chinese sufferers of leprosy (Li Junchang, "Zhongguo di mafeng wenti" [The Leprosy Problem in China], *MFJK* 1, no. 3 [1927]: 9).

55. *Xiandai mafeng bing xue,* 14; Jiang Cheng, e-mail message to the author, February 22, 2005.

56. The hierarchy is clear at the top and bottom, where urban elites and the rural population are respectively concerned. The middle category of district clinics and stations are not always clearly defined. It is even said that villages can also be organized on the district level (*Dangdai Zhongguo di weisheng shiye,* 409). There are probably variations in the middle category for different provinces. For Jiangxi province, for instance, leper villages are organized by district governments, whereas rural commune production teams accommodate local rural patients (*Jiangxi sheng zhi,* 183).

57. *Zhejiang sheng weisheng ting guangyu kaizhan mafengbing fangzhi gongzuo di zhishi* (*Directive of the Promulgation of Leprosy Control Given by the Bureau of Health of Zhejiang Province*), Zhejiang Provincial Archives, doc. no. 31-5-4 (November 8, 1957), 188–191. Another official document of the Bureau of Health of the province indicated that there were two provincial leprosy hospitals, one, Zhejiang No. 1 Leprosy Hospital, had been established by the provincial government, and the other, Guangji Hospital, had been taken over from the British missionaries and renamed Zhejiang No. 2 Leprosy Hospital. The former took in military patients, and the latter mainly cadres (Zhejiang Provincial Archives, doc. no. J176-1-46 [January 25, 1954]).

58. *Kaiping xian weisheng zhi,* 261; *Jieyang xian weisheng zhi* (*Materials on Public Health in Jieyang*) (Guangzhou: Guangdong renmin chubanshe, 1992), 222–224; *Sanshui xian weisheng zhi,* 288.

59. "Guangdong mafeng fangzhi shinian licheng," 3.

60. *Fujian sheng weisheng zhi,* 209–210.

61. He, "Jixu guzhu ganjing," 199–201.

62. *Fujian sheng weisheng zhi,* 209.

63. "Guangdong mafeng fangzhi shinian licheng," 6.

64. Jiangsu Provincial Archives, doc. no. 3119-3-214; Zhejiang Provincial Archives, doc. no. 31-5-4. In Hubei the natural separation of sufferers and the healthy was emphasized; the authorities literally forbade the mixing of the two (*Hubei sheng zhi: Weisheng zhi xia* [*Gazetteer of Hubei Province, 2: On Public Health*] [Wuhan: Hubei renmin chubanshe, 2000], 408).

65. *Dangdai Zhongguo di weisheng shiye,* 409.

66. *Anhui sheng zhi,* 54.

67. Zhejiang Provincial Archives, doc. no. 31-5-4.

68. "Luoding xian gongshe ban mafeng cun di shijian" (Experience of the Organization of the Leper Village of the Luoding Commune), *Xing bing mafeng fangyan gongzuo* 4 (1959): 31–32.

69. "Huiyang bailu cun yijiu wuba nian gongzuo gaikuang" (The Work of Bailu Village in Huiyang County), *Mafeng bing fangzhi jianbao* 9–10 (1958): 10–17, especially 10–11.

70. *Renmin ribao,* April 11, 1960, 22.

71. Ibid.

72. A Cantonese doctor wrote, in an article of 1957, that acupuncture was rarely applied in the fight against leprosy, despite its effectiveness (Yan Bingchang, "Zhenjiu liaofa yingyong yu mafeng bing suo yinqi di shenjing fanying xing shenjing tong ji houyizheng di yidian tihui" [Some Observations on the Application of Acupuncture in Treating Pain of the Nerves Caused by Leprosy and Its Side Effects], *Guangdong zhongyi* 2 [1957]:7–9).

In handbooks for barefoot doctors, however, acupuncture was one of the techniques explained for the treatment of leprosy. Barefoot doctors were also taught to inject Chinese drugs into certain meridian points of patients (*Chijiao yisheng jiaocai: Gong nanfang diqu cankao yong* [*Teaching Handbook for Barefoot Doctors for the Southern Regions*] [Shanghai: Renmin weisheng chubanshe, 1973], 929–930).

73. Jiangsu Provincial Archives, doc. no. 3119-2-277, 29–34. According to an article by Cao Bu (*Renmin ribao,* September 6, 1956, 7), several of the recipes given by Chen Yan, of the Southern Song, and Zhu Zhenheng, of the Yuan, and compiled in the *Golden Mirror* were used by the leprosy hospital of Liaoning province and proved to be effective.

74. Many such reports can be found in *zhongyi* (Chinese medicine) journals of the various provinces, especially *Fujian zhongyi, Fujian zhongyiyao zazhi, Guangdong zhongyi, Jiangxi zhongyiyao, Shanghai zhongyiyao zazhi,* and the more general *Zhongyi zazhi* from 1956 onward. The components of *saofeng wan* and its origin are given in an article by the famous leprologist Yue Meizhong ("Zuguo yixue dui mafeng bing di renshi ji qi zhiliao"

[Knowledge on and Treatment of Leprosy in Chinese Medicine], *Fujian zhongyiyao zazhi* 2, no. 4 [1957]: 11–13), which also describes a number of frequently used old formulas. An article specifically on the effectiveness of *saofeng wan,* by the leprosy hospital in Shanghai ("Yong zhongyao 'saofeng wan' zhiliao shiba li mafeng bing di chubu zongjie" [Preliminary Conclusion on the Eighteen Cases of Leprosy Cured by the Chinese Drug Saofeng Wan]), was published in the *Shanghai zhongyiyao zazhi* 11 (1958): 27–29.

75. *Fujian sheng weisheng zhi,* 210–211. This herb is now often used to treat different types of arthritis.

76. Xinhua xian yiyao weisheng kexue yanjiusuo (Research Institute of Public Health Science of Xinhua County), "Daxue teng heji zhiliao shi li mafeng bing di chubu liaoxiao guancha baodao" (Report on the Observations on the Therapeutic Efficacy of *Caulis Sargentodoxae* Used in Recipes to Treat Ten Cases of Leprosy), *Guangdong zhongyi* 5, no. 7 (1960): 322–324.

77. Some lists were even more exhaustive: besides those foods listed, patients were also forbidden to eat dog, rabbit, duck, scaleless fish, scallions, garlic, chives, broccoli, soy products, red potatoes, alcohol, vinegar, shrimp oil, and others (Fujian sheng mafeng fangzhi yuan mafeng zhiliao yanjiu xiaozu [Group on Leprosy Treatment Research of the Leprosy Control Hospital of Fujian Province], "Fujian sheng mafeng fangzhi yuan yingyong zhongyao zhiliao mafeng yinian lai di zongjie" [Conclusion After One Year of Using Chinese Drugs to Control Leprosy in Fujian Province], *Fujian zhongyiyao zazhi* 3, no. 1 [1958]: 10).

78. *Chijiao yisheng jiaocai: Gong beifang diqu cankao yong* (*Teaching Handbook for Barefoot Doctors for the Northern Regions*) (Jilin: Renmin weisheng chubanshe, 1977), 2:1336. In the *Chijiao yisheng jiaocai: Gong nanfang diqu cankao yong,* 929–930, acupuncture and injection of Chinese drugs into the meridian points are recommended.

79. Jiang Cheng, e-mail message to author, March 31, 2005.

80. *Hubei sheng zhi,* 410.

81. Patients at the Mingyue Yan village, Xingshan county, Hubei province, for example, not only left the site in 1966 but had violent confrontations with local healthy villagers over the cutting of trees for firewood. The conflict lasted for more than a year and required several high-ranking cadres to solve the problem (Xingshan xian zhengxie wenshi ziliao weiyuanhui, Xingshan xian mafang yuan [Committee on Culture and History of Xingshan County, Leprosy Control Hospital of Xingshan County], eds., *Mingyue Yan: Hubei sheng Xingshan xian mafeng fangshi zhuanji* [*Clear Moon Rock: Collections of Papers on Leprosy Control in Xingshan County of Hubei Province*], 1994, 264). Such conflicts could have been suppressed by the authorities before the Cultural Revolution, which actually triggered long-standing social conflict.

82. Jiashan xian Sishan cun Yiyuan "Yuanzhi" bianxie zu (Editorial Group on the "History of the Sishan Village Hospital)," ed., *Anhui sheng Jiashan xian Sishan cun yiyuan*

zhi (1956–1986) (*Hospital Gazetteer of Sishan Village of Jiashan County in Anhui Province, 1956–1986*) (Jiashan, 1986), 27–28.

83. The confusion was not definitely settled until the early 1970s. In 1969 the hospital was still governed by a "revolutionary committee" made up of cadres and "representatives from the masses" (*Anhui sheng zhi,* 53).

84. Chen Yonghua, "Mafeng fangzhi zhong di chengbao zeren zhi" (Contract and Responsibility System in Leprosy Control), *Zhongguo mafeng zazhi* 2, no. 3 (1986): 49.

85. Wang Shaoguang, "Zhongguo gonggong weisheng di weiji yu zhuanji" (Crisis and Turning Point of Public Health in China), http://www.ccrs.org.cn, 4 (accessed June 22, 2003).

86. *Xiandai mafeng bing xue,* 15.

87. One of the first international conferences on leprology was held in Canton in November 1985; see the announcement in the inaugural issue of the *Zhongguo mafeng zazhi* (*China Leprosy Journal*), 1985, page 47. The journal is an organ of the China Leprosy Association and the China Leprosy Control and Research Center.

88. *Qian dongnan Miaozu Dongzu zizhi zhouzhi weisheng zhi* (*Gazetteer of Public Health in the Autonomous Regions of the Miao and the Dong in Southeastern Guizhou*) (Guiyang: Guizhou renmin chubanshe, 1993), 129.

89. Reports on Zhejiang and Anhui provinces, for instance, show that, after 1986, treatment of leprosy shifted outside the hospital and other institutions and patients were increasingly treated at home (Li Yulin et al., "Zhejiang sheng mafeng fangzhi sishiwu nian di huigu" [Review of Leprosy Control in Zhejiang Province in the Past Forty-five Years], *Zhongguo mafeng zazhi* 14, no. 3 [1998]: 174–175; *Anhui sheng zhi,* 347).

90. This was also the year the journal *Zhongguo mafeng zazhi* (*China Leprosy Journal*), publishing mostly mainstream medical reports on the leprosy situation in various districts and provinces, was created. The decision to implement MDT was made after three years of testing, as the plan to test the use of MDT was decided in a 1982 national meeting on leprosy control (Jiang Cheng, "Zhongguo mafeng fangzhi,"85–86).

91. *Cixi weisheng zhi* (*Materials on Public Health in Cixi*) (Ningpo: Ningpo chubanshe, 1994), 224; *Dantu xian weisheng zhi* (*Materials on Public Health in Dantu*), 2001, 171 provided almost identical information; other local gazetteers record similar implementation of the MDT treatment (*Kaiping xian weisheng zhi,* 266; *Henan sheng zhi weisheng zhi* [*Gazetteer of Henan Province: On Public Health*] [Zhengzhou: Henan renmin chubanshe, 1993], 221; *Changzhou shi weisheng zhi* [*Materials on Public Health in Changzhou City*], 1989, 50; *Dali Bai zu zizhizhou weisheng zhi* [*Materials on Public Health in the Bai Autonomous Region in Dali*] [Kunming: Yunnan minzu chubanshe, 1996], 136; *Gansu sheng zhi,* 469; *Sanshui xian weisheng zhi,* 288–291).

92. "Mafeng fangzhi zhong di chengbao zeren zhi," 49.

93. Zhao Z. and Zhang X., "Jiushi niandai Guangdong sheng di mafeng fangzhi duice" (Leprosy Control Strategy in Guangdong Province in the 1990s), *Zhongguo mafeng zazhi* 9, no. 1 (1993): 39.

94. Wang Quanpei et al., "Xizang zizhi qu mafeng bing liuxing ji fangzhi jinkuang baogao" (Report on the Recent Epidemiological Situation of Leprosy and Its Control in the Tibet Autonomous Region), *Zhongguo mafeng pifu bing zazhi* 19, no. 6 (2003): 584; Cun Shouming, "Kunming shi mafeng yuan wai zhiliao wunian qingkuang" (The Outpatient Treatment of Leprosy in Kunming City During the Past Five Years), *Zhongguo mafeng zazhi* 2, no. 3 (1986): 44.

95. It was apparently official policy to reinforce cooperation with foreign countries and foundations during this period (Jiang Cheng, "Mafeng fangzhi shi kua shiji di shiye" [Leprosy Control Is a Cross-Century Enterprise], *Zhongguo mafeng zazhi* 12, no. 1 [1996]: 42).

96. *Kunming weisheng zhi,* 263; *Dali Bai zu zizhizhou weisheng zhi,* 136; *Jiangxi sheng zhi,* 183; Mou H. et al., "Xiaochu mafeng yundong hou xin bingli faxian qingkuang fenxi" (Analysis of the Newly Discovered Cases After LEC), *Zhongguo mafeng pifu bing zazhi* 19, no. 5 (2003): 463; *Fujian sheng zhi weisheng zhi* (*Part on Public Health of the Gazetteer of Fujian Province*) (Beijing: Zhonghua shuju, 1995), 84.

97. Other provinces with similar experiences include Guangdong, Jiangsu, and Tibet (*Jieyang xian weisheng zhi,* 1992, 224; *Jiangsu sheng zhi weisheng zhi,* 325; *Changtaixian weisheng zhi, 1955–1994* [*Materials on Public Health in Changtai County, 1955–1994*] [Changtai, 1998], 69; Wang Quanpei et al., "Xizang zizhi qu mafeng bing liuxing ji fangzhi jinkuang baogao," 584; Chen, Li, Jiang and Ye, "Leprosy in China").

98. *Dali Bai zu zizhizhou weisheng zhi,* 36.

99. *Fujian sheng weisheng zhi,* 209–210.

100. *Jiangxi sheng zhi,* 183, with most cases in the southern part of the province.

101. *Gansu sheng zhi,* 467–468.

102. *Kaiping xian weisheng zhi,* 263.

103. Huang, "Shaoguan mafeng fangzhi shiji," 61, 133.

104. *Nantong xian weisheng zhi,* 117.

105. *Jiangdu xian weisheng zhi* (*Gazetteer on Public Health of Jiangdu*) (Nanjing: Jiangsu kexue jishu chubanshe, 1992), 217.

106. *Guangxi tongzhi,* 138–139.

107. "Zhejiang mafeng zhi dagai" (The General Situation of Leprosy in Zhejiang Province) (1955, mimeographed), Zhejiang Provincial Archives, doc. no. J165-5-64, 14–15.

108. Li M. and Gu B., "Shilun woguo mafeng yuan (cun) di gaige" (On the Reform of Leper Asylums and Villages in Our Country), *Zhongguo mafeng zazhi* 10, no. 1 (1994): 37.

109. *Hubei sheng zhi,* 409.

110. *Fujian sheng weisheng zhi,* 210. The 1995 *Fujian sheng zhi* (*Gazetteer of Fujian Province*) recorded that the report system was instituted in 1962.

111. *Kaiping xian weisheng zhi,* 264.

112. *Jiangsu sheng zhi weisheng zhi,* 324.

113. *(Hunan sheng) Anhua xian weisheng zhi* (*Materials on Public Health of Anhua County of Hunan Province*) (Anhua, 1989), 211.

114. *Fujian sheng weisheng zhi,* 207. It is reported in this text that more than thirty patients were lured to an island and starved to death in 1949. Stories of sufferers being buried alive were frequent throughout the 1950s, and, in 1964, there was even the case of a mother burning her sick son alive.

115. Ibid., 210; *Zhoushan shi weisheng zhi* (*Materials on Public Health of Zhoushan City*) (Beijing: Zhonghua shuju, 2002), 442–443.

116. *Qian dongnan Miaozu Dongzu zizhi zhouzhi weisheng zhi,* 128.

117. *Nanchang xian weisheng zhi* (*Materials on Public Health in Nanchang*) (Nanchang, 1988), 19.

118. *Guangxi tongzhi,* 138.

119. *Gansu sheng zhi,* 467.

120. *Dali Bai zu zizhizhou weisheng zhi,* 136; *Qian dongnan Miaozu Dongzu zizhi zhouzhi,* 128. Toward the end of the 1950s, Guizhou province was reported to have segregated only some 30 percent of patients (Guizhou sheng weisheng ting minzheng ting [Public Health and Civil Affairs Departments of Guizhou Province], "Guanyu wosheng dui mafeng bingren di shourong, geli, zhiliao gongzuo qingkuang he jinhou yijian" [On the Treatment, Segregation, and Accommodation of Patients of Leprosy in Our Province and Suggestions for the Future], *Xing bing mafeng fangyan gongzuo* [*Bulletin on the Prevention and Research of Venereal Disease and Leprosy*] 3 [1959]: 75–76). According to Jiang Cheng, Yunnan, Guizhou, and Sichuan did not set up enough leper villages in the 1950s and 1960s, resulting in the aggravation of the epidemic situation in this region in the 1960s and 1970s. This region, where 60 percent of new cases are found, remains much infected even today (Jiang Cheng, pers. comm. to author, August 29, 2005).

121. *Jiangsu sheng zhi weisheng zhi,* 319, 630.

122. *Jiangdu xian weisheng zhi,* 219.

123. "Zhejiang sheng mafeng fangzhi sishiwu nian di huigu," 174–175.

124. *Anhui sheng Jiashan xian Sishan cun yiyuan zhi,* 24–25.

125. This was confirmed by Dr. Li Huanying, a highly outspoken leprologist, in an interview by the author, August 2002.

126. Huang, "Shaoguan mafeng fangzhi shiji," 132–133.

127. Sihui xian mafeng zhan (Leprosy Station of Sihui County), "Zou qunzhong luxian banhao mafeng cun" (Organize Leper Villages by Taking the Mass Line), *Mafeng bing fangzhi jianbao* 9–10:3–6, especially 5.

128. "Guangdong mafeng fangzhi shinian licheng," 7.

129. Jiangsu Provincial Archives, doc. no. 3119-3-1383, 10–11.

130. Ibid., doc. no. 3119-3-1473, 15.

131. *Hubei sheng zhi*, 411.

132. *Rongchang xian weisheng zhi* (*Materials on Public Health in Rongchang*) (Rongchang, 1988), 18.

133. Huang, "Shaoguan mafeng fangzhi shiji," 133.

134. *Gansu sheng zhi*, 466.

135. You, "Wunian lai," 8–9.

136. In Jieyang district, Guangdong province, for instance, two leper villages, Xikeng and Diaoling, were to take in, respectively, male and female patients from the district. The female village at Diaoling was abolished only in 1979, with remaining patients removed to the other village (*Jieyang xian weisheng zhi*, 224).

137. Sishan village, in Anhui, is an example of the latter approach (*Anhui sheng Jiashan xian Sishan cun yiyuan zhi*, 80).

138. According to Jiang Cheng, in Hainan, patients had to be sterilized before they were allowed to get married. They were allowed to adopt children (pers. comm. to author, August 29, 2005).

139. Guangdong province announced a first set of criteria for the release of patients in 1959, which was revised as early as 1962. Patients allowed to be released received a health certificate (*jiankang zheng*) and could remain in the village if they chose to (Guangdong sheng weisheng ting pifu xing bing fangzhi chu [Unit of Venereal Disease and Skin Disease Control of the Department of Public Health of Guangdong Province], "Mafeng bingren chu yuan cun [huifu jiankang] biaozhun" [Criteria for the Release of Patients of Leprosy from Hospitals and Villages After They Have Recovered Their Health], *Pifu xing bing fangzhi tongxun* 1, no. 1 [1962]: 2–3).

140. *Shanxi tongzhi: Weisheng yiyao zhi; Weisheng bian* (*Volume on Hygiene, "Medicine and Hygiene" Section, General Gazetteer of Shanxi Province*) (Beijing: Zhonghua shuju, 1997), 486. The new case in the late 1990s was brought to my attention by Jiang Cheng (pers. comm. to author, August 29, 2005).

141. Chen Zhiping and Ruan Qihao, "Di li ping zhushe ye zhiliao mafeng chubu liaoxiao guancha baogao" (Preliminary Report on the Observations of the First Results of the Injection of Di Li Ping), *Guangdong zhongyi* 6 (1960): 269–272.

142. Fujian province, for instance, had undergone four stages in the treatment of leprosy: DDS was first used, then DDS was used together with Chinese medicine, then there was a period of combined application of Chinese and Western treatments before the use of MDT in the 1980s *Fujian sheng weisheng zhi*, 210–211.

143. *Kunming weisheng zhi*, 263.

144. *Fujian sheng weisheng zhi*, 210.

145. The following account is based on interviews made during a field trip to this asylum on August 31, 2005, guided by Dr. Jiang Cheng and with the assistance of experts from the leprosy control center of Zhejiang province.

146. Wang Lin-zei, "A Brief History of the Hangchow Leper Hospital," *Leper Quarterly* 1, no. 2 (1927): 20–22.

147. Sturton worked first as the acting superintendent of the asylum in 1928, and then as superintendent during the war period (Y. Lee, "A Visit to Hangchow Leper Home," *Leper Quarterly* 1, no. 4 [1928]: 7–9; "Hangchow Leprosarium," *Leper Quarterly* 12, no. 4 [1938]: 167; "Hangzhou Songmu chang Guangji mafeng yiyuan yuanwu jieshao" [An Introduction to the Situation of the Leper Asylum of the Hangzhou Guangji Hospital at Pine Grove] [around 1950, mimeographed, kept at the Wukang leper village], 1).

148. The elderly patient told me that the maximum number of patients was some 300, whereas the official account of the asylum recorded that there were 550 beds in 1955 (http://www.chinaderma.com.cn/view.aspx?id = 635 [accessed December 19, 2006]).

149. The regulations were published in *Jiangxi zhongyiyao* (*Journal of Chinese Medicine of Jiangxi Province*) 4, nos. 1–2 (1952): 2–6.

150. *Renmin ribao,* September 16, 1980, 2; June 6, 1992, 5; October 28, 1994, 3. Jiang Cheng wrote in opposition to such discriminatory rules in an article published in 1986, but apparently to no avail ("Mafeng bing dui hunyin jiating di yingxiang" [Leprosy's Impact on Families and Marriages], *Zhongguo mafeng zazhi* 2, no. 1 [1986]: 71–72).

151. An academic by the name of Ye Ganyun recommended the lifting of the stipulation in the summer of 2000 in the legal committee under the Executive Committee of the People's Congress, and was accepted. The declaration of the new civil law was made on April 24, 2001, by Premier Jiang Zemin (Jiang Cheng, pers. comm. to author, January 18, 2005).

152. *Renmin ribao,* May 19, 1984, 5.

153. Lei Liangzhong, "Bujie, qishi yu cunluo: Mafeng he mafeng cun di gushi" (Pollution, Discrimination, and the Village: The Story of Leprosy and a Leper Village) (master's thesis, Central University of Ethnology, Beijing, 2003), 64–65, 125. I thank Professor Jing Jun for providing me with this interesting thesis.

154. Wang et al., "Xizang zizhi qu mafeng bing," 584.

155. Dr. Li Yushang, personal communication to author, December 14, 2004, on Guangrao county, Shandong province. The asylum was apparently established after 1949 and disappeared after the Cultural Revolution.

156. A few sociological surveys on the attitudes toward cured patients of leprosy in the late 1980s and 1990s clearly show this (Lu X., "Qian tan mafeng fangzhi guangli zhong di jige wenti" [Brief Discussion on a Few Problems Regarding the Control and Management of Leprosy], *Zhongguo mafeng zazhi* 8, no. 2 [1992]: 104).

157. Jiang Cheng, "Mafeng bing dui hunyin," 70–71.

158. Jiang Cheng et al., "Shehui ge jieceng renshi dui mafeng bing renshi, taidu he xinli fanying di yanjiu" (Study on the Perception, Attitude, and Psychological Reaction to Leprosy of People of All Social Classes), in *Mafeng bing shehui yixue lunwen ji* (*Collected Essays on the Social Medicine of Leprosy*) (Beijing: Zhongguo yixue kexue yuan pifu bing yanjiu suo, 1986), 63, 66.

159. "Qian tan mafeng fangzhi guangli zhong di jige wenti," 104.

160. Ibid., 103–105.

161. Such as, in Fujian province since the 1980s, for example, the distribution of pamphlets, the use of popular plays and TV soap operas, the organization of Leprosy Day, and so on (*Fujian sheng zhi weisheng zhi,* 1995, 83).

162. The information here and in the table comes from the National Center for STD and Leprosy Control, CDC, Nanjing, China, June 15, 2005.

163. Li M. and Gu B., "Shilun woguo mafeng yuan (cun) di gaige" (On the Reform of Leper Asylums and Villages in Our Country), *Zhongguo mafeng zazhi* 10, no. 1 (1994): 37.

164. Jiang Cheng, "Zhongguo mafeng fangzhi," 85–86.

165. Wang et al., "Xizang zizhi qu mafeng bing," 584.

166. "The Lepers of Japan," *The Economist,* February 24, 1996, 64; P. Pons, "Les lépreux japonais vont retrouver la liberté," *Le Monde,* February 6, 1996.

167. In Nantong, Jiangsu province, sixty-five such patients were still living in the village of the district in 1988 (*Nantong xian weisheng zhi,* 118). In the city of Dali, Yunnan province, the leprosarium was no longer taking in new patients, but it continued to accommodate "a small number of homeless patients" (*Dali shi weisheng zhi* [*Materials on Public Health in Dali City*] [Kunming: Yunnan minzu chubanshe, 1992], 73).

168. Jiang Cheng, "Zhongguo mafeng fangzhi,"86.

169. Hu Y., "Mafeng yuan hechu qu" (Where Do Leprosaria Go?), *Zhongguo mafeng zazhi* 10, no. 3 (1994): 174.

170. This leprosarium accommodated more than 1,000 patients in its peak years in the mid-1960s. For its history and a brief account of leprosy control in Taiwan, see Chang Ping-I, *Outside the World* (Taipei: Wings of Hope, 2004). The official Web site of the leprosarium is http://www.lslp.doh.gov.tw; that of the social movement is: http://www.loshengrepublic.com.

171. Zhou D. et al., "Mafeng bingren di wailiu yu guanli" (The Emigration of Patients of Leprosy and the Problem of Management), *Zhongguo mafeng zazhi* 3, no. 3 (1987): 147.

172. Li X. and Zhang L., "Zoucheng shi jiben xiaomie mafeng hou fangzhi gongzuo mianlin di wenti ji duice" (Problems and Solutions of the Tasks Facing Leprosy Control After the First Elimination of the Disease in Zoucheng City), *Zhongguo mafeng pifu bing zazhi,* 19, no. 5 (2003): 523. The same warning was given by doctors working in Shaanxi province in the 1990s (Hu, "Mafeng yuan wang he chuqu," 174).

173. Hu, "Mafeng yuan wang he chuqu," 174; Lin B. and Ma J., "Putian shi mafeng

liuxing bingxue fenxi" (Analysis of the Epidemiology of Leprosy in Putian City), *Zhongguo mafeng pifu bing zazhi* 19, no. 6 (2003): 562

174. Nong Y., "Guangzhou shi mafeng fanzhi sishi nian" (Forty Years of Leprosy Control in Guangzhou), *Zhongguo mafeng zazhi* 15, no. 1 (1999): 54. In 1987, in another district of Guangdong, Chenghai, where leprosy has a long history, an expert recommended concentrated efforts and funding for MDT in rural areas, where the disease was believed to be rampant ("Chenghai xian mafeng yidian cun di fenxi" [Analysis of Leprosy Villages in Chenghai District], *Zhongguo mafeng zazhi* 3, no. 3 [1987]: 149).

175. Mou H. et al., "Xiaochu mafeng yundong hou xin bingli faxian qingkuang fenxi" (Analysis of the Newly Discovered Cases after LEC), *Zhongguo mafeng pifu bing zazhi* 19, no. 5 (2003): 464.

176. Jiang Cheng, "Mafeng fangzhi shi kua shiji di shiye," 43. Jiang is particularly concerned about leprosy hospitals being transformed into hospitals of dermatology, and even to institutions of lucrative plastic surgery. These changes are substantially recorded in *Zhongguo yiyuan daquan* (*Encyclopedia of Hospitals in China*), published in 1989 by Guangming ribao chubanshe, under the section on hospitals for the prevention of dermatological diseases for the different provinces. This change seems to be part of the "liberalization" of the state public health policy, as the specialties of dermatology and plastic surgery are lucrative and would ideally cover the expenditures for leprosy control, and it also implies a gradual withdrawal of the state's financial role in its control.

177. It is clear from articles written by Chinese leprologists that they are concerned by the "marketization" of public health in Chinese rural villages. Experts such as Jiang Cheng and his colleagues expressed their view that this policy is wrong and unjust (Lu, "Qian tan mafeng fangzhi guangli zhong di jige wenti," 105).

EPILOGUE

1. W. H. Jefferys and J. L. Maxwell, *The Diseases of China: Including Formosa and Korea* (Philadelphia: Blakiston's, 1911), 46. Or, as another medical missionary, L. Fowler, said in 1915, "The highest authority on Tropical Medicine has stated that in all likelihood there are more lepers in China than in any other country in the world" ("Leprosy in China," *Chinese Recorder* 46, no. 4 [1915]: 227).

2. Quoted in Susan Sontag, *AIDS and Its Metaphors* (New York: Farrar, Straus and Giroux, 1988), 58.

3. Japan Law Foundation Verification Committee, "Verification Committee Concerning Hansen's Disease Problem: Final Report" (Summary Version, March 2005), http://www.mhlw.go.jp/english/policy/health/01/pdf/01.pdf, 20–24.

4. Ibid., 133–137. Mitsuda Kensuke (1876–1964), a leading Japanese leprologist, sent

Nanba Madashi as second director of the Manchurian asylum, hoping that he would "clean up the continent" (136).

5. A. A. Mouritz, *The Path of the Destroyer: A History of Leprosy in the Hawaiian Islands and Thirty Years Research into the Means by Which It Has Been Spread* (Honolulu: Honolulu Star-Bulletin, 1916), 234–235.

6. S. Pandya, "The First International Leprosy Conference, Berlin, 1897," *História, Ciências, Saúde: Manguinhos* 10, suppl. no. 1 (2003)164–165.

7. Ibid., 174. "Troisième conférence internationale scientifique de la lèpre, Strasbourg, 28–31 juillet 1923," sect. 1, "Résolutions," *BIUM: Histoire de la médicine, et de l'art dentaire*, http://web2.bium.univ-paris5.fr/livanc/ (accessed March 24, 2008).

8. It was only at the 1923 Strasbourg conference that it was decided the League of Nations should establish statistics on leprosy in the world.

9. WHO Study Group, *Epidemiology of Leprosy in Relation to Control*, Technical Report Series 716 (Geneva: WHO, 1985); 11–14; WHO, *World Health Organization Leprosy Elimination Project Status Report 2003 Draft* (Geneva: WHO, 2004).

10. M. Monot et al., "On the Origin of Leprosy," *Science* 308 (May 2005): 1040–1042.

11. Australia is probably another example. A survey by the British doctor J. Ashburton Thompson in Australia in the late 1890s contains the following conclusion: "Although lepers were imported to Victoria steadily during a long term of years and in considerable number, and although they always remained entirely unrestricted in their movements among the whites, no Victorian native white who had never left the colony has ever been attacked. Moreover the disease died away in Victoria quite independently of restrictive measures against the liberty of lepers, which in fact were first taken only in March, 1893" ("Contribution to the History of Leprosy in Australia," *Prize Essays on Leprosy* [London: New Sydenham Society, 1897], 108).

12. According to the same report, "these observations imply that some changes that occur as a result of economic development lead to the improvement of environmental risk factors (crowding, etc.) and/or host risk factors ('resistance')" (WHO Study Group, *Epidemiology of Leprosy*, 14–15).

13. Pandya, "First International Leprosy Conference," 164, 168.

14. For recent developments in this area, visit the International Leprosy Association's Web site related to the Global Project on the History of Leprosy: http://www.leprosyhistory.org.

15. For an account of recent activities and a colonial history of leprosy on Taiwan, see Wen-Ji Wang, "Laying Out a Model Village: George Gushe-Taylor and Missionary Leprosy Work in Colonial Taiwan," *East Asian Science, Technology, and Society: An International Journal* 1, no. 1. (2007): 111–133 .

16. See G. Agamben, *Homo Sacer: Sovereign Power and Bare Life* (Stanford, Calif.: Stanford University Press, 1998), especially 135–143, on the concentration camp as paradigm.

17. R. Edmond, *Leprosy and Empire: A Medical and Cultural Study* (Cambridge: Cambridge University Press, 2006), 7.

18. Without knowing the museum at Carville, one might imagine its contents by reading Gaudet's recent book, where the author explains that "the book looks through the prism of memory at how Carville residents dealt with their quest for identity and survival with dignity in spite of their illness. What comes across to the rest of us . . . is their humanity" (*Carville: Remembering Leprosy in America* [Jackson: University Press of Mississippi, 2004], xv). Tayman's recent book gives a similar glimpse into the museum in Hawaii devoted to the survivors of Molokai (*The Colony: The Harrowing True Story of the Exiles of Molokai* [New York: Scribner, 2006]).

19. Japan's attitudes are clearly revealed in the mentioned (n. 3) final report of the Japan Law Foundation Verification Committee.

20. On the domination of public opinion by the Indian middle class for a loose confinement policy, see J. Buckingham, *Leprosy in Colonial South India: Medicine and Confinement* (New York: Palgrave, 2002), 163–169. On the decision to build the Hay Ling Chau asylum in Hong Kong in 1951, see the *Annual Reports* of the Mission to Lepers Hong Kong Auxiliary (London: Mission to Lepers, 1951–1953). In the 1951 report, it is written that "during 1950 the problem of leprosy in Hong Kong gave growing concern to the Government as it was no longer possible to refer such patients to Sheklung Leprosarum (Kwangtung); and patients in increasing numbers sought refuge here from the unsettled conditions in China" (3).

21. WHO, http://www.who.int/mediacentre/factsheets/fs101/en/index.html (accessed December 19, 2006).

22. Sontag, *AIDS,* 93.

Glossary

A Hu	亞胡
aiye	艾葉
anchashi	按察使
Anhua	安化
Anyi	安義
Aomen jilue	澳門紀略
awei	阿魏
Badie	八疊
badou	巴豆
Bailu	白路
bai qianniu	白牽牛
banmao	斑貓
Baokang	寶康
Baoning	保寧
Bao pu zi	抱朴子
Baoqing	寶慶
Baoying	寶應
baozheng	保正

Beidong yuan bilu	北東園筆錄
Beihai (Pakhoi)	北海
Beiji qianjin yaofang	備急千金要方
Bencao gangmu	本草綱目
Bijie	畢節
Bing yu yuan chuanqi	病玉緣傳奇
bixie	萆薢
Bo He	帛和
Boluo	博羅
Boniu you ji kao	伯牛有疾考
bu jin	不謹
bu ren	不仁
canji	殘疾
cao wutou	草烏頭
Cenxi	岑溪
Changle	長樂
Changshi yu	嘗試語
Chaoyang	潮陽
Chao Yuanfang	巢元方
Chaozhou	潮州
Chen Duoshou shengsi fuqi	陳多壽生死夫妻
chengbao zeren zhi	承包責任制
Chengdu	成都
Chenghai	澄海
Chen Guang	陳廣
Cheng Xuanying	成玄英
Chen Huiyan	陳徽言
Chen Kun	陳坤
Chen Qi	陳綺
Chen Shiduo	陳士鐸
Chen Shigong	陳實功
Chen Shou	陳壽
Chen Sicheng	陳司成
Chen Tianchi	陳天尺
Chen Wenzhang	陳文章
Chen Yan	陳言
Chen Yuan	陳垣
Chen Yuan zaonian wenji	陳垣早年文集
Chen Zhiping	陳治平

chi	尺
chi xiao dou	赤小豆
chong	蟲
Chongqing	重慶
Chongren	崇仁
Chou Juchuan	仇巨川
Chuangyang yingyan quanshu	瘡瘍應驗全書
chuanran	傳染
Chun zhu jiwen	春渚紀聞
Cixi	慈溪
Cui Hao	崔浩
cun	寸
cunxu yuan	存恤院
dafeng	大風
da feng zi	大風子
dafushe	大蝮蛇
Dajin (Taikam, Taikom)	大衾
Dali	大理
da mafeng	大痲風
Dangtu	當塗
dansha	丹砂
Danxi yiji	丹溪醫集
Daoji	道積
Daoxun	道舜
daxue teng	大血籐
Dayu	大庾
da yuan	大院
Deng Shining	鄧士寧
Deng Shizhang	鄧士章
Deng Yigao	鄧以誥
Deqing	德清
dibao	地保
di gu pi	地骨皮
Di li ping	敵癘平
Ding Guangdi	丁光迪
Dong	獞
Dongguan	東莞
Dongjiang	東江
Dongyuan yiji	東垣醫集

Dou Menglin	竇夢麟
du	毒
Du Guangting	杜光庭
duhuo	獨活
duji	篤疾
Du Tongda	杜通達
ebing	惡病
efeng	惡風
eji	惡疾
Ershi nian mudu zhi guai xianzhuang	二十年目睹之怪現狀
fafeng yuan	發瘋園
Fahe	法和
fan chu jihai	犯觸忌害
Fan Duan'ang	范端昂
fangfeng	防風
Fan Xingzhun	范行準
Fayuan zhulin	法苑珠林
fei	肺
Feiyue mafeng yuan	飛越痲瘋院
fen	分
fenghuang	鳳凰
Feng liu wu	風流悟
Feng Menglong	馮夢龍
Fengmen quanshu	瘋門全書
fengmu	瘋目
Fengshun	豐順
fengtu	風土
Fengxin	奉新
feng yuan	瘋院
fengzi yuan	瘋子院
Fozu lidai tongzai	佛祖歷代通載
Fozu tongji	佛祖統紀
Fucheng si	福成寺
fuling	茯苓
Fuxie xinshu	伏邪新書
Fuzhai riji	復齋日記
Fuzhou	福州
fuzi	附子
gan	肝

gan cao	甘草
Gao Lu	高魯
Gao Qixue	高其學
Ge Hong	葛洪
geng	更
Gengdao ji	庚道集
gong di	公地
Gong Tingxian	龔廷賢
gong tong	公同
gu	蠱
Guang chuang	廣瘡
Guangdong xinyu	廣東新語
Guang hongming ji	廣弘明集
Guangrao	廣饒
Guangyang	廣陽
Guanyin	觀音
gui	鬼
Guixin zashi	癸辛雜識
Gujin yitong daquan	古今醫統大全
guofeng	過瘋
guolai	過癩
Guoshi bu	國史補
Guowuzhou	郭屋州
Gu Shicheng	顧世澄
Gutian	古田
Gu Zhentao	顧震濤
hai	害
Haifeng	海豐
Haikou (Hoihow)	海口
han	寒
Hangzhou	杭州
Hanjiang	涵江
Hankou	漢口
han re	寒熱
He Biao	賀彪
hei qianniu	黑牽牛
Hengzhou	衡州
Heping Weiwai	和平圍外
heshouwu	何首烏

He Wei	何薳
hezi	訶子
Huangdi neijing	黃帝內經
Huangdi nei jing suwen ji zhu	黃帝內經素問集注
Huang Kuan	黃寬
Huang Shengbai	黃勝白
Huang Yujie	黃玉階
Huang Zhong	黃鐘
Hu Cheng'an	胡承菴
Huichang	會昌
Huilai	惠來
Huiyang	惠陽
Hunyuan shengji	混元聖紀
huo	火
huoxiang	藿香
huxiang chuanran	互相傳染
huxiang chuan zhe	互相傳者
Hu Zuoting	胡佐廷
Ishikawa Rikizan	石川力山
ji	吉
Jiang Cheng	江澄
Jiangdu	江都
Jiang Jieshi	蔣介石
Jiangle	將樂
Jiangmen	江門
Jiang Tengsheng	姜滕生
Jianyang	建陽
jiaotong	姣童
Jiewei yuansou	解圍元藪
Jieyang	揭陽
jifeng	疾風
Ji Gongjia	嵇供甲
Jinan	濟南
jing	經
Jingde chuan deng lu	景德傳燈錄
Jingning	景寧
Jingyue quanshu	景岳全書
Ji shi quanshu	濟世全書
Jiulongjiang (Kiulungkiang)	九龍江

Ji Yun	紀昀
juren	舉人
Kaiping	開平
Kangding	康定
kangfu cun	康復村
kan hu fu	看護婦
Kou Qianzhi	寇謙之
Kuizhou	夔州
kuilan	潰爛
Kunming	昆明
kushen	苦參
laibing ying	癩病營
lai chuang	癩瘡
laimin suo	癩民所
Laipi zushi miao	癩皮祖師廟
Lai Shanghe	賴尚和
Laiyang	萊陽
laizi ying	癩子營
langdu	狼毒
Lanzhou	蘭州
lao	勞(癆)
lao zhai	癆瘵
leigong teng	雷公籐
leiwan	雷丸
Leizhou	雷州
Lenglu yihua	冷廬醫話
Leping	樂平
Lesheng	樂生
Liancheng	連城
Liangban qiuyu an suibi	兩般秋雨盦隨筆
Liang Gongchen	梁恭辰
Liang Shaoren	梁紹壬
Liang Tingnan	梁廷楠
Liang Zhangchi	梁章池
Liao Fufeng	廖福俸
Liao Fuxian	廖福現
Liao Shourong	廖壽榮
Liao Zonglin	廖宗林
Lienü zhuan	列女傳

lifeng 厲風
Li Gao 李杲
Li Han 李翰
Li Jianmin 李建民
Li Jing 栗勁
li/lai 癘/癩
Li Lian 李濂
Lin Fushi 林富士
Lingbiao 嶺表
lingchi 凌遲
Lingnan weisheng fang 嶺南衛生方
Lingnan zaji 嶺南雜記
Lingnan zashi shi chao 嶺南雜事詩鈔
Lingshu 靈樞
Lingwai daida 嶺外代答
lingyan 靈驗
Lin Zhiming 林志明
liren fang 癘人坊
Li Rulan 李如蘭
Li Shizhen 李時珍
lisuo 癘所
Liu Ban (Gongfu) 劉攽(貢父)
Liu Chun 劉純
Liu Jiren 劉吉人
Liu Muzhi 劉牧之
Liu Wansu 劉完素
Liu Xiang 劉向
liu zhu 流注
Lixue zhinan 吏學指南
liyang 癘瘍
Liyang jiyao 癘瘍機要
Longchuan lue zhi 龍川略志
Longxi 龍溪
Longzhou 龍州
Lunyu 論語
Luoding 羅定
Lu Shizhong 路時中
Lu Yitian 陸以湉
mafeng 麻風(痲瘋)

mafeng bao bing zhidu	痲瘋報病制度
mafeng bing fangyi zhan	痲瘋病防疫站
mafeng bing fangzhi jianbao	痲瘋病防治簡報
mafeng cun	痲瘋村
Mafeng jikan	麻瘋季刊
mafeng liao	麻風寮
Mafeng nü Qiu Liyu chuanqi	麻風女邱麗玉傳奇
mafeng yuan	麻風院(痲瘋院)
mafeng zhimindi	痲瘋殖民地
Ma Haide (George Hatem)	馬海德
mahuang	麻黃
mahuang gen	麻黃根
maifeng	脈風
mai feng zhe	賣瘋者
Mai shu	脈書
Ma Jixing	馬繼興
mamo	痲魔
manyijiu	蠻夷酒
Mao Qiling	毛奇齡
Meichuang milu	霉瘡秘錄
mei jun wei shengwu	黴菌微生物
Miao	苗
miezhong	滅種
Minfeng zaji	閩風雜記
ming	皿
Mingshan	名山
Mingyue Yan	明月岩
Minxian	閩縣
Mitsuda Kensuke	光田健輔
Modengxian zhai zhuren	莫等閒齋主人
Moximian	磨西面
Muling shu	牧令書
Nagamata Yoshirō	長又與郎
Nan'an	南安
Nanchang	南昌
Nanfeng	南豐
Nanhai	南海
Nanning	南寧
Nanping	南平

Nantong	南通
Nanyue youji	南越遊記
Neige daku	內閣大庫
neishi	內室
Niida Noboru	仁井田陞
Ningyuan	寧遠
niuhuang	牛黃
nongye she	農業社
nü se	女色
paochuang	疱瘡
pi	脾
Pifu xing bing fangzhi tongxun	皮膚性病防治通訊
pilong	疲癃
pinzi yuan	貧子院
Puji fang	普濟方
Puji tang	普濟堂
Puning	普寧
Pu Songling	蒲松齡
Putian	莆田
Qianjin yifang	千金翼方
Qi hui guzhu	氣穢蠱注
Qi Kun	祁坤
Qing bai lei chao	清稗類鈔
Qingchengzi	青城子
Qingdao	青島
qingfen	輕粉
Qingjiangpu	清江浦
Qing shi duo	清詩鐸
Qingyuan (Tsingyuen)	清遠
Qingzhou	青州
Qipo	耆婆
Qiu Xi	邱熺
qiwei	氣味
qu	區
Quanzhou	泉州
Qu Dajun	屈大均
Qujiang	曲江
Ran Boniu	冉伯牛
Renmin ribao	人民日報

Renzhai zhizhi	仁齋直指
Rongchang	榮昌
Rugao	如皋
Rumen shiqin	儒門事親
ruyi	儒醫
Sakura Magozou	佐倉孫三
Sanshui	三水
San yin ji yi bingzheng fang lun	三因極一病證方論
saofeng wan	掃風丸
shan dou gen	山豆根
Shangbo	上柏
shangkou liang	商口糧
Shantou (Swatow)	汕頭
Shaoguan	韶關
Shaowu	邵武
Shaozhou	韶州
Sha xian	沙縣
she gu	蛇蠱
shen	腎
sheng	生
Shengji zonglu	聖濟總錄
Shen Zhiwen	沈之問
shi	濕
shi chong	尸蟲
Shilong (Sheklong, Sheklung)	石龍
Shima	石碼
Shishi milu	石室秘錄
shi tiaoli	失調理
Shitou	石頭
shouling	首領
Shouyu shenfang	壽域神方
shu dihuang	熟地黃
Shunde	順德
Si fen lü	四分律
Sihui	四會
Sishan	四山
Songmu chang	松木廠
Song Xiangfeng	宋翔鳳
Su Che	蘇轍

Suilu	綏碌
Sun Simiao	孫思邈
Su Shi (Dongpo)	蘇軾(東坡)
Suwen	素問
Suwen bingji qi yi baoming ji	素問病機氣宜保命集
Taihan ji	太函集
Taiping jing hejiao	太平經合校
Taiping shenghui fang	太平聖惠方
Taiping yulan	太平御覽
Taishang dongyuan shenzhou jing	太上洞淵神咒經
Taishang zhuguo jiumin zongzhen biyao	太上助國救民總真秘要
Taishō shinshū daizōkyō	大正新修大藏經
Taizhou	泰州
Tang Changru	唐長儒
Tang lü shuyi	唐律疏議
Tangling shiyi	唐令拾遺
Tan guolai	談過癩
Tang Zijie	唐自傑
Tengxian	滕縣
Tianmen	天門
tian pao chuang	天疱瘡
tianxing	天刑
Tianxin zhengfa	天心正法
Tongmeng hui	同盟會
tongnian	同年
waijiang	外江
waike	外科
Waike dacheng	外科大成
waike xinfa yaojue	外科心法要訣
Waitai miyao fang	外臺秘要方
Wang Daokun	汪道昆
Wang Jimin	王吉民
Wang Linheng	王臨亨
Wang Tao	王燾
Wang Wen	王溫
Wangye	王爺
Wang Zhi	王植
wei sheng wu	微生物
weisheng xueli	衛生學理

Weixian	濰縣
Wei Yuansong	衛元嵩
wen	溫
Wenyi lun buzheng	溫疫論補証
Wu Chichang	吳熾昌
Wudu	武都
Wu Jianren	吳趼人
Wukang	武康
Wu Liande (Lien-teh)	伍連德
Wumen biao yin	吳門表隱
Wuning	武寧
Wu Qian	吳謙
Wushang xuanyuan santian yutang dafa	无上玄元三天玉堂大法
wu she	烏蛇
Wuwei Handai yijian	武威漢代醫簡
wu xing	五行
Wu Youxing	吳有性
Wu Zhenfang	吳震方
Wu Zhijian (T. C. Wu)	鄔志堅
Xiamen	廈門
xian	縣
Xianchuan waike bifang	仙傳外科秘方
xiang	鄉
xiangchuan	相傳
xianyi junguan	現役軍官
Xianyuan bianzhu	仙苑編珠
Xiaogan	孝感
xiaoshi	消石
Xiaosi	效思
Xiao Xi	蕭熙
Xiao Xiaoting	蕭曉亭
Xiao Yunchun	蕭運春
Xiashan Dongshan	峽山東山
Xie Guan	謝觀
Xiehe	協和
Xie Hui	謝晦
Xie Lipu (Lansheng)	謝澧浦(蘭生)
xin	心
Xincheng	新城

Xing bing mafeng fangyan gongzuo	性病痲風防研工作
Xinghua	興化
Xingke tiben	刑科提本
Xingshi heng yan	醒世恆言
Xingshi yinyuan	醒世姻緣
Xinhua	新華
Xinhua (Sinhwa)	新化
Xinhui	新會
Xinxing	新興
xiong	凶
xionghuang	雄黃
Xishi	西施
Xi Wang Mu	西王母
Xuan Ding	宣鼎
Xu Chunfu	徐春甫
Xu Dachun	徐大椿
Xu Dong	徐楝
Xue Ji	薛已
Xue shi yi an xuan	薛氏醫案選
Xu gao seng zhuan	續高僧傳
Xu Hao	徐浩
Xu Ke	徐珂
Xu Kechuang xianhua	續客窗閒話
Xu ping waike zhengzong	徐評外科正宗
Xu Yanchun	徐彥純
Xu yishuo	續醫說
Xu Yuanrui	徐元瑞
Xuyong	敘永
Xuzhou	敘州
Ya'an	雅安
Yan	顏
yang	瘍
Yangcheng guchao	羊城古鈔
Yangjiang	陽江
yangji yuan	養濟院
yanglian yin	養廉銀
yangmei chuang	楊梅瘡
Yang Shiying	楊士瀛
Yangyi daquan	瘍醫大全

Yanping 延平
Yanshi jiaxun 顏氏家訓
Yan Yuan ji 顏元集
yanzhang 煙瘴
Yan Zhitui 顏之推
Yanzhou 兗州
Ye Ganyun 葉干雲
Yeyu qiudeng lu 夜雨秋燈錄
yi 移
Yifang leiju 醫方類聚
Yifen wenji 夷氛聞紀
yiji tang 義濟堂
Yili zhushu 儀禮注疏
yin 淫
Yin Guangren 印光任
Yi shi 醫史
Yizhou 益州
Yizong jinjian 醫宗金鑑
Yongna jushi 慵納居士
Yongnian 永年
You Jiajun 尤家駿
You Shaoan 游紹安
yuan 元
Yuan Ji 袁機
yuanliu chuanran suo xi 源流傳染所繫
Yuan Shikai 袁世凱
Yu Bin 俞弁
Yuedong wenjian lu 粵東聞見錄
Yue jian lu 粵劍錄
Yue Meizhong 岳美中
Yueweicao tang biji 閱微草堂筆記
Yue zhong jianwen 粵中見聞
Yu Ji 于吉
yujin 鬱金
Yuji weiyi 玉機微義
Yunji qiqian 雲笈七籤
Yu Rang 豫讓
Yu Shenchu 俞慎初
Yutang dafa 玉堂大法

zao	燥
zaojiaoci	皂角刺
zaqi	雜氣
zeifeng	賊風
Zengcheng	增城
Zezhou	澤州
Zhang Congzheng	張從正
Zhanghua	彰化
Zhang Jiebin	張介賓
Zhang Jixian	張繼先
zhangli	瘴癘
Zhangpu	漳浦
zhangqi	瘴氣
Zhang Qu	張渠
Zhang Rulin	張汝霖
Zhang Yingchang	張應昌
Zhangzhen	章軫
Zhang Zhicong	張志聰
Zhangzhou	漳州
Zhaoqing	肇慶
Zhao Qu	趙瞿
Zhaotong	昭通
Zhao Ying	趙瑛
Zhenghe	政和
Zheng Rong	鄭榮
Zhengtong Daozang	正統道藏
Zhengyi fawen jing zhangguan pin	正一法文經章官品
Zhennan	鎮南
Zhihui	智暉
zhiqiao	櫶殼
Zhiwen lu	咫聞錄
Zhiyan	智巖
Zhiyi xubian	志異續編
Zhong Hongliang	鍾宏亮
zhongdian di xiansuo diaocha	重點的線案調查
zhongguo	中國
Zhongguo laibing shi	中國癩病史
Zhongguo mafeng pifubing zazhi	中國麻風皮膚病雜誌
Zhongguo mafeng zazhi	中國麻風雜誌

Zhongguo yixue dacheng	中國醫學大成
Zhonghua mafeng jiuji hui	中華痲瘋救濟會
Zhonghua pifuke zazhi	中華皮膚科雜誌
zhong tu	中土
zhongtu ren	中土人
Zhong Xuanwen	鍾選文
Zhou Chufei	周處非
Zhou hou beiji fang	肘後備急方
Zhou Mi	周密
Zhou Xingsi	周興嗣
Zhou Yuan	周鵷
Zhou Zuoren	周作人
Zhu	朱
zhu	注
Zhubing yuanhou lun	諸病源候論
Zhubing yuan hou lun jiaozhu	諸病源侯論校注
zhulian	注連
Zhu Xiu	朱橚
Zhu Zhenheng	朱震亨
Zizhi tongjian	資治通鑑
zui yi chuanran	最易傳染

Bibliography

PRIMARY SOURCES

Anderson, W. H. P. "The World Leprosy Situation." *Chinese Medical Journal* 47 (1933): 223–226.

Anhui sheng zhi weisheng zhi (*Gazetteer of Anhui Province: On Public Health*). Hefei: Anhui renmin chubanshe, 1996.

Band, E. *Working His Purpose Out: The History of the English Presbyterian Mission, 1847–1947.* 1947. Reprint, Taipei; Ch'eng Wen, 1972.

Bei Qi shu (*History of the Northern Qi*). Taipei: Dingwen shuju, 1980.

Beishi (*History of the Northern Dynasties*). Taipei: Dingwen shuju, 1980.

Cantlie, J. "Report on the Conditions under Which Leprosy Occurs in China, Indo-China, Malaya, the Archipelago, and Oceania: Compiled Chiefly during 1894." In *Prize Essays on Leprosy,* 239–413. London: New Sydenham Society, 1897.

Changsun Wuji et al. *Tang lü shuyi* (*Interpretations of the Tang Code*). Taipei: Xinwenfeng shuju, 1986.

Changtaixian weisheng zhi, 1955–1994 (*Materials on Public Health in Changtai County, 1955–1994*). Changtai, 1998.

Changzhou shi weisheng zhi (*Materials on Public Health in Changzhou City*). 1989.

Chao Yuanfang. *Zhubing yuan hou lun jiaozhu* (*General Treatise on the Origins and Symptoms of Disorders*). Edited by Ding Guangdi. Beijing: Renmin weisheng chubanshe, 1996.

Chaozhou fu zhi (*Gazetteer of Chaozhou Prefecture*). 1893 (1762).

Chenghai xian zhi (*Gazetteer of Chenghai*). 1815.

Chen Huiyan. *Nanyue youji* (*Records on a Voyage in the Southern Yue Region*). 1851.

Chen Kun. *Lingnan zashi shi chao* (*Poems Related to Miscellaneous Matters in Guangdong Province*). Guangzhou: Yiyuanlou, 1876.

Chen Shiduo. *Shishi milu* (*Secret Record of the Stone Chamber*). Beijing: Zhongguo zhongyiyao chubanshe, 1986.

Chen Sicheng. *Meichuang milu* (*Secret Account of the "Corrupt Sores" Disorder*). Beijing: Xueyuan chubanshe, 1994. Based on the 1885 edition.

Chen Yan. *San yin ji yi bingzheng fang lun* (*A Treatise on the Three Categories of Pathogenic Factors of Disorders*). Wenyuange Siku quanshu edition. Taipei: Shangwu yinshuguan, 1983. Vol. 743.

Chen Yonghua. "Mafeng fangzhi zhong di chengbao zeren zhi" (Contract and Responsibility System in Leprosy Control). *Zhongguo mafeng zazhi* 2, no. 3 (1986): 49–50.

Chen Yuan. "Song Zheng xueshi zhi Bai Er Gen wanguo mafeng hui xu" (Preface to Bid Bon Voyage to Bachelor Zheng, Who Is Attending the International Conference on Leprosy in Bergen). In *Chen Yuan zaonian wenji* (*Early Writings by Chen Yuan*), 298–302. 1909. Reprint, Taipei: Academia Sinica, 1992.

Chen Zhiping and Ruan Qihao. "Di Li Ping zhushe ye zhiliao mafeng chubu liaoxiao guancha baogao" (Preliminary Report on the Observations of the First Results of the Injection of Di Li Ping). *Guangdong zhongyi* 6 (1960): 269–272.

Chijiao yisheng jiaocai: Gong beifang diqu cankao yong (*Teaching Handbook for Barefoot Doctors for the Northern Regions*). Jilin: Renmin weisheng chubanshe, 1977.

Chijiao yisheng jiaocai: Gong nanfang diqu cankao yong (*Teaching Handbook for Barefoot Doctors for the Southern Regions*). Shanghai: Renmin weisheng chubanshe, 1973.

China Medical Journal (CMJ). Shanghai: Medical Missionary Association of China, 1907–1931.

Chinese Medical Journal. Beijing: China Medical Assciation, 1932–.

Chinese Medical Missionary Journal (*CMMJ*) Shanghai: Kelly & Walsh, 1887–1907.

Chinese Repository. Canton: Printed for the proprietors, 1832–1851.

Chou Juchuan. *Yangcheng guchao* (*Old Manuscript of Canton City*). 1806. Reprint, Guangzhou: Guangdong renmin chubanshe, 1993.

Chunqiu Gongyang zhuan jiaokan ji (*Corrected Edition of the Gongyang Tradition of the "Spring and Autumn Annals"*). Edited by Ruan Yuan. Taipei: Yiwen yinshuju, 1959.

Cixi weisheng zhi (*Materials on Public Health in Cixi*). Ningpo: Ningpo chubanshe, 1994.

Da Dai liji (*Book of Rites by Elder Dai*). Sibu congkan edition. Shanghai: Shanghai shudian, 1989.

Dali Bai zu zizhizhou weisheng zhi (*Materials on Public Health in the Bai Autonomous Region in Dali*). Kunming: Yunnan minzu chubanshe, 1996.

Dali shi weisheng zhi (*Materials on Public Health in Dali City*). Kunming: Yunnan minzu chubanshe, 1992.

Dantu xian weisheng zhi (*Materials on Public Health in Dantu*). 2001.

Dayu xian zhi (*Gazetteer of Dayu*). 1748.

Dongguan xian zhi (*Gazetteer of Dongguan*). 1639.

Doolittle, J. *Social Life of the Chinese: With Some Account of Their Religious, Governmental, Educational, and Business Customs and Opinions; With Special but Not Exclusive Reference to Fuhchau.* New York: Harper, 1865. Reprint, Taipei: Cheng-wen, 1966.

Dou Menglin. *Chuangyang yingyan quanshu* (*Complete Book on Sores and Skin Diseases Based on Experience*). Kangxi edition. 1697.

Douthwaite, A. W. "Leprosy." *Chinese Medical Missionary Journal (CMMJ)* 4 (1892): 251–256.

Duan Yucai, ed. *Shuo wen jie zi* (*Etymological Dictionary*), by Xu Shen. Shanghai: Shanghai guji chubanshe, 1988.

Du Guangting, ed. *Taishang dongyuan shenzhou jing* (*Scriptures of Divine Incantations of the Abyssal Caverns*). In *Zhengtong Daozang* (*Orthodox Daoist Canon*). Taipei: Xinwenfeng chubanshe, 1985. Reprint of the 1607 long edition, based on the 1445 edition.

Durand-Fardel, M. "Pathologie médicale: La lèpre en Chine." *Gazette médicale de Paris* (1877). Vols. 26:318–319; 28:341–343; 30:367–368; 33:402–404; 34:414–415.

Fan Duan'ang. *Yue zhong jianwen* (*Things Seen and Heard in Guangdong*). 1730. Reprint, Guangzhou: Guangdong gaodeng jiaoyu, 1988.

Farwell, W. *The Chinese at Home and Abroad.* San Francisco: Bancroft, 1885.

Fayuan zhulin (*Forest of Gems in the Garden of Law*). Vol . 53 of *Taishō shinshū daizōkyō* (*The Tripitaka in Chinese*), edited by Takakusu Junjirō and Watanabe Kaigyoku. Tokyo: Taishō issaikyō kankōkai, 1924–1934. Reprint, Taipei: Xinwenfeng chuban gongsi, 1983.

Fengxin xian zhi (*Gazetteer of Fengxin*). 1824

Fowler, L. "Leprosy in China." *Chinese Recorder* 46, no. 4 (1915): 227–230.

Fozu lidai tongzai (*Records of Buddhas Throughout History*). In vol. 49 of *Taishō shinshū daizōkyō* (*The Tripitaka in Chinese*), edited by Takakusu Junjirō and Watanabe Kaigyoku. Tokyo: Taishō issaikyō kankōkai, 1924–1934. Reprint, Taipei: Xinwenfeng chuban gongsi, 1983–.

Fozu tongji (*General Biographies of Buddhas*). In vol. 49 of *Taishō shinshū daizōkyō* (*The Tripitaka in Chinese*), edited by Takakusu Junjirō and Watanabe Kaigyoku. Tokyo:

Taishō issaikyō kankōkai, 1924–1934. Reprint, Taipei: Xinwenfeng chuban gongsi, 1983–.

Fujian sheng weisheng zhi (*Gazetteer on Public Health in Fujian Province*). Fuzhou: Fujian sheng weisheng zhi bianzhuan weiyuanhui, 1989.

Fujian sheng zhi weisheng zhi (*Part on Public Health of the Gazetteer of Fujian Province*). Beijing: Zhonghua shuju, 1995.

Fujian tongzhi (*General Gazetteer of Fujian*). 1737.

Fujian tongzhi (*General Gazetteer of Fujian*). 1868.

Gansu sheng zhi (*Gazetteer of Gansu Province*). Vol. 67, *Yiyao weisheng zhi* (*On Medicine and Public Health*). Lanzhou: Gansu wenhua chubanshe, 1999.

Gaoyao xian zhi (*Gazetteer of Gaoyao*). 1826.

Ge Hong. *Zhou hou beiji fang* (*Handy Recipes for Urgent Use*). Beijing: Renmin weisheng chubanshe, 1983. Based on the Ming Wanli edition.

Gengdao ji (*Collected Texts on the Way of Refining Gold*). In *Daozang yaoji xuankan* (*Selections of Important Texts in the Daoist Canon*), 9: 63–134. Shanghai: Shanghai guji chubanshe, 1989.

Gong Tingxian. *Jishi quanshu* (*A Complete Book to Save the World*). 1616. Reprint, Beijing: Zhongguo zhongyiyao chubanshe, 1999.

Gordon, C. A., comp. *An Epitome of the Reports of the Medical Officers to the Chinese Imperial Maritime Customs Service, from 1871 to 1882: With Chapters on the History of Medicine in China; Materia Medica; Epidemics; Famine; Ethnology; and Chronology in Relation to Medicine and Public Health.* London: Baillière, Tindell, and Cox, 1884.

Gray, J. *China: A History of the Laws, Manners and Customs of the People.* London: Macmillan, 1878. Reprint, New York: AMS Press, 1974.

——. *Walks in the City of Canton.* Hong Kong: De Souza, 1875.

Guangdong sheng weisheng ting pifu xing bing fangzhi chu (Unit of Venereal Disease and Skin Disease Control of the Department of Public Health of Guangdong Province). "Mafeng bingren chu yuan cun (huifu jiankang) biaozhun" (Criteria for the Release of Patients of Leprosy from Hospitals and Villages After They Have Recovered Their Health). *Pifu xing bing fangzhi tongxun* 1, no. 1 (1962): 2–3.

Guangdong tongzhi (*General Gazetteer of Guangdong*). 1864.

Guang hong ming ji (*The Enlarged Hong Ming Collection*). In vol. 52 of *Taishō shinshū daizōkyō* (*The Tripitaka in Chinese*), edited by Takakusu Junjirō and Watanabe Kaigyoku. Tokyo: Taishō issaikyō kankōkai, 1924–1934. Reprint, Taipei: Xinwenfeng chuban gongsi, 1983–.

Guangxi tongzhi: Yiliao weisheng zhi (*General History of Guangxi Province: On Medicine and Public Health*). Nanning: Guangxi renmin chubanshe, 1999.

Guerra, F. *El hospital en Hispanoamérica y Filipinas, 1492–1898*. Madrid: Ministerio de Sanidad y Consumo, 1994.

Guiot, L. *La mission du Su-Tchuen au 18e siècle* (*The Mission in Sichuan Province in the Eighteenth Century*). Paris: Téqui, 1892.

Guo Aichun, ed. *Huangdi neijing lingshu* (*The Yellow Emperor's Inner Canon: Celestial Lancets*). Tianjin: Tianjin kexue chubanshe, 1992.

Guoshi bu (*Supplement to the History of the Dynasty*). In *Biji xiaoshuo daguan*, ser. 21, vol. 2. Taipei: Xinxing shuju, 1977.

Gu Shicheng. *Yangyi daquan* (*Complete Book on the Medicine for Sores*). Shanghai: Shanghai guji chubanshe, 1997. Facsimile of the 1760 Gushi mishu edition.

Gu Zhentao. *Wumen biao yin* (*Record of Obscure Things in the Wu Area*). Nanjing: Jiangsu guji chubanshe, 1999.

"Hangzhou Songmu chang Guangji mafeng yiyuan yuanwu jieshao" (An Introduction to the Situation of the Leper Asylum of the Hangzhou Guangji Hospital at Pine Grove). Around 1950, mimeographed, kept at the Wukang leper village.

Han Shu (*The Book of Han*). Taipei: Dingwen shuju, 1981.

Hanyang xian zhi (*Gazetteer of Hanyang*). 1868.

He Biao. "Jixu guzhu ganjing wei quan jian xingbing, kongzhi mafeng er douzheng" (Continue to Strive in Order to Eliminate Venereal Disease, and to Control Leprosy). *Renmin baojian* 3 (1959): 199–210

Henan sheng zhi weisheng zhi (*Gazetteer of Henan Province: On Public Health*). Zhengzhou: Henan renmin chubanshe, 1993.

He Wei [Yuan]. *Chun zhu jiwen* (*Records of Things Heard on a Spring Islet*). Shanghai: Shanghai shudian, 1990.

Hobson, B. "On the Leprosy of the Chinese: Letter from Dr. Hobson." *Medical Times and Gazette* (London) 1 (June 2, 1860): 558–559.

Hou Hanshu (*Book of the Later Han*). Taipei: Dingwen shuju, 1979.

Huang Huakai. "Shaoguan mafeng fangzhi shiji" (On the History of Leprosy Control in Shaoguan). In *Shaoguan wenxian ziliao* (*Historical Materials on Shaoguan*). Vols. 1–2. 1983.

Huang Zhangjian, ed. *Ming shilu* (*A Veritable Record of the Ming*). Taipei: Institute of History and Philology, Academia Sinica, 1984.

Hubei sheng zhi: Weisheng zhi xia (*Gazetteer of Hubei Province, 2: On Public Health*). Wuhan: Hubei renmin chubanshe, 2000.

Huizenga, L. "Fourth International Leprosy Congress." *Leper Quarterly* 12, no. 2 (1938): 79–85.

(Hunan sheng) Anhua xian weisheng zhi (*Materials on Public Health of Anhua County of Hunan Province*). Anhua, 1989.

Hunan sheng zhi: Yiyao weisheng zhi (*Gazetteer on Medicine and Public Health of Hunan Province*). Changsha: Hunan renmin chubanshe, 1988.

Hunyuan shengji (*Annals of the Sage of Undifferentiated Beginning*). In vol. 30 of *Zhengtong Daozang* (*Orthodox Daoist Canon*), 1–160. Taipei: Xinwenfeng chubanshe, 1985. Reprint of the 1607 long edition, based on the 1445 edition.

Hutchinson, J. *On Leprosy and Fish-Eating: A Statement of Facts and Explanations*. London: Archibald Constable, 1906.

Jarossay, E. *Une âme d'apôtre, Mgr Foucard, du diocèse d'Orléans, premier évêque de Kouang-si'(Chine), 1830–1889*. Orléans: Séjourné, 1907.

Jefferys, W. H., and J. L. Maxwell. *The Diseases of China: Including Formosa and Korea*. Philadelphia: Blakiston's, 1911.

Jiangdu xian weisheng zhi (*Gazetteer on Public Health of Jiangdu*). Nanjing: Jiangsu kexue jishu chubanshe, 1992.

Jiangsu sheng zhi weisheng zhi (*Gazetteer of Jiangsu Province: On Public Health*). Nanjing: Jiangsu guji chubanshe, 1999.

Jiangxi sheng zhi: Jiangxi sheng weisheng zhi (*Gazetteer of Public Health of Jiangxi Province*). Hefei: Huangshan shushe, 1997.

Jiangxi tongzhi (*General Gazetteer of Jiangxi*). Taipei: Shangwu yinshuguan, 1983. Siku quanshu edition, based on the 1732 edition.

Jiangxi zhongyiyao (*Journal of Chinese Medicine of Jiangxi Province*) 4, nos. 1–2 (1952).

Jiashan xian Sishan cun Yiyuan "Yuanzhi" bianxie zu (Editorial Group on the "History of the Sishan Village Hospital"), ed. *Anhui sheng Jiashan xian Sishan cun yiyuan zhi (1956–1986)* (*Hospital Gazetteer of Sishan Village of Jiashan County in Anhui Province, 1956–1986*). Jiashan, 1986.

Jieyang xian weisheng zhi (*Materials on Public Health in Jieyang*). Guangzhou: Guangdong renmin chubanshe, 1992.

Jihong, ed. *Lingnan weisheng fang* (*Life-Preserving Recipes for the Lingnan Region*). Beijing: Zhongyi guji chubanshe, 1983. Facsimile of the1841 Japanese edition.

Jingde chuan deng lu (*The Transmission of the Lamp of the Jingde Era*). In vol. 51 of *Taishō shinshū daizōkyō* (*The Tripitaka in Chinese*), edited by Takakusu Junjirō and Watanabe Kaigyoku. Tokyo: Taishō issaikyō kankōkai, 1924–1934. Reprint, Taipei: Xinwenfeng chuban gongsi, 1983–.

Jingning xian zhi (*Gazetteer of Jingning*). 1872.

Jinjiang xian zhi (*Gazetteer of Jinjiang*). 1765.

Ji Yun. *Yueweicao tang biji* (*Notes on the "Yueweicao" Study*). Chengdu: Bashu shushe, 1995.

Kaiping xian weisheng zhi, 1885–1985 (*Materials on Public Health in Kaiping, 1885–1985*). 1988.

Kunming weisheng zhi (*Gazetteer of Public Health of Kunming*). Kunming: Yunnan renmin chubanshe, 1998.

Lagarde. "Lettre de M. Lagarde, conseiller de la Légation de France en Chine, à M. Wilden, ministre, Canton, le 17 juillet, 1932 , sur la léproserie de Chéklong." Archives du Ministère des Affaires Étrangères, France, série SND, vol. 1583.

Lai Shanghe. *Zhongguo laibing shi* (*The History of the* Lai *Disease in China*). Taipei, 1952.

Lamson, H. *Social Pathology in China: A Source Book for the Study of Problems of Livelihood, Health, and the Family.* Shanghai: Commercial Press, 1935. Reprint, Taipei: Ch'eng Wen, 1974.

Leizhou xian zhi (*Gazetteer of Leizhou*). 1614.

Leprosy Mission. *The Spreading Tree: The Story of the Leprosy Mission from 1918 to 1970.* London: Leprosy Mission, 1974.

Lewis, T. R., and. D. D. Cunningham. *Leprosy in India: A Report.* Calcutta: Office of the Superintendent of Government Printing, 1877.

Liancheng xian zhi (*Gazetteer of Liancheng*). 1938.

Liang Gongchen. *Beidong yuan bilu* (*Notes of the Northeastern Garden*). Kaifeng: Xu Yi wenzhai, 1866. Series 4, vol. 8.

Liang Shaoren. *Liangban qiuyu an suibi* (*Random Notes in the Autumn Rain Study*). 1837. Reprint, Shanghai: Guji chubanshe, 1982. Based on the 1895 edition.

Liang Tingnan. *Yifen wenji* (*Records of Things Heard in an Atmosphere of Barbarism*). Beijing: Zhonghua shuju, 1959.

Li Gao. *Dongyuan yiji* (*Medical Works of Li Gao*). Beijing: Renmin weisheng chubanshe, 1993.

Li Jing et al., trans. *Tangling shiyi* (*Supplementary Amplifications of the Tang Code*), by Niida Noboru. Changchun: Changchun chubanshe, 1989.

Li Junchang. "Zhongguo di mafeng wenti" (The Leprosy Problem in China). *MFJK* 1, no. 3 (1927): 3–11.

Li Lian. *Yi shi* (*History of Medicine*). Xiamen: Xiamen daxue chubanshe, 1992.

Li Shizhen. *Bencao gangmu.* Taipei: Wenguang tushu gongsi, 1955. Facsimile of the 1885 Guangxu edition.

Liu Botang and Liu Zhongru. "Mafeng zheng gailun"(A General Discussion on Leprosy). *Guangdong yiyao yuebao* 1, no. 2 (1929): 4–10.

Liu Chun, ed. *Yuji weiyi* (*The Subtle Meanings of the Precious Machine*), by Xu Yanchun. 1396. In *Liu Chun yixue quanshu.* Beijing: Zhongguo zhongyiyao chubanshe, 1999. Based on the 1439 edition.

Liu Hengrui [Jiren]. *Fuxie xinshu* (*A New Book for Overcoming Pathogens*). In vol. 4 of *Zhongguo yixue dacheng.* Changsha: Yuelu shushe, 1990.

Liu Wansu. *Suwen bingji qi yi baoming ji* (*Lifesaving Book on the Pathogenesis and Qi Mechanism of "Plain Questions"*). In *Congshu jicheng xinbian.* Taipei: Xinwenfeng chuban gongsi, 1985. Vol. 45.

Liu Xiang. *Lienü zhuan* (*Biographies of Virtuous Women*). Taipei: Guangwen shuju, 1981. Reprint of the 1591 illustrated edition.

——. *Zhanguo ce* (*Record of the Warring States*). Shanghai: Guji chubanshe, 1978.

Liu Xu. *Jiu Tang shu* (*Old Book on the Tang Dynasty*). Taipei: Wending shuju, 1979.

Li Zuwei. "Laibing yange shuo lue" (Brief History of Leprosy). *Xin yiyao* 4, no. 7 (1934): 1007–1022.

Ljungstedt, A. *An Historical Sketch of the Portuguese Settlements in China: And of the Roman Catholic Church and Mission in China.* Hong Kong: Viking, 1992. Reprint of the 1836 edition.

Lockhart, W. *Medical Missionary in China.* London: Hurst and Blackett, 1861.

Longxi xian zhi (*Gazetteer of Longxi*). 1762.

"Luoding xian gongshe ban mafeng cun di shijian" (Experience of the Organization of the Leper Village of the Luoding Commune). *Xing bing mafeng fangyan gongzuo* 4 (1959): 31–32.

Lu Shizhong. *Wushang xuanyuan santian yutang dafa* (*Great Method of the Jade Hall of the Three Heavens, of the Supreme Mysterious Origin*). 30 *juan,* ca. 1158. In vol. 30 of *Zhonghua Daozang* (*Orthodox Daoist Canon*), edited by Zhang Jiyu. Beijing: Huaxia chubanshe, 2004.

Lu Yitian. *Lenglu yihua* (*Medical Talks by Lu Yitian*). Taiyuan: Shanxi kexue jishu chubanshe, 1993.

Mafeng jikan (*Leper Quarterly*). Shanghai: Chinese Mission to Lepers, 1927–1944.

Manson, P. *Tropical Diseases: A Manual of the Diseases of Warm Climates.* 1898. 6th ed., London: Cassell, 1918.

Maxwell, J. "Leprosy in China." *Chinese Recorder* 64 (1933): 544–545.

——. "Ridding China of Leprosy." *China Medical Journal* 44 (1930): 759–767.

——. "Zhongguo mafeng yu yimin wenti" (Leprosy in China and the Question of Emigration). Translated by Hong Zhongdao. *MFJK* 4, no. 2 (1930): 2–4.

Medical Reports (of the Imperial Maritime Customs). Shanghai: Statistical Department of the Inspectorate General, 1871–1911.

Mission to Lepers Hong Kong Auxiliary. *Annual Reports.* London: Mission to Lepers, 1951–1953.

Mitsuda Kensuke. *Mitsuda Kensuke to Nihon no rai yobō jigyū: Rai yobōhō gojūshūnen kinen* (*Mitsuda Kensuke and Japan's Leprosy Prevention Enterprise: Fiftieth Anniversary of the Leprosy Prevention Law*). Tokyo: Tōfū kyōkai, 1958.

Modengxian zhai zhuren. *Bing yu yuan chuanqi* (*Drama of the Love Story of the Sick Beauty*). Shanghai: Zhonghua shuju, 1932. Includes 1913 preface; first edition, 1907.

Mouritz, A. A. *The Path of the Destroyer: A History of Leprosy in the Hawaiian Islands and Thirty Years Research into the Means by Which It Has Been Spread.* Honolulu: Honolulu Star-Bulletin, 1916.

Nagamata Yoshirō, trans. "Mafeng" (Leprosy) *Yiyao pinglun* 84 (1932):19–30.

Nan'an fu zhi buzheng (*Supplementary Gazetteer of Nan'an Prefecture*). 1875.

Nanchang fu zhi (*Gazetteer of Nanchang Prefecture*). 1873.

Nanchang xian weisheng zhi (*Materials on Public Health in Nanchang*). Nanchang, 1988.

Nanhai xian zhi (*Gazetteer of Nanhai*). 1609.

Nanhai xian zhi (*Gazetteer of Nanhai*). 1691.

Nanning shi weisheng zhi (*Gazetteer on Public Health in Nanning City*) Nanning: Nanning shi weisheng ju, 1996. Internal document.

Nanshi (*History of the Southern Dynasties*). Taipei: Dingwen shuju, 1980.

Nantong xian weisheng zhi (*Materials on Public Health in Nantong*). 1988.

Neige daku [NGDK] (Archives of the Grand Secretariat), Ming-Qing Archives of the Institute of History and Philology, Academia Sinica, Taipei.

Newman, G., E. Ehlers, and S. Impey. *Prize Essays on Leprsoy.* London: New Sydenham Society, 1895.

Oribase. *Oeuvres d'Oribase.* Edited by U. C. Bussemaker and C. Daremberg. Paris: Imprimerie Impériale, 1862.

Pu Songling. *Xingshi yinyuan* (*Marital Relations Awakening the World*). Taipei: Lianjing chubanshe, 1986.

Qian dongnan Miaozu Dongzu zizhi zhouzhi weisheng zhi (*Gazetteer of Public Health in the Autonomous Regions of the Miao and the Dong in Southeastern Guizhou*). Guiyang: Guizhou renmin chubanshe, 1993.

Qi Kun. *Waike dacheng* (*General Work on External Medicine*). Shanghai: Shanghai weisheng chubanshe, 1957.

Qingchao wenxian tongkao (*Official Documents of the Qing Dynasty*). 1936. Reprint, Taipei: Shangwu yinshuguan, 1987.

Qingchengzi. *Zhiyi xubian* (*Sequel to the Account of Extraordinary Things*). Early Qing facsimile in *Biji xiaoshuo daguan,* ser. 1, vol. 6. Taipei: Xinxing shuju, 1962.

Qingdai Aomen zhongwen dangan huibian (Collection of Chinese Archival Materials on Macao in the Qing Period). Macao: Aomen jijin hui, 1999.

Qu Dajun. *Guangdong xinyu* (*New Stories on Guangdong Province*). Beijing: Zhongguo shuju, 1985.

Report on Leprosy by the Royal College of Physicians. London: George Edward Eyre and William Spottiswoode, 1867.

Rongchang xian weisheng zhi (*Materials on Public Health in Rongchang*). Rongchang, 1988.

Sakura Magozou. *Minfeng zaji* (*Miscellaneous Records of Fujian Customs*). Fuzhou: Meihua shuju, 1904.

Sanshui xian weisheng zhi (*Gazetteer on Public Health in Sanshui*). Sanshui: Sanshui xian weisheng ju xiuzhi bangongshi, 1989.

Shanxi tongzhi: Weisheng yiyao zhi; Weisheng bian (*Volume on Public Health, "Medicine and Public Health" Section, General Gazetteer of Shanxi Province*). Beijing: Zhonghua shuju, 1997.

Shaowu fu zhi (*Gazetteer of Shaowu Prefecture*). 1900.

Sha xian zhi (*Gazetteer of Sha*). 1928.

Shengji zonglu (*General Record of Imperial Charity*). 1962. Reprint, Beijing: Renmin weisheng chubanshe, 1992.

Shengzu Ren Huangdi [Kangxi] shilu (*Veritable Records of the Reign of Emperor Kangxi*). Taipei: Huawen yinshuguan, 1969.

Shen Zhiwen. *Jiewei yuansou* (*Sources of Relief*). Shanghai: Shanghai guji chubanshe, 1997. Facsimile of the 1816 Wuxi edition.

Shizong Xian Huangdi [Yongzheng] shilu (*Veritable Records of the Reign of Emperor Yongzheng*). Taipei: Huawen yinshuguan, 1969.

Shouyu shenfang (*Miraculous Recipes for Achieving Longevity*). In *Yifang leiju* (*Compilation of Medical Recipes by Kind*). Beijing: Renmin weisheng chubanshe, 1981. Based on the 1852 Japanese edition.

Si fen lü (*The Four-Part Regulations*). In vol. 22 of *Taishō shinshū daizōkyō* (*The Tripitaka in Chinese*), edited by Takakusu Junjirō and Watanabe Kaigyoku. Tokyo: Taishō issaikyō kankōkai, 1924–1934. Reprint, Taipei: Xinwenfeng chuban gongsi, 1983–.

Sima Guang. *Zizhi tongjian* (*Comprehensive Mirror to Aid in Government*). Beijing: Guji chubanshe, 1956. Based on the thirteenth-century Yuan annotated edition.

Sima Qian. *Shiji* (*Records of the Grand Historian*). Beijing: Zhonghua shuju, 1982.

Song Lian. *Yuanshi* (*History of the Yuan Dynasty*). Taipei: Dingwen shuju, 1980.

Su Che. *Longchuan lue zhi* (*A Brief History of Longchuan*). Beijing: Zhonghua shuju, 1982.

Sun Simiao. *Beiji qianjin yaofang* (*Essential Recipes for Urgent Use Worthy of a Thousand Gold Pieces*). Beijing: Renmin weisheng chubanshe, 1982. Reprint of the Edo igaku facsimile of the Northern Song edition.

——. *Qianjin yifang* (*Supplementary Recipes Worthy of a Thousand Gold Pieces*). Beijing: Renmin weisheng chubanshe, 1955. Based on the 1307 edition.

Taiping shenghui fang (*Recipes of the Imperial Grace During the Great Peace*). Taipei: Xinwenfeng chuban gongsi, 1969. Facsimile of the Japanese manuscript edition, National Central Library).

Taiping yulan (*Imperial Overview of the Era of Great Peace* [976–983]). Taipei: Shangwu yinshuguan, 1975. Facsimile of the 1922 Sibu congkan edition).

Taishang zhuguo jiumin zongzhen biyao (*Secret Essentials of the Highest Zhenren Assisting the Country and Saving the People*). In vol. 54 of *Zhengtong Daozang* (*Orthodox Daoist Canon*). Taipei: Xinwenfeng chubanshe, 1985. Reprint of the 1607 long edition, based on the 1445 edition.

Taishō shinshū daizōkyō (*The Tripitaka in Chinese*). Edited by Takakusu Junjirō and Watanabe Kaigyoku. Tokyo: Taishō issaikyō kankōkai, 1924–1934. Reprint, Taipei: Xinwenfeng chuban gongsi, 1983–.

Tan Dihua, ed. *Guangdong beike ji* (*Texts on Steles in Guangdong Province*). Guangzhou: Guangdong gaodeng jiaoyu chubanshe, 2001.

Thompson, J. A. "Contribution to the History of Leprosy in Australia." In *Prize Essays on Leprosy*, 1–238. London: New Sydenham Society, 1897.

——. "Leprosy in Hawaii: A Critical Enquiry." In *Mittheilungen und Verhandlungen der internationalen wissenschaftlichen Lepra-Conferenz zu Berlin im October 1897.* Berlin, 1897–1898), part 2:274–281.

"Troisième conférence internationale scientifique de la lèpre, Strasbourg, 28–31 juillet 1923," sect. 1, "Résolutions." *BIUM: Histoire de la médecine, et de l'art dentaire*, http://web2.bium.univ-paris5.fr/livanc/ (accessed March 24, 2008).

Tuotuo. *Songshi* (*History of the Song Dynasty*). Taipei: Dingwen shuju, 1979.

Van den Wyngaert, A., ed. *Sinica Franciscana: Relationes et Epistolas Fratrum Minorum Saeculi XVII et XVIII.* Florence: Collegium S. Bonaventurae, 1942.

Waley, A. *The Analects of Confucius.* London: Allen and Unwin, 1938. Reprint, Taipei: Jinshan tushu chubanshe, 1970.

Wang Daokun. *Taihan ji* (*Collection of Writings by Wang Daokun*). 1591 Wanli edition.

Wang Linheng. *Yue jian lu* (*Records on Guangdong*). Beijing: Zhonghua shuju, 1987. Based on the 1601 Wanli edition.

Wang Ming, ed. *Taiping jing hejiao* (*Collated Edition of the Taiping Canon*). Beijing: Zhonghua shuju, 1960.

Wang Tao. *Waitai miyao fang* (*Secret Essentials from the Imperial Collections*). Osaka: Toyo igaku, 1981.

Wang Zhi. *Changshi yu* (*Pronouncements on Things Tried*). 1800 engraving, with 1762 preface.

Watson, B., trans. *Chuang Tzu: Basic Writings.* New York: Columbia University Press, 1968.

"Weisheng gongzuo dayaojin quanmin juban mafeng cun" (Great Leap Forward in Public Health: The Entire People Organize Leper Villages). *Mafeng bing fangzhi jianbao* (*Bulletin of Leprosy Control*) (Shandong province). Vols. 9–10 (1958).

Wei Zheng. *Suishu* (*Book of the Sui Dynasty*). Taipei: Dingwen shuju, 1980.

Wong Foon [Huang Kuan]. "Dr. F. Wong's Memorandum on Leprosy." In "Medical Reports for the Half Year Ended 30th September 1873, Forwarded by the Surgeons to the Customs at the Treaty Ports of China: Being No. 6 of the Series and Forming the Sixth Part of the Customs Gazette for July-September 1873," 41–51. Shanghai: Imperial Maritime Customs Statistical Department, 1874.

Wright, H. P. *Leprosy: An Imperial Danger.* London: Churchill, 1889.

Wu Chichang. *Xu kechuang xianhua* (*Sequel to "Miscellaneous Stories Told by Guests"*). Beijing: Wenhua yishu chubanshe, 1988.

Wu Jianren. *Ershi nian mudu zhi guai xianzhuang* (*Strange Phenomena Observed During the Past Twenty Years*). Taipei: Guangya chuban youxian gongsi, 1984. Based on the 1909 edition.

Wu Qian et al. *Yizong jinjian* (*Golden Mirror of Medical Orthodoxy*). Beijing: Renmin weisheng chubanshe, 1990. Based on the 1742 Wuyingdian edition.

Wuxian weisheng zhi (*Materials on Public Health in Wuxian*). Shanghai: Shanghai shehui kexue yuan chubanshe, 1992.

Wuxi Jingui xian zhi (*Gazetteer of Wuxi and Jingui*). 1813.

Wu Youxing. *Wenyi lun buzheng* (*Treatise on Epidemics Caused by the Warm Factor, with Supplementary Verifications*). Taipei: Xinwenfeng shuju, 1985. Facsimile of the 1895 edition by Zheng Chongguang.

Wu Zhenfang. *Lingnan zaji* (*Miscellaneous Records on the Lingnan Region*). In *Biji xiaoshuo daguan*, ser. 3, vol. 10. Taipei: Xinxing shuju, 1974.

Xianchuan waike bifang (*Secret Formulas of External Medicine Transmitted by Immortals*). In *Daozang yaoji xuankan* (*Selections of Important Texts in the Daoist Canon*), 9:589–598. Shanghai: Shanghai guji chubanshe, 1989.

Xianyuan bianzhu (*Garden of Immortals: A Pearl Treasury*). In vol. 18 of *Zhengtong Daozang* (*Orthodox Daoist Canon*), 411–447. Taipei: Xinwenfeng chubanshe, 1985. Reprint of the 1607 long edition, based on the 1445 edition.

Xiao Xiaoting. *Fengmen quanshu* (*A Complete Work on the Feng Disorder*). Guangzhou: Jingye tang. 1845 engraving of the 1836 Wu Yunlou edition.

——. *Fengmen quanshu.* Zhenben yishu jicheng. Beijing: Zhongguo yiyao chubanshe, 1999.

Xing bing mafeng fangyan gongzuo (*Bulletin on the Prevention and Research of Venereal Disease and Leprosy*). Vol. 3 (1959).

Xingke tiben (*Documents of the Ministry of Punishment*), Number 1 Archives (Ming-Qing dynasties), Beijing.

Xinhua xian yiyao weisheng kexue yanjiusuo (Research Institute of Public Health Science of Xinhua County). "Daxue teng heji zhiliao shi li mafeng bing di chubu liaoxiao guancha baodao" (Report on the Observations on the Therapeutic Efficacy of *Caulis Sargentodoxae* Used in Recipes to Treat Ten Cases of Leprosy). *Guangdong zhongyi* 5, no. 7 (1960): 322–324.

Xinhui xian zhi (*Gazetteer of Xinhui*). 1690.

Xiong Dongliang. "Tianzhujiao Kangding jiaoqu Moximian mafeng yuan shilue ji qi jiefang hou jianzhi yange" (The History of the Leper Asylum in Moximian of the Kangding Diocese and Its Reforms after the Liberation). Unpublished document, June 1995.

Xuan Ding. "Mafeng nü Qiu Liyu chuanqi" (Story of Qiu Liyu, the *Mafeng* Girl). In *Yeyu qiudeng lu* (*Records of Night Rain and Autumn Lamp*). Reprinted in *Bing yu yuan chuanqi* (*Drama of the Love Story of the Sick Beauty*). Shanghai: Zhonghua shuju, 1932. Includes 1913 preface; first editon, 1907.

Xu Chunfu. *Gujin yitong daquan* (*A Complete Book of Old and New Medical Traditions*). 10 vols. Taipei: Xinwenfeng chubanshe, 1978. Facsimile of the 1570 Ming edition.

Xu Dachun. *Xu ping waike zhengzong* (*Comments by Xu Dachun on Chen Shigong's "Orthodoxy of External Medicine"*). Vol. 5 of *Zhongguo yixue dacheng*, edited by Cao Bingzhang. Changsha: Yuelu, 1990.

Xu Dong, ed. *Muling shu* (*Collected Writings by Magistrates*). 1838.

Xue Ji. *Liyang jiyao* (*Keys and Essentials to Skin Disorders of the* Li *Category*). In vol. 1 of *Xue shi yi an xuan* (*Selections of Xue Ji's Medical Cases*). Beijing: Renmin weisheng chubanshe, 1986.

Xu gao seng zhuan (*Further Biographies of Eminent Monks*). In vol. 50 of *Taishō shinshū daizōkyō* (*The Tripitaka in Chinese*), edited by Takakusu Junjirō and Watanabe Kaigyoku. Tokyo: Taishō issaikyō kankōkai, 1924–1934. Reprint, Taipei: Xinwenfeng chuban gongsi, 1983–.

Xu Hao. *Fuzhai riji* (*Diary of Xu Hao*). In *Ming-Qing shiliao huikan,* ser. 8, vol. 4. Taipei: Wenhai shuju, 1967–1969.

Xu Ke. *Qing bai lei chao* (*Collection of Popular Customs of the Qing*). 1917. Reprint, Beijing: Zhonghua shuju, 1984.

Xu Yuanrui. *Lixue zhinan* (*Instructions to Bureaucrats*). *Juan* 15 of *Jujia biyong shilei* (*Necessary Things in Daily Life*). Taipei: Zhongwen chubanshe, 1984. Facsimile of the 1673 Japanese print of the Ming edition.

Yan Bingchang. "Zhenjiu liaofa yingyong yu mafeng bing suo yinqi di shenjing fanying xing shenjing tong ji houyizheng di yidian tihui" (Some Observations on the Application of Acupuncture in Treating Pain of the Nerves Caused by Leprosy and Its Side Effects). *Guangdong zhongyi* 2 (1957): 7–9.

Yang Shiying. *Renzhai zhizhi* (*Easy and Direct Formulas of Mr. Yang Shiying*). Siku quanshu wenyuange edition. Taipei: Shangwu yinshuguan, 1983. Vol. 744.

Yan Yuan. *Yan Yuan ji* (*Collected Writings of Yan Yuan*). Beijing: Zhonghua shuju, 1987.

Yan Zhitui. *Yanshi jiaxun* (*Family Precepts of the Yan Lineage*). Shanghai: Guji chubanshe, 1980.

Yao Silian. *Liangshu* (*Book of the Liang Dynasty*). Taipei: Dingwen shuju, 1980.

Yifang leiju (*A Collection of Medical Recipes*). 1861. Reprint, Beijing: Renmin weisheng chubanshe, 1981.

Yili zhushu (*Annotations of Etiquette and Ceremonies*). Taipei: Yiwen yinshuju, 1955. Based on the 1815 edition.

Yin Guangren and Zhang Rulin. *Aomen jilue* (A Sketch of the History of Macao). 1751. Reprint, Guangzhou: Guangdong gaodeng jiaoyu chubanshe, 1988.

Yongna Jushi. *Zhiwen lu* (*Records of Things Heard from Near and from Afar*). In *Biji xiaoshuo daguan,* ser. 2, vol. 6. 1817. Reprint, Taipei: Xinxing shuju, 1978. Based on the 1817 edition.

Yu Bin. *Xu yishuo* (*Sequel to "On Medicine"*). Shanghai: Shanghai kexue jishu chubanshe, 1984. Reprint of the 1598 Japanese edition.

Yunji qiqian (*Bookcase of the Clouds with the Seven Labels*). In vol. 38 of *Zhengtong Daozang* (*Orthodox Daoist Canon*). Taipei: Xinwenfeng chubanshe, 1985. Reprint of the 1607 long edition, based on the 1445 edition.

Zengcheng xian zhi (*Gazetteer of Zengcheng*). 1801.

Zeng Huichou. "Wo wanquan tongyi dongyuan rucun buyao kuada xuanchuan" (I Totally Agree That We Should Not Exaggerate the Propaganda to Mobilize Patients to Enter [Leper] Villages). *Mafeng bing fangzhi jianbao* 2, no. 3 (1958): 73.

Zhang Congzheng. *Rumen shiqin* (*How Confucian Scholars Should Care for Their Parents*). In *Zihe yiji,* edited by Deng Tietao et al. Beijing: Renmin weisheng chubanshe, 1994.

Zhanghua xian zhi (*Gazetteer of Zhanghua*). Daoguan edition. In *Taiwan wenxian congkan,* no. 156. Taipei: Taiwan yinhang jingji yanjiushi, 1962.

Zhang Jiebin. *Jingyue quanshu* (*The Complete Works of Zhang Jiebin*). Shanghai: Shanghai kexue jishu chubanshe, 1991. Facsimile of the 1711 Kangxi edition.

Zhang Qu. *Yuedong wenjian lu* (*A Record of Things Heard and Seen in Eastern Guangdong*). Guangzhou: Guangdong gaodeng jiaoyu chubanshe, 1990. Preface, 1739.

Zhang Tingyu. *Ming shi* (*History of the Ming Dynasty*). Taipei: Dingwen shuju, 1979.

Zhang Yingchang, ed. *Qing shiduo* (*Collection of Qing Poems*). Beijing: Zhonghua shuju, 1960.

Zhang Zhicong. *Huangdi nei jing suwen ji zhu* (*Annotated Plain Questions of the "Yellow Emperor's Inner Canon"*). Vol. 1 of *Zhongguo yixue dacheng,* edited by Cao Bingzhang. Shanghai: Shanghai kexue chubanshe, 1990.

Zhao Erxun et al., eds. *Qing shi gao* (*Draft of the History of the Qing Dynasty*). Taipei: Hongshi chubanshe, 1981.

Zhengtong Daozang (*Orthodox Daoist Canon*). Taipei: Xinwenfeng chubanshe, 1985. Reprint of the 1607 long edition, based on the 1445 edition.

Zhengyi fawen jingzhang guanpin (*Chapter on Petitions and Officials of the Zhengyi Canon*). In vol. 48 of *Zhengtong Daozang* (*Orthodox Daoist Canon*). Taipei: Xinwenfeng chubanshe, 1985. Reprint of the 1607 long edition, based on the 1445 edition.

Zhou Mi. *Guixin zashi* (*Miscellaneous Writings in the Guixin Neighborhood*). Beijing: Zhonghua shuju,1988.

Zhou Qufei. *Lingwai daida* (*Answers to Questions on the Deep South*). Shanghai: Gushu liutong chu, 1921. Reprint, Taipei: Xingzhong shuju, 1964.

Zhoushan shi weisheng zhi (*Materials on Public Health of Zhoushan City*). Beijing: Zhonghua shuju, 2002.

Zhou Zuoren. "Tan guolai" (On the Custom of Passing on *Lai*). In *Bing zhu ye tan* (*Night Talks in Front of a Lit Candle*), 89–96. Shijiazhuang: Hebei jiaoyu chubanshe, 2002.

Zhu Xiu. *Puji fang* (*Recipes for General Relief*). Taipei: Taiwan shangwu yinshuguan, 1983.

Zhu Zhenheng. *Danxi yiji* (*Medical Works of Zhu Zhenheng*). Beijing: Renmin weisheng chubanshe, 1993.

Zuohua san ren. *Feng liu wu* (*Reflections After Amorous Encounters*). Facsimile of ca. mid-eighteenth century editon. Shanghai: Shanghai guji chubanshe, 1990.

SECONDARY SOURCES

Acton, H., and Lee Yi-hsieh, trans. *Glue and Lacquer.* London: Golden Cockerel Press, 1941.

Agamben, Giorgio. *Homo Sacer: Sovereign Power and Bare Life.* Stanford. Calif.: Stanford University Press, 1998.

Anderson, W. *Colonial Pathologies: American Tropical Medicine, Race, and Hygiene in the Philippines.* Durham, N.C.: Duke University Press, 2006.

——. "Leprosy and Citizenship." *Positions* 6, no. 3 (1998): 707–729.

——. "Postcolonial Histories of Medicine." In *Locating Medical History: The Stories and Their Meanings,* edited by F. Huisman and J. Warner, 285–306. Baltimore: Johns Hopkins University Press, 2004.

Arnold, D. *Colonizing the Body: State Medicine and Epidemic Disease in Nineteenth-Century India.* Berkeley: University of California Press, 1993.

——. *Science, Technology and Medicine in Colonial India.* New Cambridge History of India, part 3, vol. 5. Cambridge: Cambridge University Press, 2000.

Bashford, A. *Imperial Hygiene: A Critical History of Colonialism, Nationalism and Public Health.* New York: Palgrave Macmillan, 2004.

Benedict, C. *Bubonic Plague in 19th-Century China.* Stanford, Calif.: Stanford University Press, 1996.

Biggs, R. "Medicine, Surgery, and Public Health in Ancient Mesopotamia." In *Civilizations of the Ancient Near East,* edited by J. M. Sasson,1911–1924. New York: Scribner, 1995.

Bodde, D. "Forensic Medicine in Pre-imperial China." *Journal of the American Oriental Society* 102, no. 1 (1982): 1–15.

Boxer, C. R. *Dutch Merchants and Mariners in Asia, 1602–1795.* London: Variorum Reprints, 1988.

Brothwell, D., and A. T. Sandison, eds. *Diseases in Antiquity: A Survey of the Diseases, Injuries and Surgery of Early Populations.* Springfield, Ill.: Charles Thomas, 1967.

Brunel, N. "Lèpre: Découverte franco-britannique." *Label France* 44 (2001): 48.

Buckingham, J. *Leprosy in Colonial South India: Medicine and Confinement.* New York: Palgrave, 2002.

Burns, S. "From 'Leper Villages' to Leprosaria': Public Health, Nationalism and the Culture of Exclusion in Japan." In *Isolation: Places and Practices of Exclusion,* edited by C. Strange and A. Bashford, 104–118. London: Routledge, 2003.

Carmichael, A. "Leprosy." In *The Cambridge World History of Human Disease,* edited by K. Kiple, 834–839. New York: Cambridge University Press, 1993.

Chakrabarty, D. *Provincializing Europe: Postcolonial Thought and Historical Difference.* Princeton, N.J.: Princeton University Press, 2000.

Chang Ping-I. *Outside the World.* Taipei: Wings of Hope, 2004.

Chen, K. *Buddhism in China: A Historical Survey.* Princeton, N.J.: Princeton University Press, 1964.

Chen, X., W. Li, C. Jiang, and G. Ye. "Leprosy in China: Epidemiological Trends between 1949 and 1998." *Bulletin of the WHO* 79, no. 4 (2001): 306–312.

Cheng Meibao. *Diyu wenhua yu guojia rentong: Wan Qing yilai Guangdong wenhuaguan di xingcheng* (*Regional Culture and National Identity: The Construct of the Concept of Guangdong Culture since the Late Qing*). Beijing: Sanlian shudian, 2006.

Chen Xianyi, Li Wenzhong, Chen Jiakun, eds. *Mafeng bing fangzhi shouce* (*Handbook for Leprosy Control*). Beijing: Kexue chubanshe, 2002.

Chen Yongfa. *Zhongguo gongchandang geming qishi nian* (*Seventy Years of Revolution of the Chinese Communist Party*). Taipei: Lianjing chubanshe, 1998.

Chen Yuan. *Chen Yuan zaonian wenji* (*Early Writings of Chen Yuan*). 1909. Reprint, Taipei: Academia Sinica, 1992.

Chin Hsien-yu. "Colonial Medical Police and Postcolonial Medical Surveillance Systems in Taiwan, 1895–1950s." *Osiris* 13 (1998): 326–338.

Cohen, P. *China and Christianity: The Missionary Movement and the Growth of Chinese Antiforeignism, 1860–1870.* Cambridge, Mass.: Harvard University Press, 1963.

Conrad, L., and D. Wujastyk, eds. *Contagion: Perspectives from Pre-modern Societies.* Burlington, Vt.: Ashgate, 2000.

Crossley, P. K., H. F. Siu, and D. S. Sutton, eds. *Empire at the Margins: Culture, Ethnicity, and Frontier in Early Modern China.* Berkeley: University of California Press, 2006.

Dai Wenfeng. "'*Haiguan yibao' yu Qing mo Taiwan kaigang diqu di jibing*" ("Medical Reports of the Chinese Imperial Maritime Customs Service" and Diseases in Developed Regions in Taiwan During the Latter Part of the Qing). *Si yu yan* 33, no. 2 (1995): 157–213.

Dangdai Zhongguo di weisheng shiye (*Enterprises of Public Health in Contemporary China*). Beijing: Zhongguo shehui kexue, 1986.

Davis, E. *Society and the Supernatural in Song China.* Honolulu: University of Hawai'i Press, 2001.

Demaître, L. "The Description and Diagnosis of Leprosy by 14th-Century Physicians." *Bulletin of the History of Medicine* 59, no. 3 (1985): 327–344.

Denny, O. E. " The Leprosy Problem in the United States." *National Medical Journal* (English part of the *Zhonghua yixue zazhi*) 30, no. 5 (1927): 391–398.

Diamond, N. "The Miao and Poison: Interactions on China's Southwest Frontier." *Ethnology* 27, no. 1 (1988): 1–26.

Dikotter, F. *The Discourse of Race in Modern China.* London: Hurst, 1992.

Dols, M. "The Leper in Medieval Islamic Society." *Speculum* 58, no. 4 (1983): 891–916.

——. "Leprosy in Medieval Arabic Medicine." *Journal of the History of Medicine and Allied Sciences* 34, no. 3 (1979): 314–333.

Dong Shaoxin. "Xiyang chuanjiaoshi zai Hua zaoqi xingyi shiji kaoshu" (Study on the Medical Activities of Western Missionaries in China in the Early Period). Ph.D. diss., Guangzhou Sun Yat-sen University, 2004.

Edmond, R. *Leprosy and Empire: A Medical and Cultural Study.* Cambridge: Cambridge University Press, 2006.

Ell, S. "Blood and Sexuality in Medieval Leprosy." *Janus: Revue internationale de l'histoire des sciences, de la médicine et de la technique* 71 (1984): 153–164.

Elman, B. *On Their Own Terms: Science in China, 1550–1900.* Cambridge, Mass.: Harvard University Press, 2005.

Fan Jiawei. "Han-Tang jian fojiao yu yiliao jiuji: Yi laibing wei zhongxi" (Medical Relief in the Han-Tang Periods, with Special Emphasis on the *Lai* Ailment). Unpublished document.

——. *Liu Chao Sui-Tang yixue zhi chuancheng yu zhenghe* (*Heritage and Consolidation of Medicine from the Six Dynasties to the Sui-Tang Periods*). Hong Kong: Chinese University Press, 2004.

Fan Xingzhun. *Zhongguo yixue shilue* (*A Brief History of Chinese Medicine*). Beijing: Zhongyi guji chubanshe, 1986.

Faure, B. *The Power of Denial: Buddhism, Purity, and Gender.* Princeton, N.J.: Princeton University Press, 2003.

——. *The Red Thread: Buddhist Approaches to Sexuality.* Princeton, N.J.: Princeton University Press, 1998.

Faure, D. *Emperor and Ancestor: State and Lineage in South China.* Stanford, Calif.: Stanford University Press, 2007.

Feng, H. T., and J. K. Shryock. "The Black Magic in China Known as *Ku.*" *Journal of the American Oriental Society* 55, no. 1 (1935): 1–30.

Fitzgerald, J. *Awakening China: Politics, Culture, and Class in the Nationalist Revolution.* Stanford, Calif.: Stanford University Press, 1996.

Foucault, M. *Les anormaux: Cours au Collège de France (1974–1975).* Paris: Gallimard/Seuil, 1999.

Furth, C. *A Flourishing Yin.* Berkeley: University of California Press, 1996.

Gaudet, M. *Carville: Remembering Leprosy in America.* University Press of Mississippi, 2004.

Ge Jianmin. *Daojiao yixue* (*Daoist Medicine*). Beijing: Zongjiao wenhua chubanshe, 2001.

González, J. M. *Historia de las misiones dominicanas de China.* Vol. 1. Madrid: Ediciones Studium, 1964.

Goossaert, V. "Bureaucratic Charisma: The Zhang Heavenly Master Institution and Court Taoists in Late-Qing China." *Asia Major,* ser. 3, vol. 17, no. 2 (2004): 121–160.

Guangdong sheng weisheng ting manxing bing fangzhi chu (Chronic Disease Control Unit of the Public Health Department of Guangdong Province). "Guangdong mafeng fangzhi shinian licheng, 1951–1962" (Ten Years of Leprosy Control in Guangdong Province). *Pifu xing bing fangzhi tongxun* 2, no. 2 (1963): 1–10.

Gussow, Z. *Leprosy, Racism, and Public Health: Social Policy in Chronic Disease Control.* Boulder, Colo.: Westview Press, 1989.

Gussow, Z., and G. Tracy. "Stigma and the Leprosy Phenomenon: The Social History of a Disease in the 19th and 20th Centuries." *Bulletin of the History of Medicine* 44, no. 5 (1970): 425–449.

Hanson, M. "Northern Purgatives, Southern Restoratives: Ming Medical Regionalism." *Asian Medicine: Tradition and Modernity* 2, no. 2 (2006): 115–170.

——. "Robust Northerners and Delicate Southerners: The 19th-Century Invention of a Southern Medical Tradition." *Positions* 6, no. 3 (1998): 515–550.

Harper, D. *Early Chinese Medical Literature.* London: Kegan Paul, 1998.

Haynes, D. *Imperial Medicine: Patrick Manson and the Conquest of Tropical Disease.* Philadelphia: University of Pennsylvania Press, 2001.

Henry, T. "Sanitizing Empire: Japanese Articulations of Korean Otherness and the Construction of Early Colonial Seoul, 1905–1919." *Journal of Asian Studies* 64, no. 3 (2005): 639–676.

Herman, R. D. K. "Out of Sight, out of Mind, out of Power: Leprosy, Race and Colonization in Hawai'i." *Journal of Historical Geography* 27, no. 3 (2001): 319–337.

He Shixi, ed. *Lidai wuming yijia yan'an* (*Cases Showing Medical Efficacy of Unnamed Doctors in Past Dynasties*). Shanghai: Xuelin chubanshe, 1983.

——. *Zhongguo lidai yijia chuanlu* (*Biographies of Medical People in Chinese History*). 4 vols. Beijing: Renmin weisheng chubanshe,1991.

Hirokawa Waka. "Hansen byōsha no ryōyō keitai ni kansuru kōsatsu: Gunma Ken Agatsuma Kusatsu chō Yunosawa Buraku no jirei kara" (A Study on the Care of Patients of Hansen's Disease Based on the Yunosawa Leper Village in Kusatsu, Agatsuma District, Gunma Prefecture). *Buraku mondai kenkyū* 173 (2005): 22–42.

Huang Shengbai. "Shuo li"(On *Li*). *Yiyao xue* 12 (1929).

Hummel, A. *Eminent Chinese of the Ch'ing Period.* Taipei: Cheng-wen, 1970.

Hymes, R. *Way and Byway: Taoism, Local Religion, and Models of Divinity in Sung and Modern China.* Berkeley: University of California Press, 2002.

Idema, W. "Diseases and Doctors, Drugs and Cures: A Very Preliminary List of Passages of Medical Interest in a Number of Traditional Chinese Novels and Related Plays." *Chinese Science* 2 (1977): 37–63.

Iijima Wataru. "Infectious and Parasitic Disease Studies in Taiwan, Manchuria, and Korea under the Japanese Empire: Brief History on Japanese Colonial Medicine." Paper presented at the conference Ideas and Practices of Hygiene in Han Societies from the Traditional to the Modern Periods, Academia Sinica, Taipei, November 22–24, 2004.

Ishikawa Rikizan. "Xuansha sanshu byōnin kō" (Study on the Three Kinds of Xuansha Patients). In *Kamada Shigeo hakase kanreki kinen ronshū: Chūgoku no bukkyō to bunka.* Tokyo: Ōkura shuppan kabushiki kaisha, 1988.

Japan Law Foundation Verification Committee. "Verification Committee Concerning Hansen's Disease Problem: Final Report." Summary Version, March 2005.

Jiang Cheng. "Mafeng bingren chuangban di zazhi: 'Chenguang jikan'" (A Journal Created by Patients of Leprosy: *Morning Light Quarterly*). *Zhongguo mafeng zazhi* 8, no. 1 (1992): 44–45.

——. "Sun Zhongshan xiansheng guanxin mafeng" (Mr. Sun Yat-sen Was Concerned About Leprosy). *Manxing bing fangzhi tongxun* 2 (1985): 48.

——. "Zhongguo mafeng fangzhi wushi nian hui mou" (Looking Back on the Half Century of Leprosy Control in China). *Zhongguo mafeng pifu bing zazhi* 15, no. 3 (1999): 85–86.

Jiang Zhushan. "Ming-Qing huanan diqu youguan mafeng bing di minjian liaofa" (Popular Healing of Leprosy in Southeastern China in the Ming and Qing Periods). *Dalu zazhi* (April 1995): 182–192.

Joseph, G. "Essentially Christian, Eminently Philanthropic: The Mission to Lepers in British India." *História, Ciências, Saúde: Manguinhos*10, suppl. no. 1 (2003): 247–275.

Jung Keunsik. "'Colonial Modernity' and the Hegemony of the Body Politic in Leprosy Relief Work." Unpublished document, 37 pages.

Kakar, S. "Leprosy in British India, 1860–1940: Colonial Politics and Missionary Medicine." *Medical History* 40 (1996): 215–230.

——. "Medical Developments and Patient Unrest in the Leprosy Asylum, 1860–1940." In *Health, Medicine and Empire: Perspectives on Colonial India,* edited by B. Pati and M. Harrison, 188–216. London: Sangam Books, 2000.

Katz, P. *Demon Hordes and Burning Boats: The Cult of Marshal Wen in Late Imperial Chekiang.* Albany: SUNY Press, 1995.

Kikkuchi Ichiro. "Hansen's Disease Patients: Responses to Stigma and Segregation in Kumamoto, Japan." *International Journal of Dermatology* 33, no. 2 (1994): 142–145.

Kinnier Wilson, J. V. "Leprosy in Ancient Mesopotamia." *Revue d'assyriologie* 60, no. 1 (1966): 47–58.

Kipp, R. "The Evangelical Uses of Leprosy." *Social Science and Medicine* 39, no. 2 (1944): 165–178.

Kuriyama, S. "The Imagination of Winds and the Development of the Chinese Conception of the Body." In *Body, Subject, and Power in China,* edited by A. Zito and T. Barlow, 23–41. Chicago: University of Chicago Press, 1994.

Lau Chau-mun. *The Everlasting Couple.* Taipei: Liberal Arts Press, 1975.

Lei Liangzhong. "Bujie, qishi yu cunluo: Mafeng he mafeng cun di gushi" (Pollution, Discrimination, and the Village: The Story of Leprosy and a Leper Village). Master's thesis, Central University of Ethnology, Beijing, 2003.

"The Lepers of Japan." *The Economist,* February 24, 1996, 64.

Leung, A. K. C. "The Business of Vaccination in 19th-Century Canton." *Late Imperial China* 29, no. 1, supplement (2008): 7–39.

——. "Evolution of the Idea of *Chuanran* Contagion in Imperial China." In *Health and Hygiene in Modern Chinese East Asia,* edited by A. K. C. Leung and C. Furth. Durham, N.C.: Duke University Press, forthcoming.

——. "Medical Learning from the Song to the Ming." In *The Song-Yuan-Ming Transition in Chinese History,* edited by P. Smith and R. von Glahn, 374–398. Cambridge, Mass.: Harvard University Press, 2003.

Liang Qizi [A. K. C. Leung]. "Jibing yu fangtu zhi guanxi: Yuan zhi Qing jian yijie di kanfa" (The Relations Between Diseases and Locality: The Views in Medical Books from the Yuan to the Qing). In *Xingbie yu yiliao: Di san jie guoji hanxue huiyi lunwen ji* (*Gender and Medicine: Volume of the Third International Conference on Sinology*), edited by Huang Kewu, 165–212. Taipei: Institute of Modern History, Academia Sinica, 2002.

Liang Qizi. "Ming-Qing yufang tianhua cuoshi zhi yanbian" (History of Measures to Prevent Smallpox in the Ming-Qing Period). In *Guoshi shilun,* edited by Yang Liansheng et al., 239–253. Taipei: Shihuo chubanshe, 1987.

——. *Shishan yu jiaohua* (*Philanthropy and Moral Transformation*). Taipei: Lianjing chubanshe, 1997.

Liang Zhangchi. "Zhongguo gudai mafeng shishi kaobian" (Analysis of Historical Facts on Leprosy in Ancient China). *Pifu xing bing fangzhi tongxun* 2, no. 1 (1963): 51–63.

Lieber, E. "Old Testament 'Leprosy,' Contagion and Sin." In *Contagion: Perspectives from Pre-modern Societies,* edited by L. Conrad and D. Wujastyk, 99–136. Burlington, Vt.: Ashgate, 2000.

Li Fengmao. "*Daozang* suo shou zaoqi daoshu di wenyi guan" (Views on Epidemics as Shown by Early Daoist Texts in the *Daoist Canon*). *Zhongguo wenzhe yanjiu jikan* 3 (1993): 417–454.

Li Jianmin. "Bencao gangmu huobu kaoshi" (Fire as Medicine: The "Fire" Section of the *Bencao gangmu*). *Bulletin of the Institute of History and Philology, Academia Sinica* 73, no. 3 (2002): 396–441.

——. "Contagion and Its Consequences: The Problem of Death Pollution in Ancient China." In *Medicine and the History of the Body: Proceedings of the 20th, 21st and 22nd Iternational Symposia on the Comparative History of Medicine—East and West*, 201–222. Ishiyaku EuroAmerica, 1999.

——. "Xian Qin liang Han bingyin guan ji qi bianqian: Yi xin chutu wenwu wei zhongxin" (The Etiological Concepts and Their Changes in the Qin and Han Periods: Based on Recent Archaeological Findings). Unpublished document, 2006.

Lin Bingliang. "Ji Shilong Guowuzhou mafeng yuan shimuo" (The History of the Leper Asylum at Guowuzhou of Shilong). *Guangdong wenshi ziliao* 57 (1988): 145–148.

Lin Fushi. "Jibing yu xiudao: Zhongguo zaoqi daoshi xiudao yinyuan kaoshi zhiyi" (Illness and Practicing the Dao: Analysis of the Causes Behind the Practice of the Dao in Early China). *Hanxue yanjiu* 19, no. 1 (2001): 137–166.

——. "Shi shi Shuihudi Qin jian zhong di 'li' yu 'ding sha'" (Explanations of the Terms "*Li*" and "*Ding Sha*" in Qin Bamboo Strips Discovered at Shuihudi). *Shiyuan* 15 (1986): 1–38.

Lin Zhiming. *Feiyue mafengyuan* (Fly Over the Leprosarium). Hong Kong: Legend, 2000.

Li Qinpu. "Bawan shi chong yu bawan hu chong" (On the Question of the Eighty Thousand Corpse *Chong*). *Zhonghua yishi zazhi* 26, no. 2 (1996): 108.

Li Shang-jen. "Shijiu shiji houqi Yingguo yixue jie dui Zhongguo mafeng bing qing di diaocha yanjiu" (British Medical Research on Leprosy in Late Nineteenth-Century China). *Bulletin of the Institute of History and Philology, Academia Sinica* 74, no. 3 (2003): 445–506.

Liu Muzhi. "Mafeng bing zai Zhongguo yixue ji lishi shang de jizai" (Records of Leprosy in Chinese History and Medical Works). *Zhonghua pifu ke zazhi* 4, no. 1 (1956): 3–5.

Liu Shiyong. "Qingjie, weisheng yu baojian: Ri zhi shiqi Taiwan shehui gonggong weisheng guannian zhi zhuanbian" (Sanitation, Hygiene, and Health Protection: The Changes in the Conceptualization of Public Health in Taiwan During the Japanese Occupation Period). *Taiwan shi yanjiu* 8, no. 1 (2001): 41–88.

Liu Zhiwei. *Zai guojia yu shehui zhijian: Ming-Qing lijia fuyi zhidu yanjiu* (*Between State and Society: The Study of the Household Registration and Tax System in Guangdong of the Ming-Qing Period*). Guangzhou: Zhongshan daxue chubanshe, 1997.

Li Wenzhong, ed. *Xiandai mafeng bing xue* (*Modern Leprology*). Shanghai: Shanghai kexue chubanshe, 2006.

Li Yongchun. *Shiyong zhongyi cidian* (*A Practical Dictionary of Chinese Medicine*). Taipei: Zhiyin chubanshe, 1992.

Li Yulin et al. "Zhejiang sheng mafeng fangzhi sishiwu nian di huigu" (Review of Leprosy Control in Zhejiang Province in the Past Forty-five Years). *Zhongguo mafeng zazhi* 14, no. 3 (1998): 173–175.

Lu, G.-D., and J. Needham. "Records of Diseases in Ancient China." In *Diseases in Antiquity: A Survey of the Diseases, Injuries and Surgery of Early Populations,* edited by D. Brothwell and A. T. Sandison, 222–237. Springfield, Ill.: Charles Thomas, 1967.

Mafeng bing shehui yixue lunwen ji (*Collected Essays on the Social Medicine of Leprosy*). Beijing: Zhongguo yixue kexue yuan pifu bing yanjiu suo, 1986.

Ma Jixing. *Mawangdui gu yishu kaoshi* (*Research and Explanations on Old Medical Texts Found in Mawangdui*). Changsha: Hunan kexue jishu chubanshe, 1992.

——. *Zhongyi wenxian xue* (*Studies on Traditional Chinese Medical Texts*). Shanghai: Kexue jishu chubanshe, 1990.

McGrew, R. "Leprosy." In *Encyclopedia of Medical History,* 161–165. New York: McGraw-Hill, 1985.

McLeod, K., and R. Yates. "Forms of Ch'in Law: An Annotated Translation of the *Feng-chen shih.*" *Harvard Journal of Asiatic Studies* 41, no. 1 (1981): 111–163.

Moblo, P. "Blessed Damien of Moloka'i: The Critical Analysis of Contemporary Myth." *Ethnohistory* 44, no. 4 (1997): 691–726.

——. "Institutionalizing the Leper: Partisan Politics and the Evolution of Stigma in Post-monarchy Hawai'i." *The Journal of the Polynesian Society* 107, no. 3 (1998): 229–262.

Monot, M., et al. "On the Origin of Leprosy." *Science* 308 (May 2005): 1040–1042.

Nakayama, A., and N. Sivin. *Chinese Science: Explorations in an Ancient Tradition.* Cambridge, Mass.: MIT Press, 1973.

Navon, L. "Beggars, Metaphors, and Stigma: A Missing Link in the Social History of Leprosy." *Social History of Medicine* 11, no. 1 (1998): 89–105.

Nutton, V. "Medicine in Medieval Western Europe, 1000–1500." In *The Western Medical Tradition 800 BC–AD 1800,* 139–198. Cambridge: Cambridge University Press, 1995.

Obregon, D. "Building National Medicine: Leprosy and Power in Colombia, 1870–1910." *Social History of Medicine* 15, no. 1 (2002): 89–108.

——. "La construction sociale de la lèpre en Colombie, 1884–1959." In *Les sciences hors d'Occident au XXe siècle,* edited by A.-M. Moulin, 4:159–175. Paris: Orstom, 1996.

Obringer, F. *Aconit et l'opriment: Drogues et poisons en Chine ancienne et médiévale.* Paris: Fayard, 1997.

Palmer, R. "The Church, Leprosy and Plague in Medieval and Early Modern Europe." In *The Church and Healing,* edited by W. J. Sheils, 79–99. Oxford: Blackwell, 1982.

Pandya, S. S. "Anti-contagionism in Leprosy, 1844–1897." *International Journal of Leprosy and Other Mycobacterial Diseases* 66, no. 3 (1998): 374–384.

——. "The First International Leprosy Conference, Berlin, 1897." *História, Ciências, Saúde: Manguinhos* 10, suppl. no. 1 (2003): 161–177.

Parry, S. S. "Of Vital Importance to the Community: The Control of Leprosy in the Northern Territory." *Health and History* 5, no. 1 (2003): 1–21.

Pons, P. "Les lépreux japonais vont retrouver la liberté." *Le Monde*, February 6, 1996.

Porkert, M. *The Theoretical Foundations of Chinese Medicine: Systems of Correspondence.* Cambridge, Mass.: MIT Press, 1974.

Pregadio, F. *Great Clarity: Daoism and Alchemy in Early Medieval China.* Stanford, Calif.: Stanford University Press, 2006.

Rawcliffe, C. *Leprosy in Medieval England.* Suffolk, U.K.: Boydell Press, 2006.

Ren Linhao. *Liang Song shiqi di Taizhou daojiao* (*Taizhou Daoism Under the Song*). http://www.lhinfo.net/minren/rlh/taizhoudaojiao3.htm (accessed September 10, 2006).

Rifkin, S. "Health Care for Rural Areas." In *Medicine and Public Health in the People's Republic of China*, edited by J. Quinn, 141–152. Washington, D.C.: U.S. Department of Health, Education, and Welfare, National Institutes of Health, 1973.

Rogaski, R. *Hygienic Modernity: Meanings of Health and Disease in Treaty-Port China.* Berkeley: University of California Press, 2004.

——. "Nature, Annihilation, and Modernity: China's Korean War Germ-Warfare Experience Reconsidered." *Journal of Asian Studies* 61, no. 2 (2002): 381–415.

Roland, C. "George Gushue-Taylor and the Medical Missions of Formosa." *Journal of Medical Biography* 4, no. 2 (1996): 82–93.

Roselli, A. "Les maladies d'Arétée de Cappadoce." Unpublished document, 2004.

Rosenthal, M. *Health Care in the People's Republic of China: Moving toward Modernization.* Boulder, Colo.: Westview Press, 1987.

Russell-Wood, A. J. R. *The Portuguese Empire, 1415–1808: A World on the Move.* Baltimore: Johns Hopkins University Press, 1998.

Schipper, K. *Le corps taoiste. Corps physique, corps social.* Paris: Fayard, 1982.

——. "Seigneurs royaux, dieux des épidémies." *Archives de sciences sociales des religions* 59, no. 1 (1985): 31–40.

Schipper, K., and F. Verellen, eds. *The Taoist Canon: A Historical Companion to the "Daozang."* Chicago: University of Chicago Press, 2004.

Shah, N. *Contagious Divides: Epidemics and Race in San Francisco's Chinatown.* Berkeley: University of California Press, 2001.

Sivin, N. "Huang ti nei ching." In *Early Chinese Texts: A Bibliographical Guide*, edited by Michael Loewe, 196–215. Berkeley: Society for the Study of Early China, 1993.

——. *Traditional Medicine in Contemporary China.* Ann Arbor: Center for Chinese Studies, University of Michigan, 1987.

Skinsnes, O. K. "Leprosy in Society." *Leprosy Review* 35 (1964): 21–35.

Song Xian. *Gudai Posi yixue yu Zhongguo* (*Ancient Persian Medicine and China*). Beijing: Jingji ribao chubanshe, 2001.

Sontag, S. *AIDS and Its Metaphors.* New York: Farrar, Straus and Giroux, 1988.

Souza, G. B. *The Survival of Empire: Portuguese Trade and Society in China and the South China Sea, 1630–1754.* Cambridge: Cambridge University Press, 1986.

Stol, M. "Leprosy: New Light from Greek and Babylonian Sources." *Jaarbericht Ex Oriente Lux* 30 (1987–1988): 22–31.

Stoler, A. L. *Carnal Knowledge and Imperial Power: Race and the Intimate in Colonial Rule.* Berkeley: University of California Press, 2002.

Strickmann, M. *Chinese Magical Medicine.* Stanford, Calif.: Stanford University Press, 2002.

Szonyi, M. "The Illusion of Standardizing the Gods: The Cult of the Five Emperors in Late Imperial China." *Journal of Asian Studies* 56, no. 1 (1997): 113–135.

Tang Changru. *Wei-Jin Nan-Bei Chao shi lun shiyi* (*Miscellaneous Writings on the History of the Wei-Jin Nan-Bei Dynasties*). Beijing: Xinhua shuju, 1983.

Tayman, J. *The Colony: The Harrowing True Story of the Exiles of Molokai.* New York: Scribner, 2006.

Touati, O. "Historiciser la notion de contagion: L'exemple de la lèpre dans les sociétés médiévales." In *Air, miasmes et contagion: Les épidémies dans l'Antiquité et au Moyen Age,* edited by S. Bazin-Tacchella, D. Quéruel, and É. Samama, 157–187. Langres, Fr.: Guéniot, 2001.

Tsukimoto, A. "By the Hand of Madi-Dagan, the Scribe and *Apkallu*-Priest: A Medical Text from the Middle Euphrates Region." In *Priests and Officials in the Ancient Near East,* edited by K. Watanabe, 187–200. Heidelberg: Universitätsverlag C. Winter.

Van Wettum, B. A. J. "A Chinese Opinion on Leprosy: Being a Translation of a Chapter from the Medical Standard Book, *Imperial Edition of the Golden Mirror for the Medical Class.*" *T'oung Pao,* ser. 2, vol. 2 (1901): 256–268.

Vaughan, M. *Curing Their Ills: Colonial Power and African Illness.* Stanford, Calif.: Stanford University Press, 1991.

Von Glahn, R. *Sinister Way: The Divine and the Demonic in Chinese Religious Culture.* Berkeley: University of California Press, 2004.

Wang Jimin. "Zhongguo mafeng shi zhong zhi mingren"(Famous People in the Chinese History of Leprosy). *Zhonghua yixue zazhi* 27, no. 9 (1941): 565–568.

Wang Quanpei et al. "Xizang zizhi qu mafeng bing liuxing ji fangzhi jinkuang baogao" (Report on the Recent Epidemiological Situation of Leprosy and Its Control in the Tibet Autonomous Region). *Zhongguo mafeng pifu bing zazhi* 19, no. 6 (2003): 583–585.

Wang Shaoguang. "Zhongguo gonggong weisheng di weiji yu zhuanji" (Crisis and Turning Point of Public Health in China). http://www.ccrs.org.cn (accessed June 22, 2003).

Wang Wenji. "Laibing yuan li de yixiangren" (Strangers in the Leprosy Colony). In *Gujin lunheng* (*Disquisitions on the Past and Present*), 116–124. Taipei: Academia Sinica, 2003.

Wang, Wenji. "Laying Out a Model Village: George Gushe-Taylor and Missionary Leprosy Work in Colonial Taiwan." *East Asian Science, Technology, and Society: An International Journal* 1, no. 1. (2007): 111–133.

Weinstein, S. *Buddhism under the Tang.* Cambridge: Cambridge University Press, 1987.

WHO. *World Health Organization Leprosy Elimination Project Status Report 2003 Draft.* Geneva: WHO, 2004.

WHO Regional Office for the Western Pacific. *Overview and Epidemiological Review of Leprosy in the WHO Western Pacific Region, 1991–2001.* Manila: WHO, 2003.

WHO Study Group. *Epidemiology of Leprosy in Relation to Control.* Technical Report Series 716. Geneva: WHO, 1985.

Wong, C. M., and L. T. Wu. *History of Chinese Medicine.* 1932. Reprint, Taipei: Southern Materials Center, 1985.

Worboys, M. "The Colonial World as Mission and Mandate: Leprosy and Empire, 1900–1940." *Osiris* 15 (2001): 207–218.

——. *Spreading Germs: Disease Theories and Medical Practice in Britain, 1865–1900.* Cambridge: Cambridge University Press, 2000.

Wright, D., and R. Jones. "Leprosy." In *The Anchor Bible Dictionary,* edited by D. N. Freedman, 277–282. New York: Doubleday, 1992.

Wuwei Handai yijian (*Medical Texts in Bamboo Strips of the Han Period Discovered in Wuwei*). In *Zhongguo xibei wenxian congshu: Xibei kaogu wenxian,* edited by Wu Jian et al., ser. 7, vol. 6. Lanzhou: Lanzhou guji shudian, 1990.

Xiao Fan. "Han-Song jian wenxian suojian gudai Zhongguo nanfang di dili huanjing yu difang bing ji qi yingxiang" (Geographic Environment, Endemic Diseases of China's South as Described in Texts from the Han to the Song, and Their Influences). *Bulletin of the Institute of History and Philology, Academia Sinica* 63, no. 1 (1993): 67–171.

Xiao Xi. "Boniu you ji kao" (A Philological Study on the Ailment of Boniu). *Guangdong zhongyi* 1 (1958): 25–28.

Xiao Yunchun. "Zuguo yixue duiyu mafeng zhi renshi" (Our Mother Country's Knowledge on Leprosy). *Zhongyi zazhi* 4 (1956): 170–173.

Xie Guan. *Zhongguo yixue yuanliu lun* (*On the Traditions of Chinese Medicine*). Taipei: Guting shuwu, 1970.

Xingshan xian zhengxie wenshi ziliao weiyuanhui, Xingshan xian mafang yuan (Committee on Culture and History of Xingshan County, Leprosy Control Hospital of Xingshan County), eds. *Mingyue Yan: Hubei sheng Xingshan xian mafeng fangshi zhuanji* (*Clear Moon Rock: Collections of Papers on Leprosy Control in Xingshan County of Hubei Province*). Xingshan xian, 1994.

Yang Lien-sheng. "The Concept of 'Pao' as a Basis for Social Relations in China." In *Chinese Thought and Institutions,* edited by J. K. Fairbank, 291–309. Chicago: University of Chicago Press, 1957.

Yang Lihe. "Zhongguo mafeng fangzhi sanshiwu nian ji zhanwang" (Thirty-five Years of Leprosy Control in China and Future Prospects). *Zhongguo mafeng zazhi* 2, no. 1 (1986): 13–15.

Yang Ruisong. "Xiangxiang minzu chiru: Jindai Zhongguo sixiang wenhua shi shang di 'Dongya bingfu'" (Imaging National Humiliation: "Sick Man of East Asia" in Modern Chinese Intellectual and Cultural History). *Guoli Zhengzhi daxue lishi xuebao* 23 (2005): 1–44.

You Jiajun. *Mafeng bingxue gailun* (*General Discussion on Leprosy*). Shanghai: Huadong yiwu shenghuo she, 1953.

——. "Wunian lai mafeng fangzhi gongzuo di fazhang"(Growth of the Work on Leprosy Control During the Past Five Years). *Zhonghua pifu ke zazhi* 4, no. 1 (1956): 8–9.

Yue Meizhong. "Guanyu zuguo yixue mafeng shishi ji qi zhuzuo di xushu" (On the Historical Facts of Leprosy and Its Description in Medical Texts in Our Mother Country). *Shanghai zhongyi zazhi* 9 (1956): 40–43.

——. "Zuguo yixue dui dafeng bing di renshi ji qi zhiliao bing ji xiandai yixue duiyu mafeng bing di zhishi" (Knowledge and Therapeutics of Leprosy in Our Country and Modern Medical Understanding of the Disease). *Xin zhongyi yao* 8, nos. 3–4 (1957): 5–16.

Yu Shenchu. *Zhongguo mafeng bingxue* (*Study on Leprosy in China*). Shanghai: Fuxing zhongyishe, 1941.

Yu Zongfa. *Yunmeng Qinjian zhong sixiang yu zhidu gouzhi* (*Thought and Institution Picked Up in the Qin Bamboo Strips Excavated in Yunmeng*). Taipei: Wenjin chubanshe, 1992.

Zakovitch, Y. "Miracles (Old Testament)." In *The Anchor Bible Dictionary*, edited by D. N. Freedman, 851–856. New York: Doubleday, 1992.

Zhang Jiafeng [Chang Chia-feng]. "Qingchu di bidou yu chadou zhidu" (The Institutions of Smallpox Avoidance and Inspection in the Early Qing). *Hanxue yanjiu* 14, no. 1 (27) (1996): 135–156.

Zhongguo mafeng pifu bing zazhi (*China Journal of Leprosy and Skin Diseases*). Jinan: Zhongguo mafeng fangzhi xiehui (China Association of Leprosy Control) and Shandong pifu xing bing fangzhi yanjiusuo (Shandong Institute of Leprosy and Venereal Disease Control). 1985–.

Zhongguo mafeng zazhi (*China Leprosy Journal*) Guangzhou, 1985–.

Zhongguo yiyuan daquan: Shandong fence (*Volume on Shandong Province of the Encyclopedia of Hospitals in China*). Beijing: Guangming Ribao chubanshe, 1989.

Index

Studies of the Weatherhead
East Asian Institute

Columbia University

SELECTED TITLES

(Complete list at http://www.columbia.edu/cu/weai/weatherhead-studies.html)

Mediasphere Shanghai: The Aesthetics of Cultural Production, Alexander Des Forges. University of Hawai'i Press, 2007

Kingdom of Beauty: Mingei and the Politics of Folk Art in Imperial Japan, Kim Brandt. Duke University Press, 2007

Modern Passings: Death Rites, Politics, and Social Change in Imperial Japan, Andrew Bernstein. University of Hawai'i Press, 2006

The Making of the "Rape of Nanjing": The History and Memory of the Nanjing Massacre in Japan, China, and the United States, Takashi Yoshida. Oxford University Press, 2006

The Merchants of Zigong: Industrial Entrepreneurship in Early Modern China, Madeleine Zelin. Columbia University Press, 2005

Bad Youth: Juvenile Delinquency and the Politics of Everyday Life in Modern Japan, 1895–1945, David Ambaras. University of California Press, 2005

Science and the Building of a Modern Japan, Morris Low. Palgrave Macmillan, Ltd., 2005

Kinship, Contract, Community, and State: Anthropological Perspectives on China, Myron L. Cohen. Stanford University Press, 2005

Rearranging the Landscape of the Gods: The Politics of a Pilgrimage Site in Japan, 1573–1912, Sarah Thal. University of Chicago Press, 2005

Reluctant Pioneers: China's Expansion Northward, 1644–1937, James Reardon-Anderson. Stanford University Press, 2005

Contract and Property in Early Modern China, Madeleine Zelin, Jonathan K. Ocko, and Robert P. Gardella, eds. Stanford University Press, 2004

Gutenberg in Shanghai: Chinese Print Capitalism, 1876–1937, by Christopher A. Reed. UBC Press, 2004

Japan's Colonization of Korea: Discourse and Power, by Alexis Dudden University of Hawai'i Press, 2004

Divorce in Japan: Family, Gender, and the State, 1600–2000, by Harald Fuess. Stanford University Press 2004

The Communist Takeover of Hangzhou: The Transformation of City and Cadre, 1949–1954, by James Gao. University of Hawai'i Press, 2004

Taxation Without Representation in Rural China, by Thomas P. Bernstein and Xiaobo Lü. Modern China Series, Cambridge University Press, 2003

The Reluctant Dragon: Crisis Cycles in Chinese Foreign Economic Policy, by Lawrence Christopher Reardon. University of Washington Press, 2002

Cadres and Corruption: The Organizational Involution of the Chinese Communist Party, by Xiaobo Lü. Stanford University Press, 2000

Japan's Imperial Diplomacy: Consuls, Treaty Ports, and War with China, 1895–1938, by Barbara Brooks. Honolulu: University of Hawai'i Press, 2000

China's Retreat from Equality: Income Distribution and Economic Transition, Carl Riskin, Zhao Renwei, Li Shi, eds. M. E. Sharpe, 2000

CPSIA information can be obtained at www.ICGtesting.com
Printed in the USA
BVOW07*0911141114

374784BV00001BA/3/P

9 780231 123006